T0320576

Core Topics in Anaesthesia and Peri-operative Care of the Morbidly Obese Surgical Patient

Core Topics in Anaesthesia and Peri-operative Care of the Morbidly Obese Surgical Patient

Edited by

Christopher Bouch
Leicester Royal Infirmary

Jonathan Cousins
St Mary's and Hammersmith Hospitals, London

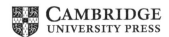

CAMBRIDGE
UNIVERSITY PRESS

CAMBRIDGE
UNIVERSITY PRESS

University Printing House, Cambridge CB2 8BS, United Kingdom

One Liberty Plaza, 20th Floor, New York, NY 10006, USA

477 Williamstown Road, Port Melbourne, VIC 3207, Australia

314-321, 3rd Floor, Plot 3, Splendor Forum, Jasola District Centre, New Delhi - 110025, India

79 Anson Road, #06-04/06, Singapore 079906

Cambridge University Press is part of the University of Cambridge.

It furthers the University's mission by disseminating knowledge in the pursuit of
education, learning and research at the highest international levels of excellence.

www.cambridge.org
Information on this title: www.cambridge.org/9781107163287
DOI: 10.1017/9781316681053

First published 2018

A catalogue record for this publication is available from the British Library

Library of Congress Cataloging in Publication data
Names: Bouch, Christopher, editor. | Cousins, Jonathan, editor.
Title: Core topics in anaesthesia and peri-operative care of the morbidly obese surgical patient / edited by
Christopher Bouch, Jonathan Cousins.
Description: New York, NY : Cambridge University Press, 2019. | Includes bibliographical references and index.
Identifiers: LCCN 2018016123 | ISBN 9781107163287 (Hardback)
Subjects: | MESH: Perioperative Care | Anesthesia | Obesity, Morbid – surgery | Surgical Procedures, Operative
Classification: LCC RD540 | NLM WO 178 | DDC 617.4/3–dc23
LC record available at https://lccn.loc.gov/2018016123

ISBN 978-1-107-16328-7 Hardback

Contents

Contributors

Marco Adamo MD FRCS
Consultant Upper GI and Bariatric Surgeon
University College London Hospital
London
United Kingdom

Ahmed R. Ahmed PhD FRCS
Consultant Upper GI and Bariatric Surgeon
St Mary's Hospital
Imperial Healthcare NHS Trust
London
United Kingdom

Vassilis Athanassoglou MB BChir FRCA
Consultant Anaesthetist
Oxford University Hospitals
Oxford
United Kingdom

Sherif Awad MB ChB FRCS
Consultant Bariatric Surgeon
Royal Derby Hospitals
Derby
United Kingdom

Paul Ayrton
Manual Handling Department
University Hospitals of Leicester NHS Trust
Leicester
United Kingdom

Ben Bailiff FRCP FRCPath
Haematology Consultant
University Hospitals Coventry and Warwick
United Kingdom

Rhodri Birtchnell MB BCh Bsc(Hons) FCARCSI MRCA EDRA
Consultant Anaesthetist
Morriston Hospital
Swansea
United Kingdom

Christopher Bouch MB ChB FRCA EDICM FFICM
Society for Obesity and Bariatric Anaesthesia (UK)
Consultant in Anaesthesia and Critical Care Medicine
Leicester Royal Infirmary
University Hospitals of Leicester NHS Trust
Leicester
United Kingdom

David Bowrey MB BCh MD FRCS MMed Ed SFHEA
Consultant Upper GI and Bariatric Surgeon
Leicester Royal Infirmary
University Hospitals of Leicester NHS Trust
Leicester
United Kingdom

Liam Brennan BSc MBBS FRCA
Consultant Paediatric Anaesthetist
Addenbrooke's Hospital
Cambridge
United Kingdom

Jay B. Brodsky MD
Department of Anesthesiology, Perioperative and Pain Medicine
Stanford University School of Medicine
Stanford, CA
USA

Adele S. Budianksy MD
Resident in Anaesthesiology and Pain Medicine
The Ottawa Hopsital
Ontario
Canada

Chris Carey MBBS FRCA
Consultant in Anaesthesia
Brighton and Sussex University Hospitals NHS Trust
United Kingdom

Michele Carron MD PhD
Department of Medicine, Anaesthesiology and
Intensive Care
University of Padova
Padova
Italy

Harvinder Chahal BMedSci (Hons) MBBS FRCP PhD
Consultant in Endocrinology and Bariatric Medicine
Imperial College Healthcare Trust
St Mary's Hospital
London
United Kingdom

Andrew Chamberlain MB ChB FRCA
Specialist Registrar in Anaesthesia
York District Hospital
York
United Kingdom

Matt Charlton MD FRCA FFICM
Higher Specialist Trainee in Anaesthesia and Critical
Care Medicine
Leicester Royal Infirmary
University Hospitals of Leicester NHS Trust
Leicester
United Kingdom

Jonathan Cousins FRCA MB BS BSc
Society for Obesity and Bariatric Anaesthesia (UK)
Consultant in Anaesthesia and Cardiac Intensive Care
St Mary's Hospital
Imperial College Healthcare NHS Trust
London
United Kingdom

Luc De Baerdemaker MD
Department of Anaesthesia
University Hospital Ghent
Belgium

Ashish Desai FRCS MCh DNB
Consultant Paediatric Surgeon
King's College Hospital
London
United Kingdom

N. Durkin
Department of Paediatric Surgery
King's College Hospital
London
United Kingdom

Naveen Eipe MBBS MD
Assistant Professor in Anesthesiology and Pain
Medicine
The Ottawa Hospital
Ontario
Canada

Naim Faikh Gomez LMS
Senior Clinical Surgical Fellow
St Mary's Hospital
Imperial College Healthcare Trust
London
United Kingdom

Khaleel Fareed MB ChB
Consultant Bariatric Surgeon
Royal Derby Hospitals
Derby
United Kingdom

Peter Gregory MB ChB BSc FRCA
Society for Obesity and Bariatric Anaesthesia (UK)
Consultant Anaesthetist
Frimley Park Hospital
United Kingdom

Andrew Hall MA BChir MB FRCP (Edin) FRCA FFICM
Consultant in Anaesthesia, Critical Care and Sleep
Medicine.
Leicester General Hospital
University Hospitals of Leicester NHS Trust
Leicester
United Kingdom

David Haslam MBBS DGM
Clinical Director of the National Obesity Forum
General Practitioner
Watton-at-Stone
Hertfordshire
United Kingdom

Chris Hebbes MBChB BSC MMedSci FRCA FFICM
Specialist Registrar and Lecturer
Leicester Royal Infirmary and University of Leicester
University Hospitals of Leicester NHS Trust
Leicester
United Kingdom

Bjorn Heyse MD
Department of Anaesthesia
University Hospital Ghent
Belgium

Nick Kennedy MBBS FRCA FFICM
Consultant Anaesthetist
Taunton and Somerset NHS Trust
United Kingdom

Brian Kent MB BCh FRCP
Consultant in Sleep and Respiratory Medicine
Guy's and St Thomas' NHS Foundation Trust
London
United Kingdom

Meera Kurup MB BS FRCA
Consultant Paediatric Anaesthetist
King's College Hospital
London
United Kingdom

Will Lester FRCP FRCPath PhD
Haematology Consultant
University Hospitals of
Birmingham
Birmingham
United Kingdom

Andrew Lewitt
Manual Handling Department
University Hospitals of Leicester NHS Trust
Leicester
United Kingdom

Neil MacDonald MB ChB FRCA
Consultant Anaesthestist
Royal London Hospital
London
United Kingdom

Iqbal S. Malik MBBCh FRCP PhD
Consultant Cardiologist
Hammersmith Hospital
Imperial College Healthcare NHS Trust
London
United Kingdom

Mike Margarson MB BS FRCA FFICM
Society for Obesity and Bariatric
Anaesthesia (UK)
Consultant in Anaesthesia and Critical Care
Medicine
St Richards Hospital
Chichester
United Kingdom

Rupert Mason BM
Specialist Anaesthetic Registrar
St Richards Hospital
Chichester
United Kingdom

Benjamin Millette BM BCh
Specialist Registrar in Anaesthesia and Critical Care
Medicine
Oxford University Hospitals
Oxford
United Kingdom

Alexander Miras MRCP PhD
Senior Lecturer in Endocrinology
Hammersmith Hospital
Imperial College Healthcare Trust
London
United Kingdom

Tiffany S. Moon MD
Assistant Professor of Anesthesiology
UT SouthWestern Medical Center
Dallas, TX
USA

S. Noor
Department of Paediatric Surgery
King's College Hospital
London
United Kingdom

Mary O'Kane FBDA
Dietitian (Adult Obesity)
The General Infirmary at Leeds
Leeds
United Kingdom

Tom Palser MA BMBCh DM FRCS
Specialist Registrar in Upper GI Surgery
Leicester Royal Infirmary
University Hospitals of Leicester NHS Trust
Leicester
United Kingdom

Anil Patel MBBS FRCA
Consultant Anaesthetist
Royal National Throat, Nose and Ear Hospital
University College Hospital
London
United Kingdom

Kanchan Patil MBBS FRCA
Society for Obesity and Bariatric Anaesthesia (UK)
Consultant Anaesthetist
St George's University Hospital
London
United Kingdom

Melanie Paul MB ChB
Specialist Registrar
Leicester Royal Infirmary
University Hospitals of Leicester NHS Trust
Leicester
United Kingdom

Belén Pérez-Pevida MD
Division of Diabetes, Endocrinology and Metabolism
Hammersmith Hospital
Imperial College Healthcare NHS Trust
London
United Kingdom

Gail Pinnock BSc (Hons) RD MBDA
Specialist Bariatric and Obesity Dietitian
Spire Hospitals
United Kingdom

Pei Kee Poh MBBS FRCA
Specialist Registrar in Anaesthesia
Leicester General Hospital
University Hospitals of Leicester NHS Trust
Leicester
United Kingdom

Jonathan Redman MB, ChB FRCA FFICM
Society for Obesity and Bariatric Anaesthesia (UK)
Consultant in Anaesthesia and Critical Care Medicine
York District Hospital
York
United Kingdom

Nick Reynolds LLM MB ChB FRCA FFICM
Consultant in Anaesthesia and Critical Care Medicine
Royal Derby Hospitals
United Kingdom

Neil Ruparelia BSc (Hons) MB BS MSc DPhil MRCP FESC
Consultant Cardiologist
Hammersmith Hospital
Imperial College Healthcare NHS Trust
London
United Kingdom

Harry Rutter MB BChir MSc PGDipLATHE FRCP Edin
Senior Clinical Research Fellow
London School of Hygiene and Tropical Medicine
Consultant and Honorary Senior Lecturer in Public Health Medicine
Oxford
United Kingdom

Roman Schumann MD
Professor of Anaesthesia
Tufts University School of Medicine
Boston, MA
USA

Paul Sharpe MB ChB FRCA
Consultant in Obstetric Anaesthesia
Leicester Royal Infirmary
University Hospitals of Leicester NHS Trust
Leicester
United Kingdom

Peter Shirley MB ChB FRCA FFICM EDIC
Consultant in Critical Care Medicine and Anaesthesia
Royal London Hospital
London
United Kingdom

Mark Skues BM BS FRCA
Consultant Anaesthetist
Countess of Chester Hospital Foundation Trust
United Kingdom

Helen Smith MBBS MA (Med Ed) FHEA FRCA
Consultant Paediatric Anaesthetist
Addenbrooke's Hospital
Cambridge
United Kingdom

Joerg Steier MD PhD
Reader in Sleep and Respiratory Medicine
Lane Fox Unit/Sleep Disorders Centre
King's College
London
United Kingdom

Jonathan Thompson Bsc (Hons) MB ChB FRCA MD FFICM
Honorary Professor and Consultant in Anaesthesia and Critical Care Medicine
Leicester Royal Infirmary and University of Leicester
University Hospitals of Leicester NHS Trust

Leicester
United Kingdom

Henna Tirmizi MD
Assistant Professor of Anaesthesia
Tufts University School of Medicine
Boston, MA
USA

Christos Tsironis MD MSc FRCS
Consultant Bariatric and Upper GI Surgeon
St Mary's Hospital
Imperial College Healthcare NHS Trust
London
United Kingdom

Nicolas Varela MD PhD EDPM DESA
Pain Management Centre at National Hospital for
Neurology and Neurosurgery
University College London
London
United Kingdom

Nathan Ware MBBS FRCA
Society for Obesity and Bariatric Anaesthesia (UK)
Consultant Anaesthetist
Leicester Royal Infirmary
University Hospitals of Leicester NHS Trust
United Kingdom

Elinor Wighton MB ChB FRCA
Consultant in Anaesthesia

Leicester Royal Infirmary
University Hospitals of Leicester NHS Trust
Leicester
United Kingdom

Marcus Wood FRCA
Consultant Anaesthetist
Leicester Royal Infirmary
University Hospitals of Leicester NHS Trust
Leicester
United Kingdom

Hsiu L. Yap MB, ChB
Specialist Registrar in Endocrinology
Imperial College Healthcare Trust
St Mary's Hospital
London
United Kingdom

K. T. Yeung MBBS, FRCS
Department of Upper GI and Bariatric Surgery
St Mary's Hospital
Imperial Healthcare NHS Trust
London
United Kingdom

Francesco Zarantonello MD
Department of Medicine, Anaesthesiology and
Intensive Care
University of Padova
Padova
Italy

Preface

The aim of this book is to cover the essential components in the peri-operative care of the obese patient for anaesthetists, intensivists, surgeons, physicians, nursing staff, medical students and other healthcare support staff. We have specifically not written a textbook to cover the care of the patient undergoing weight loss surgery. There are plenty of well-established texts on this already. There is, however, a section on this specialist area within the book.

This book has been driven by the Society for Obesity and Bariatric Anaesthesia Key Issues meetings that cover the key points in caring for this ever-increasing group of patients. The book chapters, however, are not simply a replication of the lectures delivered as part of this course. These are new chapters written by experienced practitioners and applying their experience to the obese patient.

Peri-operative care for obese patients is associated with a lot of myth and conjecture regarding a number of aspects of care. We hope that this book provides readers from all disciplines, not just anaesthesia, with information to prepare them to manage these patients in the peri-operative period.

This is a brand new book. We have put it together with content that we feel leads the reader through a logical pathway for obesity peri-operative care. However, if you the reader feel areas are missing or could be improved, please let us know and we can plan for future editions.

We hope that this book becomes a popular choice for those wishing to improve their knowledge and therefore care of obese patients. We are extremely grateful to all authors who have contributed to the book and the publishers who have facilitated and supported us through what, at times, has seemed like a never-ending task.

Abbreviations

6MWT	six-minute walk test
11βHSD-1	11-beta-hydroxysteroid dehydrogenase type 1
AAGBI	Association of Anaesthetists of Great Britain and Ireland
ABW	adjusted body weight
ACE	angiotensin-converting enzyme
ADA	American Diabetes Association
ADH	anti-diuretic hormone
AES	anti-embolism stockings
AF	atrial fibrillation
AHI	apnoea/hypopnea index
AKI	acute kidney injury
ALI	acute lung injury
AMPK	adenosine monophosphate kinase
ANP	atrial natriuretic peptide
APAP	autoadjusting positive airway pressure
ARDS	acute respiratory distress syndrome
ASA	American Society of Anesthesiology
ASMBS	American Society for Metabolic and Bariatric Surgery
ASPEN	American Society for Parenteral and Enteral Nutrition
AT	anaerobic threshold
ATP	adenosine triphosphate
AFOI	awake fibre optic intubations
BAPEN	British Association for Parenteral and Enteral Nutrition
BET	bolus, elimination, transfer
BIS	bi-spectral index
BMI	body mass index
BNP	B-type natriuretic peptide
BPD	biliopancreatic diversion
CABG	coronary artery bypass graft
CAD	coronary artery disease
CDS	Chinese Diabetes Society
CKD	chronic kidney disease
CMACE	Centre for Maternal and Child Enquiries
CO	cardiac output
COPD	chronic obstructive pulmonary disease
CPAP	continuous positive airway pressure
CPET	cardiopulmonary exercise testing
CPR	cardiopulmonary resuscitation
CPSP	chronic post-surgical pain
CRP	C-reactive protein
CSE	combined spinal epidural
CT	computed tomography
CTA	computed tomography angiography
CVD	coronary vascular disease
CVP	central venous pressure
DA	difficult airway
DAS	Difficult Airway Society
DBS	double-burst stimulation
DI	Diabetes India
DKA	diabetic ketoacidosis
DMV	difficult mask ventilation
DOA	depth of anaesthesia
DOAC	direct oral anti-coagulant
DS	duodenal switch
DSS-II	Second Diabetes Surgery Summit
DUK	Diabetes UK
DVT	deep venous thrombosis
ECG	electrocardiogram
ECMO	extracorporeal membrane oxygenation
EDC	endocrine-disrupting chemical
EDR	ECG-derived respiration
EDS	excessive daytime sleepiness
EEG	electroencephalogram
EN	enteral nutrition
ERCP	endoscopic retrograde cholangiopancreatography
ERV	expiratory reserve volume
EOSS	Edmonton obesity staging system
ERAS	enhanced recovery after surgery
ESG	endoscopic sleeve gastroplasty
ESS	Epworth sleepiness score

ETAG	end tidal anaesthetic concentration guided	LBW	lean body weight
EuSOS	European Surgical Outcome Study	LH	leteinising hormone
EWS	early warning score	LMWH	low molecular weight heparin
FEV$_1$	forced expiratory volume in 1 second	LPL	lipoprotein lipase
FFM	fat free mass	LV	left ventricle
FFR	fractional flow reserve	LVH	left ventricle hypertrophy
FiO$_2$	fraction inspired oxygen concentration	MAC	minimum alveolar concentration
FONA	front of neck access	MACE	major adverse cardiac event
FRC	functional residual capacity	MAPK	mitogen-activated protein kinase
FSH	follicle-stimulating hormone	MCP-1	monocyte chemoattractant protein
FVC	forced vital capacity	MDT	multidisciplinary team
GA	general anaesthesia	MET	metabolic equivalent
GALT	gut-associated lymphoid tissue	MetS	metabolic syndrome
GI	gastro-intestinal	MGB	mini gastric bypass
GIP	gastric inhibitory polypeptide	MMIF	macrophage migration inhibiting factor
GLP-1	glucagon-like peptide 1	MMT	methadone maintenance therapy
GOJ	gastro-oesophageal junction	MO	morbid obesity
GORD	gastro-oesophageal reflux disease	MP	Mallampati
GP	general practitioner	MRI	magnetic resonance imaging
HDL	high-density lipoprotein	NAFLD	non-alcoholic fatty liver disease
HDU	high dependency unit	NAP	National Audit Project
HEE	Health Education England	NASH	non-alcoholic steatohepatitis
HELP	head-elevated laryngoscopy position	NBSR	National Bariatric Surgery Register
HFNO	high-flow nasal oxygenation	NC	neck circumference
HR	heart rate or hazard ratio	NCMP	National Child Measurement Programme
HRT	hormone replacement therapy	nCPAP	nocturnal continuous positive airway pressure
IAP	intra-abdominal pressure		
IBW	ideal body weight	NCEPOD	National Confidential Enquiry into Patient Outcome and Death
IC	indirect calorimetry		
ICD	International Classification of Diseases	NGT	nasogastric tube
		NIBP	non-invasive blood pressure
ICU	intensive care unit	NICE	National Institute for Health and Care Excellence
IDF	International Diabetes Federation		
iFR	instantaneous wave free ratio	NIH	National Institutes of Health
IGB	intra-gastric balloon	NIPPV	non-invasive positive pressure ventilation
IGF-1	insulin-like growth factor 1		
IH	intermittent hypoxaemia	NIV	non-invasive ventilation
IL	interleukin	NMBA	neuromuscular blocking agent
IOTF	International Obesity Task Force	NMJ	neuromuscular junction
IRS	insulin receptor substrate	NPV	negative predictive value
ISWT	incremental shuttle walk test	NSAIDs	non-steroidal anti-inflammatory drugs
ITU	intensive therapy unit		
IV	intravenous	NT-proBNP	N-terminal pro-B-type natriuretic peptide
IVC	inferior vena cava		
IVPCA	intravenous patient-controlled analgesia	OAT	opioid antagonist therapy
		ODI	oxygen desaturation index
JIB	jejunoileal bypass	OHS	obesity hypoventilation syndrome
LAGB	laparoscopic adjustable gastric band	OR	odds ratio

OSA	obstructive sleep apnoea	SBO	small bowel obstruction
OSAS	obstructive sleep apnoea syndrome	SDB	sleep disordered breathing
OSDS	obesity supine sudden death syndrome	SIRS	systemic inflammatory response syndrome
OS-MRS	obesity surgery mortality risk score	SNS	sympathetic nervous system
$PaCO_2$	partial pressure of arterial carbon dioxide	SOBA	Society for Obesity and Bariatric Anaesthesia
PACU	post-anaesthesia care unit	SpO_2	oxygen saturation
PAI-1	plasminogen activator inhibitor 1	SUFE	slipped upper femoral epiphysis
PaO_2	partial pressure of arterial oxygen	SV	stroke volume
PCA	patient-controlled analgesia	SWL	safe working load
PCOS	polycystic ovary syndrome	T2DM	type 2 diabetes mellitus
PE	pulmonary embolism	TAP	transversus abdominus plane
PEEP	positive end expiratory pressure	TBI	traumatic brain injury
PI3 K	phosphatidylinositol-3'-kinase	TBW	total body weight
PICC	peripherally inserted central catheter	TCI	target-controlled infusion
PICU	paedeatric intensive care unit	THRIVE	transnasal humidified rapid-insufflation ventilatory exchange
PK	pharmacokinetic		
PN	parenteral nutrition	TIVA	total intravenous anaesthesia
PONV	post-operative nausea and vomiting	TLC	total lung capacity
PORC	post-operative residual curarisation	TMD	thyromental distance
POSSUM	physiological and operative severity score for the enumeration of mortality and morbidity	TNF-α	tumour necrosis factor alpha
		TOF	train of four
		TOT	transdermal opioid therapy
PPI	proton pump inhibitor	TPS	transitional pain service
PPV	positive predictive value	TTE	transthoracic echocardiography
PR	per rectal	UFH	unfractionated heparin
PRAE	peri-operative adverse events	UDCA	urosdeoxycholic acid
PSG	polysomnography	UK	United Kingdom
PSV	pressure support ventilation	ULBT	upper lip bite test
RAS	renin–angiotensin system	VC	vital capacity
RBP4	retinol binding protein 4	V_D	volume of distribution
RCRI	revised cardiac risk index	VE	minute ventilation
RCT	randomised controlled trial	VEGF	vasoactive endothelial growth factor
RM	recruitment manoeuvre	VLDL	very low-density lipoproteins
ROS	reactive oxygen species	VO_2 peak	peak oxygen consumption
RRT	renal replacement therapy	Vt	tidal volume
RSI	rapid sequence induction	VTE	venous thromboembolism
RSII	rapid sequence induction-intubation	VV-ECMO	veno-venous extracorporeal membrane oxygenation
RTA	road traffic accident		
RV	right ventricle or residual volume	WC	waist circumference
RYGB	Roux-en-Y gastric bypass	WLS	weight loss surgery
SaO_2	oxygen saturation	WHO	World Health Organization
SAP	safe apnoea period	WHtR	waist-to-height ratio

The Obesity Problem and its Relationship to Healthcare

Harry Rutter

Introduction

Obesity is defined by the World Health Organization (WHO) as 'abnormal or excessive fat accumulation that may impair health.' Body mass index (BMI), is the most widely used measure to classify overweight and obesity. It is calculated as a person's weight in kilograms divided by the square of their height in meters (kg/m^2). In adults, WHO defines overweight as a BMI greater than or equal to 25, and obesity as a BMI greater than or equal to 30.

The global prevalence of obesity more than doubled between 1980 and 2014, and there are now almost two million people with overweight or obesity worldwide. The problem has increased rapidly across most high-income countries and is now growing in many low- and middle-income countries as well. In the UK, around 60% of adults are either overweight or obese, and around a quarter are obese. The problem is linked to deprivation, with the highest levels in the most deprived groups.

Obesity is implicated in many health conditions, including cardiovascular disease, some cancers (such as breast cancer and liver cancer), musculoskeletal problems and poor mental health. It is also a stigmatised condition, and people with obesity may find themselves discriminated against in public, in education, employment and elsewhere.

Despite significant media and political attention in many countries, for at least a decade, there has been little progress in reversing the global epidemic of obesity. Although the prevalence is stabilising in some countries, and some population groups, no country has yet successfully turned the tide and seen a persistent reduction in population prevalence. Tackling the complex problem of obesity will require a major increase in both the extent and intensity of prevention, and in the delivery of treatment. Bariatric surgery is an essential ingredient in this mix.

The Scale of the Problem

A proportion of the population has always been overweight, but the numbers started to climb slowly during the latter part of the twentieth century. In England adult obesity prevalence has increased steadily, rising from 15% in 1993 to 27% in 2015. The combined prevalence of both overweight and obesity is 68% in men and 58% in women. The geographical distribution shows a higher prevalence in the Midlands and the North of England, and the lowest in London and the South. There is relatively little variation by socioeconomic status in men, but in women the range is from 17% in the highest-income quintile to 39% in the second lowest.

The patterns are different in children. In 1984 only 1.2% of boys were obese, compared to 6.0% in 2002–2003, while in girls the figures ranged from 1.8% in 1984 to 6.6% in 2002–2003. This compares with obesity prevalence in 2015–2016 of 9% in 4–5-year-olds and 20% among 10–11-year-olds.

These figures are linked to stark socioeconomic differences, with an obesity prevalence of 13% among 4–5-year-olds living in the most deprived areas of the country compared to 5% among those in the least deprived. In 10–11-year-olds the figures were 26% in the most deprived areas, compared to 12% in the least deprived areas. In both age groups the size of these inequalities has increased over time and continues to widen. These differences are reflected in appreciable geographical variation, which is largely driven by differences in socio-economic status between different parts of the country.

There are wide differences between countries, with a prevalence of almost 40% in the United States of America, and high levels in countries such as Mexico, Canada, Australia and New Zealand, as well as the UK. Japan and Korea, however, both have an adult obesity prevalence of less than 5%, and countries such as Norway, Switzerland and the Netherlands all have low levels of around 10% prevalence.

The Burden of Obesity

Obesity is very closely associated with type 2 diabetes mellitus, and hypertension is twice as common among obese adults as it is in those of normal weight – around 40% of the former compared to around 20% of the latter. Obesity-related liver disease is increasing rapidly, and although the progression of the condition is not yet fully understood there is a high likelihood that it will become a major problem in the coming years.

Obesity is increasingly classified as a disease in its own right, although this remains contentious. The American Medical Association adopted the classification in 2013, and the World Obesity Federation followed suit in 2017. The World Obesity Federation took an epidemiological approach, in which food is viewed as the primary disease agent, acting on the body to produce disease. Positioning obesity in this way may be helpful in a healthcare context as a strong argument in favour of allocating resources towards prevention and treatment of the condition. This approach is not, however, without its critics, who have voiced concerns that obesity is primarily a risk factor for other conditions, rather than a disease in its own right, and medicalising a condition that is largely driven by the circumstances in which people live may place undue focus on individual-level rather than population-level responses.

Effects on Morbidity and Life Expectancy

In 2001, a report by the National Audit Office estimated that approximately 6% of all deaths in England in 1998 were caused by obesity – amounting to 30 000 excess deaths in that year. This is comparable to another study that found that 8.7% of deaths in the UK were attributable to obesity, the highest proportion in Europe.

Adults with severe obesity (with a BMI greater than 40) have increased risks of dying at a young age from many causes, including cancer, heart disease, stroke, diabetes and kidney and liver diseases, and experience dramatically reduced life expectancy compared with people of normal weight.

A major meta-analysis of data from long-term cohort studies involving almost 900 000 participants found that mortality was lowest at about 22·5–25 kg/m^2 in both men and women, and each 5 kg/m^2 BMI above this was on average associated with increased mortality of around 30%. Median life expectancy was reduced by 2–4 years in the BMI range 30–35 kg/m^2, and by 8–10 years in the BMI range 40–50 kg/m^2.

Effects on Healthcare Costs and the Wider Economy

A 2014 report found that obesity is a greater burden on the UK's economy than armed violence, war and terrorism, costing the country nearly £47bn a year and generating an annual loss equivalent to 3% of GDP. More than 2.1 billion people around the world – or nearly 30% of the global population – are overweight or obese, with the figure set to rise to almost half of the world's adult population by 2030.

Estimates of the direct costs to the NHS for treating overweight and obesity, and related morbidity in England, have ranged from £479.3 million in 1998 to £4.2 billion in 2007. Estimates of the indirect costs (those costs arising from the impact of obesity on the wider economy, such as loss of productivity) over the same time ranged between £2.6 billion and £15.8 billion.

Modelled projections suggest that indirect costs could be as much as £27 billion by 2015. In 2006–2007, obesity and obesity-related illness was estimated to have cost £148 million in inpatient stays in England. In Scotland, the total societal cost of obesity and overweight in 2007–2008 was estimated to be between £600 million and £1.4 billion; the NHS cost may have contributed as much as £312 million.

Drivers of Obesity

At the most basic level, overweight and obesity are the result of long-term overconsumption of food energy relative to energy expenditure through physical activity. Even a small excess of under 100 kcal/day can result in appreciable weight loss when maintained over the medium to long term.

Underpinning these outcomes is a multitude of factors, ranging from the behaviour of multinational food companies, through urban design and patterns of travel, to individual level preferences, behaviours, physiology and genetics. The common outcome of excess body fat may be driven by widely varied factors in different individuals and across different population groups.

The dominant framing of obesity is of a condition that is driven by a failure of self-control on the part of individuals, but the overwhelming scientific consensus is that this is not an appropriate conceptualisation of the problem. There is no evidence of a decline in levels of willpower or self-control across populations that have experienced large rises in the prevalence of obesity, but the environments in which people live have changed hugely in recent decades. It is unquestionably possible to eat a healthy diet and engage in adequate levels of physical activity, but the ubiquity of cheap, appealing, energy-dense food, and widespread barriers to regular physical activity, stack the odds against many of us. Obesity is in large part driven by these kinds of factors, which are collectively known as the 'obesogenic environment'. Individual-level factors still play a part, but they have played a much smaller part in the rise in prevalence of obesity over recent decades than these environmental factors. Effective responses to obesity thus need to take account of these underpinning drivers of the problem, striking a balance between upstream population-level actions and downstream individual-level interventions.

Prevention and Treatment

A balance is also needed between prevention and treatment of obesity, which overlap considerably. Obesity in childhood has a tendency to track through into adulthood and once excess weight is established it is very hard to lose it. There is thus a strong rationale for policy to focus on preventing children from becoming overweight or obese in the first place, and for minimising the likelihood of weight gain across the population. There are, however, large numbers of people who are already obese, many of whom might benefit from treatment, as well as ongoing prevention of further increases in weight.

Obesity is a complex problem. The choices we make about the food we buy, cook and eat, and the physical activity we engage in, are shaped by multiple factors that interact in often unpredictable non-linear ways across dynamic systems, ranging, for example, from agricultural policy and the price of fuel, to density of fast food restaurants and the availability of cycle lanes on one's commute. Effective responses to obesity will need to act across all levels of these systems, using many different mechanisms, and it is likely to take several decades for all the required changes for a comprehensive response to be in place.

Despite overwhelming scientific consensus on the need for strong, upstream action, and political endorsement of this, there is a consistent bias towards downstream individual-level actions, which tend to require high levels of agency for maximal effect; this is known as 'lifestyle drift'. This needs to be recognised, and strong and effective upstream actions taken to reverse these biases.

A wide range of actions is needed across food and physical activity systems. These should address the physical, socio-cultural, economic and political environments within which people live. This could lead to a range of responses, such as infrastructure for safe cycling, restrictions on advertising and marketing of unhealthy foods to children, taxes on sugar-sweetened drinks and national planning policy on walkable cities. Achieving a comprehensively healthy environment that truly promotes healthy eating and adequate physical activity will take many years, and steady progress will be required, with sustained action across these and other domains at global, national, regional and local levels.

Treatment options range from weight management programmes to drugs and bariatric surgery. There is evidence of effectiveness of some commercial weight-loss programmes in adults, but the evidence of effectiveness of these kinds of interventions in children is weaker.

A number of medications have been used for weight loss, but as a result of safety concerns most have either not been licensed for use in the UK or have been withdrawn from sale. Orlistat, which reduces dietary absorption of fat, is available at the time of writing and other medications may well be developed in the future.

The mainstay of treatment of severe obesity is bariatric surgery, which is addressed in detail later in this book (see Section 6). Bariatric surgery is a major undertaking for the person concerned, requiring life-long changes to eating habits in ways that many people find challenging, but in appropriately selected individuals it can lead to rapid resolution of type 2 diabetes, effective and maintained weight loss, and improvement or resolution of hyperlipidaemia, hypertension, obstructive sleep apnoea and musculoskeletal disorders, with improved quality of life.

Guidance from the National Institute for Health and Care Excellence (NICE) recommends bariatric surgery for people with a BMI greater than 40 kg/m^2 and people with a BMI between 35 and 40 kg/m^2 with other significant disease. It may also be beneficial in people with a BMI greater than 30 who have poorly controlled type 2 diabetes and people of Asian origin with recent-onset type 2 diabetes, as Asian people are more vulnerable to complications of diabetes than people from other population groups.

The NICE guidance is very clear about the need for support from a multidisciplinary team that is able to conduct thorough pre-operative assessment, regular post-operative assessment, including specialist dietetic and surgical follow-up, and psychological support before and after surgery. In order to be eligible for bariatric surgery in England an individual should have exhausted all appropriate non-surgical measures, and have received intensive weight loss support.

Although bariatric surgery is expensive (around £6000 per procedure in 2015) it is cost-effective because of the significant health benefits it can lead to. However, despite its importance as an individual-level intervention, it has limited impact at population level: there are well over a million people with a BMI over 40 in the UK, but only around 6000 bariatric procedures are conducted each year.

Conclusions

Obesity represents one of the most pressing health problems of our time. It has increased rapidly across the world over recent decades, and shows no signs of abating. Almost two-thirds of the population of the United Kingdom is overweight or obese at a level that increases the risk of multiple health problems. This not only carries major personal and financial costs for those individuals, it also has significant impacts on health systems and society as a whole.

Despite widespread policy attention, and some investment, no country has yet reversed this trend. But there are positive signs in some high-income countries that the increase in prevalence is slowing, and perhaps even stopping. However, even if there is a major decline in population prevalence over the coming years, a large proportion of the population will remain overweight and obese, and many of these people would stand to benefit from treatment.

Bariatric surgery is a cost-effective procedure that has the potential to transform the lives of severely obese individuals, attenuating or even reversing many of the important health consequences of the condition. Well under 1% of potentially eligible patients receive this procedure each year, but as the obesity epidemic progresses it seems highly likely, not only that the level of activity in bariatric surgery will increase, but that the case mix is also likely to change and include greater numbers of severely obese individuals. Greater knowledge and understanding of how best to respond to this is essential, across the health system and among the professionals who will have to deliver this care.

Further Reading

Banegas JR, Lopez-Garcia E, Gutierrez-Fisac JL, Guallar-Castillon P, Rodriguez-Artalejo F. A simple estimate of mortality attributable to excess weight in the European Union. *Eur J Clin Nutr*. 2003;**57**(2):201–8.

Bray GA. Medical consequences of obesity. *J Clin Endocrinol Metab*. 2004;**89**(6):2583–9.

Bray GA, Kim KK, Wilding JPH, on behalf of the World Obesity Feferation. Obesity: a chronic relapsing progressive disease process. A position statement of the World Obesity Federation. *Obes Rev*. 2017;**18**(7):715–23.

Brownell KD, Kersh R, Ludwig DS, et al. Personal responsibility and obesity: a constructive approach to a controversial issue. *Health Aff (Millwood)*. 2010;**29**(3):379–87.

Buchwald H, Avidor Y, Braunwald E, et al. Bariatric surgery: a systematic review and meta-analysis. *JAMA*. 2004;**292**(14):1724–37.

Butland B, Jebb SA, Kopelman P, et al. *Tackling Obesities: Future Choices*. London: Government Office for Science and Department of Health and Social Care; 2007.

Dobbs R, Sawers C, Thompson F, et al. *Overcoming Obesity: An Initial Economic Analysis*. London: McKinsey Global Institute; 2014.

Hachem A, Brennan L. Quality of life outcomes of bariatric surgery: a systematic review. *Obes Surg*. 2016;**26**(2):395–409.

Hartmann-Boyce J, Johns DJ, Jebb SA, et al. Behavioural Weight Management Review G. Behavioural weight management programmes for adults assessed by trials conducted in everyday contexts: systematic review and meta-analysis. *Obes Rev*. 2014;**15**(11):920–32.

Hunter D, Popay J, Tannahill C, Whitehead M, Elson T. *Learning Lessons from the Past: Shaping a Different Future*. London: Marmot Review; 2009.

Kitahara CM, Flint AJ, Berrington de Gonzalez A, et al. Association between Class III Obesity (BMI of 40–59 kg/m2) and Mortality: A Pooled Analysis of 20 Prospective Studies. *PLOS Med*. 2014;**11**(7):e1001673.

National Audit Office. *Tackling Obesity in Britain*. London: National Audit Office; 2001.

National Institute of Health and Care Excellence. *Obesity: Indentification, Assessment and Management: Clinical Guideline [CG189]*. London: National Institute of Health and Care Excellence; 2014.

NHS Digital Statistics Team. Statistics on Obesity, Physical Activity and Diet – England 2017. London: NHS; 2017

Prospective Studies Collaboration. Body-mass index and cause-specific mortality in 900000 adults: collaborative analyses of 57 prospective studies. *Lancet*. 2009;**373** (9669):1083–96.

Roberto CA, Swinburn B, Hawkes C, et al. Patchy progress on obesity prevention: emerging examples, entrenched barriers, and new thinking. *Lancet*. 2015;**385**(9985):2400–9.

Rutter HR, Bes-Rastrollo M, de Henauw S, et al. Balancing upstream and downstream measures to tackle the obesity epidemic: a position statement from the European

Association for the Study of Obesity. *Obes Facts*. 2017;**10** (1):61–3.

Swinburn BA, Sacks G, Hall KD, et al. The global obesity pandemic: shaped by global drivers and local environments. *Lancet*. 2011;**378**(9793):804–14.

Swinburn B, Egger G, Raza F. Dissecting obesogenic environments: the development and application of a framework for identifying and prioritizing environmental interventions for obesity. *Prev Med*. 1999; **29**(6 Pt 1): 563–70.

The Scottish Government. *Preventing Overweight and Obesity in Scotland: A Route Map Towards Healthy Weight*. Edinburgh: The Scottish Government; 2010.

2 Drivers of Obesity, Nutrition and Dietary Considerations

David Haslam

Introduction

The global obesity epidemic is a recent phenomenon, but existence of obesity was recorded at least 30 000 years ago, as shown by prehistoric statues such as the Venus of Hohle Fels and the Venus of Willendorf, considered to be amongst the oldest examples of figurative art on Earth. The Neolithic era also yielded numerous artefacts displaying obesity, found in Anatolia (now Turkey) and Malta. Basic drivers for obesity must have always existed; the question is, what new drivers have caused a quarter of the population to become obese over the last 30 years?

Drivers of Obesity

The description, causes and basic management of obesity have been known for thousands of years. In 500BC Sushruta, the Indian Priest and physician wrote 'A person afflicted with obesity develops such symptoms as shortness of breath, thirst, ravenous appetite, excessive sleepiness, perspiration, fetid odours in the body, wheezing sound in the throat during sleep, or sudden suspension of breath,...'. A century later, Hippocrates described the energy balance equation: 'It is very injurious to health to take in more food than the constitution will bear, when at the same time, one uses no exercise to carry off this excess. For as aliment fills, and exercise empties the body, the result of an exact equipoise between them must be to leave the body in the same state they found it, that is, in perfect health'. Galen, the physician to the Roman Emperors treated patients with exercise, diet and rubbing, and produced insightful case studies on obese patients, although his theory that the condition was caused by an imbalance in the four bodily humours – specifically an excess of blood – had no merits. Obesity was well known to Avicenna, the Arabic physician, born in 980AD, who devoted a large section of his Canon of Medicine to the condition and its management. Maimonades, the

twelfth-century Iberian physician followed Galen's principles, recognising that obesity had repercussions on bodily health, and treating it with medication, massage, exercise and baths. Many other physicians, too numerous to mention, studied and managed obesity, including George Cheyne, Morgagni, Thomas Willis and Tobias Venner – the first person to use the word 'obesity' in print. But special mention for progressing the science of drivers of obesity is Philip Theophrastus Aureolus Bombastus von Hohenheim (1493–1541) better known as Paracelsus, a highly unpopular figure who fell out with the Church and the medical profession, and burnt a pile of Galen's and Avicenna's books in the street, stating, 'The stubble on my chin knows more than you and all your scribes, my shoe buckles are more learned than your Galen and Avicenna, and my beard has more experience than all your high colleges!' He introduced the concept of a 'microcosm' and a 'macrocosm', i.e. an internal and an external environment that both contribute to illness, rather than Galen and Hippocrates four internal humours. Thus obesity is at least somewhat due to external drivers. A great believer in alchemy, he also had unusual beliefs on how nature is governed, writing in 1515 *A Book on Nymphs, Gnomes, Giants, Dwarves, Incubi and Succubae, Stars and Signs*, proving that however great a person's reputation might be, their evidence base should be carefully scrutinised.

If physicians practising 3000 years ago could introduce and initiate treatment for obesity, there's no reason present day practitioners can't do similar.

Just as there is a genetic reason why some smokers get carcinoma of the bronchus and others don't, there are similar reasons why some overeaters get fat and others stay lean. Obesity was historically rare, and only now that food is plentiful and unhealthy, and technology reduces our need to exercise, has the condition become an epidemic. This proves that there are environmental drivers behind the epidemic, but we now recognise the multifactorial nature of the disease.

In 1973 Ethan Sims and his team devised an experiment to study 'experimental human obesity'. Instead of laboratory rats, he used laboratory humans, force feeding healthy young male prisoners, controlling for exercise levels and observing weight gain to an average BMI of 28, alongside a deterioration in glycaemic control, leading him to coin the word 'diabesity'. However, a more interesting finding was that different individuals required vastly different quantities of calories to achieve the weight gain, proving that there is more to weight gain than calories and the energy balance equation alone. We are genetically programmed to eat whenever food is available in case of future famine, and rest whenever possible, to conserve energy for hunting for food, or escape from attack from sabre tooth tigers. There is no in-built instinct to stop eating, or to perform scheduled or formal exercise, so our natural default tendency is to eat and remain stationary, and a huge effort of mind and body is needed to do the opposite. In summary, factors other than diet and physical activity contribute to the increase in BMI over time.

Energy intake that exceeds energy expenditure has traditionally, and still is broadly considered to be the main driver of weight gain, although quality of nutritional intake may exert its effect on energy balance through other complex hormonal, metabolic and neurological pathways that influence satiety. The food environment, marketing of unhealthy foods and urbanisation, increase in sedentary behaviours and reduced physical activity play important roles, but many more drivers are being identified. Emerging risk factors include environmental contaminants, chronic psycho-social stress, neuroendocrine dysregulation and genetic/epigenetic mechanisms.

A recent International workshop in Uppsala, Sweden discussed environmental contaminants in relation to obesity and concluded: 'there is an urgent need to reduce the burden of environmental contaminants so that obesity does not become the normal outlook in the future'. The workshop attendees concluded that public health efforts should focus on the importance of early obesity prevention by means of reducing chemical exposures, rather than only treating the established disease. 'Just as a bad start can last a lifetime and beyond, a good start can last a lifetime as well.' During the workshop, delegates discussed human studies showing that exposure of pregnant mothers to environmental contaminants are linked with increased weight gain in their offspring. Studies have also demonstrated that prenatal exposure to dichlorodiphenyldichloroethylene (DDE, a DDT metabolite), is linked with rapid weight gain in children, and that higher levels of DDE in the blood of pregnant women is associated with obesity in adult offspring. Furthermore, several pollutants, e.g. polychlorinated biphenyls, dioxins, bisphenol A and other pesticides, are associated with mitochondrial dysfunction, lipid disturbances, insulin resistance, diabetes and hypertension in human studies. Also, there is growing appreciation that development during the critical period is particularly vulnerable to the effects of exogenous endocrine-disrupting chemicals (EDCs) that can reprogramme essential signalling/differentiation pathways and lead to lifelong consequences.

Factors activating stress in the body include psycho-social and socio-economic handicaps, depressive and anxiety traits, alcohol and smoking, and it has been suggested that environmental, perinatal and genetic factors induce neuroendocrine perturbations that are followed by abdominal obesity and co-morbidities. There is considerable evidence from clinical to cellular and molecular studies that elevated cortisol, particularly when combined with secondary inhibition of sex steroids and growth hormone secretions, is causing accumulation of fat in visceral adipose tissues. It has been postulated that a continuously changing and sometimes threatening external environment may activate central pathways that stimulate the adrenals to release glucocorticoids, which may mediate a pathogenetic role in the metabolic syndrome. However, a recent study was unable to support a causal link between psycho-social factors and abdominal obesity. Although individuals with permanent stress were slightly more obese, there was no overall independent effect and no evidence that abdominal obesity or its consequences increased with higher levels of stress or depression.

A person's genes play an important role in determining their health and physiological status, including insulin sensitivity and blood pressure. Single nucleotide polymorphisms in the genome are related to the occurrence and severity of cardiovascular disease (CVD), diabetes, obesity and dysfunctional metabolism, reproduction and endocrine systems. The developmental origins of health and disease (DOHaD) hypothesis, explains how this may increase the risk of disease later in life. As originally formulated, the DOHaD paradigm initially focused on multiple studies that documented links between poor nutrition *in utero* and increased risk in offspring of obesity, CVD and diabetes mellitus over a lifespan. Among the mechanisms underlying obesity, epigenetics – the science of heritable changes in gene expression that occur without a change in the DNA sequence – is emerging as an important factor.

Primary Care Management of Obesity

Patients understand the complex nature of their condition, expect the healthcare professional to raise the topic of their weight in a positive manner and want to be fully and expertly assessed and treated, not just told to 'eat less, move more'. A recent study revealed that:

- the patient–physician relationship plays an important role in the adequacy of obesity management;
- patients have clear expectations of substantive conversations with their primary care team;
- complex conditions affect weight and patients require assistance tailored to individual obesity drivers;
- current services provide support in important ways (accessibility, availability, accountability, affordability, consistency of messaging), but are not yet meeting patient needs for individual plans, advanced education and follow-up opportunities.

Unfortunately, in practice, attitudes are very different to patient expectations. Few medical practitioners report having received training in weight management. Many regard weight management as unsuccessful and lack confidence owing to lack of teaching. A Pulse survey of over 1000 GPs saw 32% of respondents answering 'yes' to a question about whether they have offended a patient by raising the issue of them being overweight.

However, where funding, training and facilities are available, GPs experienced an increase in their confidence and self-efficacy in managing excess weight. In an Australian study, GPs described changing their usual practice with the aid of a structured management tool for obesity, and felt more confident to discuss obesity with their patients. Care in general practice can improve GP confidence and self-efficacy in managing obesity; enhancing GP's 'professional self-efficacy' is a step in improving obesity management within primary care. Management of children in primary care remains difficult and often unrewarding.

Primary care management of obesity begins the moment the individual walks through the surgery door, and down the corridor into the physician's office. Identification of excess weight doesn't require any science or gadgets, merely observation; if a person looks as though they have a weight problem, they have a weight problem. Precise measurements can be useful in the primary care setting, including weight, height, BMI, bio-impedance for percentage fat to monitor improvements, but, unlike most bio-medical assessments, patients are perfectly capable of, and often prefer, measuring their own weight. Every house has a set of scales. Roughly a quarter of the population of the UK suffers from obesity, and obese individuals utilise services more than lean individuals according to studies such as Counterweight, because of multiple co-morbidities, therefore it is reasonable to assume that almost one-third of patients who access their GP surgery are obese, and many more overweight. Consequently, the majority of individuals in CVD, diabetes and sleep apnoea clinics will be obese, providing a significant clinical and financial burden to practices, and ensuring that obesity management is a priority in primary care. An obese person, consulting for whatever reason, should not be allowed to finish the consultation without the topic of weight being raised, otherwise the future likelihood of diabetes, heart disease, sleep apnoea and cancer will not have been alleviated. There is a common misperception that approaching the topic of obesity is difficult and time-consuming, but bearing in mind that all GPs have, during their careers, had to tell mothers that their baby has died, and wives that their husband has been killed in a traffic accident, telling someone they have some excess weight is not daunting.

Management of obesity in primary care begins with lifestyle interventions. Promotion of physical activity is crucial for reduction in cardio-metabolic risk, and resolution of pre-diabetes, as well as improving general health, including cancer risk, but on its own is unlikely to induce weight loss. Percentage body fat is likely to reduce, and improvements can be tracked using relatively inexpensive scales. Accelerometers, including fitness trackers, and also pedometers are useful for some individuals, but it must be remembered that the ideological target of 10000 steps or more per day is inappropriate for someone with poor mobility who only manages 200 steps daily, in whom an initial increase to 400 is a boost to their health. Exercise on prescription has gained a poor reputation, possibly because a positive referral doesn't mean that an individual is suitable for a scheme, or even that they will turn up.

A discussion with patients around dietary intervention is important. This can be done with the aid of tier 2 interventions provided by commercial enterprises, including slimming clubs, meal replacement therapies or very low-calorie diets; however, there is mounting evidence that low carbohydrate diets have the edge over low fat regimes. Studies that insist on assessing isocaloric low-carbohydrate versus low-fat diets, are misguided, and only reflect the academic environment rather than real life. In real clinical life, patients on low-carbohydrate regimes will choose to eat less due to earlier satiation; therefore only studies that involve ad libitum diets are of interest to primary care rather than academia. Clinically relevant ad libitum diets, including studies such as Diogenes, reveal that higher protein content in an ad libitum diet improves weight loss maintenance after weight loss, in overweight and obese adults over 12 months. The A to Z diet replaced the word 'ad libitum' with 'free living', concluding that 'overweight and obese women assigned to follow the Atkins diet, which had the lowest carbohydrate intake, lost more weight at 12 months than women assigned to follow the Zone diet, and had experienced comparable or more favourable metabolic effects than those assigned to the Zone, Ornish, or LEARN diets'. Similarly the Direct study found that the Mediterranean and low-carbohydrate diets are effective alternatives to the low-fat diet for weight loss and appear to be just as safe as the low-fat diet. In addition to producing weight loss, the low-carbohydrate and Mediterranean diets had some beneficial metabolic effects, a result suggesting that these dietary strategies might be considered in clinical practice and that diets might be individualised according to personal preferences and metabolic needs. In summary, it is naïve to believe that a calorie is just a calorie; the body responds to a calorie of fat, a calorie of protein, a calorie of carbohydrate, or alcohol in completely different ways physiologically and metabolically, so simple mathematic equations based on heat chambers don't apply. Therefore only ad libitum or 'free-living' diets reveal the truth. Laboratory conditions do not apply to the real world, outside and beyond academic ivory towers.

Pharmaceutical interventions are beyond the scope of this text, but it is important that primary care is primed to provide such medications and monitor them effectively, and be aware of the side effects and 'stopping' rules; this includes older drugs such as orlistat, and possibly phentermine, and newer agents such as saxenda and mysimba, not forgetting pipeline agents not yet licensed in the UK.

Anyone who undergoes bariatric surgery will have encountered their GP as their first port of call, so primary care practitioners must have a working knowledge of the range of procedures available, referral guidelines, operative techniques, side effects and what to do in an emergency situation or unsuspected event.

Conclusion

'The body was never meant to be treated as a refuse bin, holding all the foods that the palate demands.' – Mahatma Gandhi.

Further Reading

Björntorp P. Do stress reactions cause abdominal obesity and comorbidities? *Obes Rev.* 2001;**2**(2):73–86.

Brown RE, Sharma AM, Ardern CI, et al. Secular differences in the association between caloric intake, macronutrient intake, and physical activity with obesity. *Obes Res Clin Pract.* 2015; **10**(3): 243–55.

Ford ND, Patel SA, Narayan KM. Obesity in low-and middle- income countries: burden, drivers and emerging challenges. *Ann Rev Publ Health.* 2017;**38**:145–164.

Iszatt N, Stigum H, Verner MA, et al. Prenatal and postnatal exposure to persistent organic pollutants and infant growth: a pooled analysis of seven European birth cohorts. *Environ Health Perspect.* 2015;**123**(7):730–6.

Karmaus W, Osuch JR, Eneli I, et al. Maternal levels of dichlorodiphenyl-dichloroethylene (DDE) may increase weight and body mass index in adult female offspring. *Occup Environ Med.* 2009;**66**(3):143–9.

Lind P, Lind PM, Lejonklou MH, et al. Uppsala consensus statement on environmental contaminants and the global obesity epidemic. *Environ Health Perspect.* 2016;**124**(5): A81–3.

Papavramidou NS, Papavramidis ST, Christopoulou-Aletra H. Galen on obesity: etiology, effects and treatment. *World J Surg.* 2004;**28**(6):631–5.

Romieu I, Dossus L, Barquera S, et al. Energy balance and obesity: what are the main drivers? *Cancer Causes Contr.* 2017; **28**(3):247–58.

Shai I, Schwarzfuchs D, Henkin Y, et al. Weight loss with a low-carbohydrate, Mediterranean or low-fat diet. *N Engl J Med.* 2008;**359**(3):229–41.

Sturgiss E, Haesler E, Elmitt N, et al. Increasing general practitioners' confidence and self-efficacy in managing obesity: a mixed methods study. *BMJ Open.* 2017;7(1):e014314.

Body Morphology and Fat Distribution

Henna Tirmizi and Roman Schumann

Introduction

Not all fat is created equal. Two different people can have the exact same body weight with varying percentages of body fat and can carry that fat in different areas of their body. The study of body morphology and fat distribution helps not only define the way fat is arranged on a person, but how fat deposits on different parts of the body differ physiologically and lead to varying cardio-metabolic risk profiles.

Scales of Measurement

BMI

Body mass index (BMI) is calculated as a person's weight in kilograms divided by height in meters squared. It is the most widely used and well-recognized measure of adiposity, both in clinical practice and the medical literature. The National Heart, Lung and Blood Institute in the United States uses BMI ranges to categorise individuals within a population. These ranges include a BMI below 18.5 (underweight), 18.5–<25 (normal weight), 25–<30 (overweight), 30–<35 (grade 1 obesity), 35–<40 (grade 2 obesity) and BMI >40 (grade 3 obesity). While the use of BMI as a measure of obesity is attractive for its simplicity, it is unable to account for the more detailed and important information of adipose tissue distribution. For example, three different individuals with grade 1 obesity could have very different body fat distributions: one with an even distribution of weight, one with central (also known as abdomino-visceral) obesity and a third with most of their weight located around the hips and thighs (gluteo-femoral obesity). These types of adipose tissue distributions carry substantially different cardiac and metabolic risk profiles for the afflicted individual, indicating the limitations of BMI alone as a measure of obesity. Examination of the all-cause mortality of

overweight and obese individuals has shown a greater risk of mortality with higher obesity BMI grades. Yet, grade 1 obesity was not associated with higher mortality, and being overweight was linked with lower all-cause mortality. Adults with central obesity have the worst long-term survival, regardless of BMI category. This evidence suggests that scales of measurement other than BMI may be important to appropriately assess an individual's obesity-associated health risk profile.

Waist Circumference

With increasing recognition of the link between visceral body fat and metabolic complications of obesity, waist circumference (WC) has been used as a marker of visceral adiposity. WC can be measured from several different anatomical locations, resulting in varying values. The anatomical landmark 2.5 cm above the umbilicus has been shown to correlate well with abdominal fat mass. Obesity-associated risk assessed by WC is almost identical in whites and African Americans, indicating its reliability across ethnic backgrounds. The latter is not necessarily the case, as other measures of adiposity (including BMI and waist-to-height ratio) have shown correlations with mortality in white adults, but not African Americans.

Waist-to-Hip Ratio, Waist-to-Thigh Ratio and Waist-to-Height Ratio

Adiposity indices that contain the waist circumference in relation to additional anthropomorphic measurements have shown promise as reliable indicators of metabolic and cardiovascular risk. The waist-to-thigh ratio (WTR) for both genders and the waist-to-hip ratio (WHR) in women have been positively associated with mortality in middle-aged adults. These ratios of body measurement offer additional prognostic information beyond BMI and WC in this patient population (See Table 3.1).

Table 3.1 Common scales of measurement and their methods of calculation. Circumference measured in cm.

Scale of Measurement	Calculation
Body Mass Index (BMI)	Weight in kilograms/ (height in m)^2
Waist-to-Hip Ratio (WHR)	Waist circumference/ hip circumference
Waist-to-Thigh Ratio (WTR)	Waist circumference/ thigh circumference
Waist-to-Height Ratio (WHtR)	Waist circumference/ height in cm

While BMI overestimates fat in muscular individuals and does not provide information about fat distribution, waist-to-height ratio (WHtR) is a better indicator of central adipose tissue. This ratio is believed to be more useful than BMI and WC alone because it not only incorporates the visceral fat prediction of WC, but it also adjusts for height, giving an unbiased estimate of WC. Waist-to-hip ratio is a more sensitive predictor of mortality than BMI for men and women and it may also be the best indicator for undiagnosed type 2 diabetes and impaired fasting glucose. Even in obese children and adolescents, WHtR has been a significant predictor of metabolic syndrome.

Radiological Assessment of Adiposity

The utility of imaging modalities in defining differences in body composition and differentiating between adipose and lean tissue has been increasingly recognised. Computed axial tomography (CT), magnetic resonance imaging (MRI), ultrasound and dual-energy X-ray absorptiometry (DXA) have all been described. Advances in sensitivity and quality have not only allowed distinction between lean and adipose tissue, but recognition of various fat deposits within tissue beds, improving our understanding of the functional roles of adipose tissue in different body types.

CT and MRI are both considered gold standards for measuring, with accuracy and reproducibility, visceral adipose tissue (VAT). While MRI has limiting factors of cost and time required for imaging, CT is associated with ionising radiation. In order to decrease time and radiation dose, estimating whole-body adipose and lean tissue volumes from extrapolation across multiple isolated 2D slices has been used for both MRI and CT. The risk of significant error, however, remains prevalent as volumes from unscanned regions of the body are extrapolated.

Compared to CT and MRI, DXA offers the advantage of significantly less ionising radiation, less cost and decreased risk of errors in calculating tissue volumes. VAT volume measured by DXA strongly correlates with VAT volume measured by MRI. Lack of radiation exposure and widespread availability and portability have popularized ultrasound assessment of adiposity. VAT measures strongly correlate with MRI and CT measurements. However, subcutaneous adipose tissue assessments with ultrasound have shown less accuracy and reliability. Overall, advances in technology have increased the availability of imaging in clinical and research settings, while reducing scanning time and injurious exposures for patients.

Considerations of Adiposity and Drug Dosing

With the physiologic changes and pharmacologic implications of obesity, a reliable method for drug dosing is desirable. Obesity increases both the lean and fat masses of the person with obesity. Although an obese person has more lean mass than a non-obese person of the same age, height and sex, the percentage of fat mass per kilogram of total body weight (TBW) increases more than the lean mass. This results in a relative decrease of the percentage of lean mass and water in the obese compared to the non-obese.

Ideal body weight (IBW) is calculated with the equation: IBW (kg) = 45.4 kg (49.9 kg for men) + 0.89 ×(height in cm − 152.4). Although, it contains more information (sex of patient) than other body scalars, IBW is not an ideal metric for all drug dosing. Regardless of body composition, all patients of the same sex and height would receive the same dose of any given drug.

Predicted normal weight (PNWT) was developed to predict the expected normal weight of an obese individual. PNWT is equal to the sum of an individual's lean body weight (LBW) and a fraction of the individual's excess fat content that represents predicted normal fat mass. LBW consists of a person's weight without almost all adipose tissue. PNWT has a separate formula for males and females, and is unique in that is was specifically developed to characterise the pharmacokinetics of drugs.

The reader is referred to Chapter 9 for more information on drug dosing.

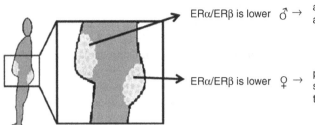

ERα/ERβ is lower ♂ → accelerates visceral adipose tissue deposition

ERα/ERβ is lower ♀ → promotes gluteo-femoral subcutaneous adipose tissue deposition

Figure 3.1 Oestrogen receptors alpha and beta (Erα, Erβ) are important regulators of adipose tissue depot distribution and accumulation.

Toxic versus Benign Fat: Anatomical Differences

The study of regional differences in adipose tissue distribution is expanding. Fat in different areas of the body can have distinctive cellular composition, microvasculature, innervation and metabolic characteristics. Not only does fat in various parts of the body respond differently to hormones and drugs, the distinct actions of these adipose tissue depots result in unique physiologic states. There is strong evidence to show that a predominantly gluteal-femoral compared with abdominal/central fat distribution is associated with a lower metabolic risk.

Sexual Dimorphism in Body Fat Distribution

Pre-menopausal women tend to store fat on the hips, thighs and buttocks. This gives them a pear shape, also known as a gluteal-femoral body fat distribution. Men, on the other hand, store fat predominantly over the abdomen. This results in an apple shape or abdominal/central fat distribution. Oestrogen is involved in the maintenance of the gluteal-femoral body fat distribution. The loss of circulating oestrogen in women undergoing menopause is associated with increases in central obesity. Oestrogen receptor alpha (ERα) and oestrogen receptor beta (ERβ) are receptors present in human adipose tissue. These receptors influence adiposity and modulate the distribution of fat between depots. ERα is found in higher concentrations in abdominal subcutaneous than gluteal subcutaneous fat, whereas ERβ is more abundant in gluteal than abdominal fat. The ratios of these receptors have proven to be important as well. The alpha receptor has the primary role of adiposity regulation by limiting fat accumulation. The beta receptor counteracts ERα effects. The ratio of ERα/ERβ expression in the abdominal and gluteal areas leads to different phenotypes. A greater ratio of ERα/ ERβ in abdominal fat serves to limit adipose accumulation in this depot, whereas a lower ERα/ ERβ ratio in gluteal fat results in conditions for accumulation of gluteal fat (see Figure 3.1). Men, in general, have a relative lack of ERα in the visceral adipose tissue depot, and are therefore predisposed to store more fat viscerally. Deletion of ERα from adipocytes in males and females causes increased visceral adiposity. Sexual differences in adipose tissue distribution are further accentuated by suppressive effects of testosterone on lipoprotein lipase activity in femoral subcutaneous tissue in men. This limits the deposition of fat from free fatty acids and triglycerides in the gluteal area of men.

Genetics

Abdominal and gluteal adipose tissue aspirates have shown differential expression of genes that regulate fatty acid and glucose uptake. This genetic variation contributes to differences in cardio-metabolic risk based on a person's body fat distribution. These genes have been identified as the so-called homeobox (HOX) genes that differ in human gluteal and abdominal adipose tissue. HOX genes control morphogenesis and several HOX genes are regulated by gender-specific steroid hormones, hence accounting for many of the differences in fat distribution between men and women. Variations in genetic expression result in differing responses from adipose tissue depots, depending on anatomical location. For example, growth hormone receptor is expressed 75% more in abdominal adipose tissue than it is in gluteal adipose tissue. Growth hormone receptor expression correlates significantly with the expression of critical regulators of lipolysis. Therefore, growth hormone preferentially decreases central obesity, and this is at least partially mediated by a greater sensitivity to growth hormone action at the level of the growth hormone receptor.

Adipocyte Generation

Central and gluteal-femoral fat differ in cellular generation rates. Pre-adipocytes are correlated with the formation of both abdominal and femoral fat. However, adipocytes are formed at a higher rate in femoral fat. The gluteo-femoral area is believed to be more effective at storing excess fat than the abdomen. Evidence suggests that abdominal adipose tissue has a limited ability to store excess lipid energy substrate. This, combined with heightened lipolysis from abdominal adipose tissue increases free fatty acid delivery to the liver. Impaired adipogenesis and the resultant lipotoxicity from free fatty acids lead those with an abdominal body fat distribution to be more likely to have specific disease states such as metabolic syndrome, insulin resistance and type 2 diabetes. In summary, fat tissue depot heterogeneity influences metabolic health.

Fat Distribution and Metabolic Syndrome

There are significant differences in the functional characteristics of subcutaneous abdominal, intra-abdominal and gluteo-femoral fat depots. Intra-abdominal/visceral adipose tissue has been a known contributor to metabolic risk, but there is increasing evidence that subcutaneous abdominal fat plays a major role in obesity-related insulin resistance in comparison to visceral fat. Correspondingly, men with non-insulin-dependent diabetes mellitus (NIDDM) have been found to have a fat distribution pattern that favours abdominal subcutaneous deposition rather than peripheral subcutaneous or intra-peritoneal fat deposition. Women with lower-body fat have been found to have lower fasting glucose and lipid concentrations. In contrast to abdominal fat, lower-body fat has been described as a reservoir for metabolic storage, retaining extra free fatty acids when there is excess energy. This can be credited to its lower lipolytic activity and higher lipoprotein lipase activity compared to abdominal fat.

Obesity is associated with a chronic low-grade inflammatory state. This is secondary to increased production of pro-inflammatory cytokines in adipose tissue. Intrinsic developmental differences between glutco-fcmoral and abdominal adipose tissue result in a consistently weaker expression of genes related to inflammation from gluteo-femoral adipose tissue.

Body Morphology and Cardiac Risk

Body fat distribution has shown strong positive correlations with cardiac risk factors. Markers of hypertension, dyslipidemia and inflammation are all associated with each other. Studies on healthy postmenopausal women are particularly revealing. Transitioning through menopause, women lose protective oestrogens and gain a subsequent excess of androgens resulting in upper body fat accumulation. This is considered a major mediator of menopause-related cardiac morbidity and mortality. Indices of central and peripheral fat distribution have shown opposite patterns of associations with cardio-metabolic risk factors.

Atrial Fibrillation

Epicardial fat is a distinct adipose tissue depot that is associated with the presence, severity and recurrence of atrial fibrillation. Multiple proposed mechanisms exist for this influence. There are no fascial boundaries between epicardial fat and the myocardium. Adipocyte infiltration into underlying atrial myocardium results in conduction slowing. Epicardial fat is metabolically active; rich in adipokines, this promotes fibrosis in atrial myocardium. Inflammation caused by cytokines secreted by epicardial fat (such as C-reactive protein, interleukins and tumour necrosis factor alpha (TNF-α)) could facilitate arrhythmogenesis. The role of fat in the development and severity of atrial fibrillation becomes particularly important when the effects of ageing, metabolic disorders and systemic disease on fat are considered.

Heart Failure

Obesity is associated with an increased risk of heart failure, even after correcting for other risk factors such as hypertension, coronary artery disease and diabetes. Both visceral fat and subcutaneous fat have been associated with increased left ventricular (LV) mass. However, only visceral fat is associated with an increased LV mass-to-volume ratio (a measure of concentricity), which is a precursor to heart failure. Gluteal-femoral obesity, in contrast, has been associated with eccentric remodelling (increased LV end-diastolic volume with reduced LV mass, concentricity and wall thickness) and a higher cardiac output and lower systemic vascular resistance.

Waist circumference and visceral fat mass are associated with arterial stiffness. Similarly, the presence of higher amounts of visceral adipose tissue has been associated with higher systolic blood pressure, whereas lower body fat is associated with lower mean blood pressure.

Body Morphology and Atopy

Asthma

Patterns of body fat distribution significantly influence the function of the respiratory system. Fat accumulation causes changes in respiratory physiology, causing impairment of various lung function parameters. Thoracic and abdominal infiltration directly affects the downward movement of the diaphragm and chest wall mechanics. Obesity is associated with reduced respiratory system compliance and abdominal fat facilitates the development of restrictive lung disease.

Abdominal obesity has not only been shown to have adverse effects on asthma prevalence, but does so even when accounting for the effect of general obesity. Abdominal adiposity by WHtR correlates with poorer asthma control in adults. Adolescents with excess abdominal adiposity, as determined by WHtR have been shown to have a higher risk of asthma compared to non-obese adolescents. Research generated results that are difficult to unify, and show a negative association between asthma control and visceral adipose tissue measured by ultrasound, but not anthropometric measures such as WHtR, WHR and BMI. Altered lung mechanics, airway inflammation, and oxidative stress are all thought to be the responsible factors for the development of the obese–asthma phenotype.

Atopic Dermatitis

There is strong evidence for the association of obesity and clinical manifestations of asthma. The link between obesity and atopic dermatitis remains vague. Women, particularly those with abdominal obesity, have a significantly higher propensity for atopic dermatitis than those without. This association was not seen in men.

Interventions in Fat Distribution

While bariatric surgery is an accepted and effective method to reduce adiposity and cardio-metabolic risk, the effects of liposuction are conflicting. Abdominal subcutaneous liposuction has shown no effects on liver, muscle and adipose tissue insulin sensitivity in some studies, while a reduction in systolic blood pressure and fasting insulin was evident in others. Scarce research exists on lipectomy specifically in the lower body, with some evidence that removal of femoral fat leads to increased triglyceride levels in women. Significant metabolic improvements can be seen when adiposity is reduced by lifestyle interventions. Diet and exercise have effects on all adipose tissue depots as well as other metabolically active tissues. Various pharmacologic interventions alter body shape in expected ways, with increased abdominal depots correlating with worsening metabolic profile and decreased abdominal depots showing improvement. With pharmacologic weight loss interventions, multiple fat depots are usually affected in the form of generalised weight loss.

Summary

Our understanding of body morphology and fat distribution has reached a significant turning point. Fat distribution has been better defined with specific scalars of measurement. Adipose tissue depots are accurately visualized with various imaging modalities. In this setting, knowledge of the genetic and physiologic differences between abdominal and gluteal adipose tissue is growing. While correlation with cardio-metabolic risk has not been entirely elucidated, a protective effect of gluteo-femoral fat is apparent. Further investigation of interventions that influence fat distribution may provide solutions for patients with elevated risk profiles.

Further Reading

Abate N, Garg A, Peshock RM, et al. Relationship of generalized and regional adiposity to insulin sensitivity in men with NIDDM. *Diabetes*. 1996;**45**(12):1684–93.

Abbasi SA, Hundley WG, Bluemke DA, et al. Visceral adiposity and left ventricular remodeling: The Multi-Ethnic Study of Atherosclerosis. *Nutr Metab Cardiovasc Dis* . 2015;**25**(7):667–76.

Bennasar-Veny M, Lopez-Gonzalez AA, Tauler P, et al. Body adiposity index and cardiovascular health risk factors in Caucasians: a comparison with the body mass index and others. *PLoS One*. 2013;**8**(5):e63999.

Celebi Sozener Z, Aydin O, Mungan D, et al. Obesity-asthma phenotype: Effect of weight gain on asthma control in adults. *Allergy Asthma Proc*. 2016;**37**(4):311–17.

Cornier MA, Despres JP, Davis N, et al.; American Heart Association Obesity Committee of the Council on Nutrition, Physical Activity and Metabolism, Council on Arteriosclerosis, Thrombosis and Vascular Biology, Council on Cardiovascular Disease in the Young, Council on Cardiovascular Radiology and Intervention, Council on Cardiovascular Nursing, Council on Epidemiology and Prevention & Council on the Kidney in Cardiovascular Disease, and Stroke Council 2011. Assessing adiposity: a scientific statement from the American Heart Association. *Circulation.* 2011;**124**(18):1996–2019.

Davis KE, Neinast, DM, Sun K, et al. The sexually dimorphic role of adipose and adipocyte estrogen receptors in modulating adipose tissue expansion, inflammation, and fibrosis. *Molec Metab.* 2013;**2**(3):227–42.

Flegal KM, Kit BK, Orpana H, et al. Association of all-cause mortality with overweight and obesity using standard body mass index categories: a systematic review and meta-analysis. *JAMA.* 2013;**309**(1):71–82.

Gavin KM, Cooper EE, Hickner RC Estrogen receptor protein content is different in abdominal than gluteal subcutaneous adipose tissue of overweight-to-obese premenopausal women. *Metab Clin Exper.* 2013;**62**(8):1180–8.

Giese SY, Bulan EJ, Commons GW, et al. Improvements in cardiovascular risk profile with large-volume liposuction: a pilot study. *Plastic Reconstruct Surg.* 2001;**108** (2):510–9.

Guerra RS, Amaral TF, Marques EA, et al. Anatomical location for waist circumference measurement in older adults: a preliminary study. *Nutr Hosp.* 2012;**27**(5):1554–61.

Hatem SN, Redheuil A, Gandjbakhch E. Cardiac adipose tissue and atrial fibrillation: the perils of adiposity. *Cardiovasc Res.* 2016;**109**(4):502–9.

Hernandez TL, Bessesen DH, Cox-York KA, et al. Femoral lipectomy increases postprandial lipemia in women. *Am J Physiol Endocrinol Metabol.* 2015;**309**(1):E63–71.

Jensen MD. Role of body fat distribution and the metabolic complications of obesity. *J Clin Endocrinol Metabol.* 2008;**93** (11 Suppl 1):S57–63.

Benedetti FJ, Bosa VL, Giesta JM, et al. Anthropometric indicators of general and central obesity in the prediction of asthma in adolescents: central obesity in asthma. *Nutr Hosp.* 2015;**32**(6):2540–8.

Karastergiou K, Bredella MA, Lee MJ, et al. Growth hormone receptor expression in human gluteal versus abdominal subcutaneous adipose tissue: association with body shape. *Obesity.* 2016;**24**(5):1090–6.

Karastergiou K, Fried SK, Xie H, et al. Distinct developmental signatures of human abdominal and gluteal subcutaneous adipose tissue depots. *J Clin Endocrinol Metabol.* 2013;**98**(1):362–71.

Katzmarzyk PT, Mire E, Bray GA, et al. Anthropometric markers of obesity and mortality in white and African American adults: the Pennington center longitudinal study. *Obesity.* 2013;**21**(5):1070–5.

Lee MJ, Wu Y, Fried SK. Adipose tissue heterogeneity: implication of depot differences in adipose tissue for obesity complications. *Molec Aspects Med.* 2013;**34**(1):1–11.

Lv N, Xiao L, Camargo CA, Jr, et al. Abdominal and general adiposity and level of asthma control in adults with uncontrolled asthma. *Ann Am Thorac Soc.* 2014;**11**(8):1218–24.

Neeland IJ, Gupta S, Ayers CR, et al. Relation of regional fat distribution to left ventricular structure and function. *Circul Cardiovasc Imag.* 2013;**6**(5):800–7.

Obeid NR, Malick W, Concors SJ, et al. Long-term outcomes after Roux-en-Y gastric bypass: 10- to 13-year data. *Surg Obes Related Dis.* 2016;**12**(1):11–20.

Peppa M, Koliaki C, Hadjidakis DI, et al. Regional fat distribution and cardiometabolic risk in healthy postmenopausal women. *Eur J Intern Med.* 2013;**24**(8):824–31.

Pramyothin P, Karastergiou K. What can we learn from interventions that change fat distribution? *Curr Obes Rep.* 2016;**5**(2):271–81.

Reis JP, Macera CA, Araneta MR, et al. Comparison of overall obesity and body fat distribution in predicting risk of mortality. *Obesity.* 2009;**17**(6):1232–9.

Sahakyan KR, Somers VK, Rodriguez-Escudero JP, et al. Normal-weight central obesity: implications for total and cardiovascular mortality. *Ann Intern Med.* 2015;**163**(11):827–35.

Seabolt LA, Welch EB, Silver HJ. Imaging methods for analyzing body composition in human obesity and cardiometabolic disease. *Ann NY Acad Sci.* 2015;**1353**:41–59.

Wong CX, Ganesan AN, Selvanayagam JB. Epicardial fat and atrial fibrillation: current evidence, potential mechanisms, clinical implications, and future directions. *Eur Heart J.* 2017;**38**(17):1294–302.

Reports and Guidelines Related to the Morbidly Obese Patient

Kanchan Patil

During the last 20 years, obesity has reached epidemic proportions in the United Kingdom (UK). In England, the prevalence of obesity (BMI 30) among adults rose from 14.9% to 25.6% between 1993 and 2014. There are many studies and reports published in recent times focusing on this complex issue of obesity. Each report gives an insight into the management of obese patients from differing perspectives. For the peri-operative management of obese patients, the following reports are particularly important and 'set the scene' for providing care:

1. Too Lean a Service NCEPOD report 2012
2. 4th National Audit Project NAP4 2011
3. 5th National Audit Project NAP5 2014
4. Maternal Obesity in the UK: Findings from a National Project 2010
5. Measuring Up 2013

Too Lean a Service: A Review of the Care of Patients who Underwent Bariatric Surgery

The National Confidential Enquiry into Patient Outcome and Death (NCEPOD) published this report in 2012. Bariatric surgery is used to promote health in those who suffer from severe or complex obesity. The complexity of surgical procedures varies from simple gastric balloon insertion to a multiple-staged duodenal switch operation. This report described the variability in UK practice and identified correctable factors in the care process (from referral to follow-up) for patients undergoing bariatric surgery. All adult patients (>16 years old) who underwent bariatric surgery from 1 June 2010 to 31 August 2010 were included. Cases were limited to a maximum of three per surgeon per hospital. For each patient a clinical questionnaire and organisational questionnaire for each hospital participating in the study was completed. A multidisciplinary group of advisors reviewed all the cases.

Key Findings

- 48% of hospitals that performed gastric banding carried out 10 or less operations in the 2010–2011 financial year. Furthermore 40% of these hospitals performed no other bariatric procedures and 22% were also low volume sites for other surgical weight loss procedures.
- Just over half (55%) of the hospitals in the study ran multidisciplinary team (MDT) meetings for bariatric surgical patients.
- Bariatric physicians and anaesthetists only attended MDT meetings in around 55% of cases.
- 82% of private hospital undertaking elective bariatric surgery did not deliver special training to their staff.
- 43% of hospitals undertaking weight loss surgery did not have critical care beds.
- 24% of institutions did not have appropriate anti-embolic stockings, 18% lacked special surgical equipment, e.g. extra-long laparoscopic instruments, and 54% were unable to provide appropriate imaging modalities for morbidly obese patients.
- Only 32% of patients had documented evidence of anaesthetic review prior to admission for surgery.
- 19% of patients were considered to have had a less than adequate pre-assessment.
- In 24% of cases, consent forms did not contain appropriate information.
- For 12% of patients nursed on level 0/1 wards, no 'track-and-trigger' system was in place.
- 20% of discharge summaries were judged to be poor or unacceptable, often providing insufficient clinical detail and drug information.

Key Recommendations

1. Bariatric surgery is not for the occasional operator. The specialist associations involved with

bariatric surgery should provide guidance regarding the numbers of procedures that both independent operators and institutions should achieve in order to optimise outcomes.

2. All hospitals that undertake weight loss surgery on morbidly obese patients or admit patients as an emergency must have appropriate equipment, such as anti-embolic stockings, ability to weigh a patient, hoists, blood pressure cuffs and imaging facilities.

3. Patients should have access to all the necessary professional experts required for their care. This should be provided through MDT assessment.

4. An agreed MDT peri-operative plan should be documented in each individuals medical notes.

5. All bariatric patients should have an assessment of the predicted difficulty of intubation recorded.

6. A deferred two-stage consent process with sufficient time lapse between the episodes should be adopted for all patients.

7. All patients should have a physiological 'track-and-trigger' system as part of their peri-operative care to record observations.

8. On discharge home, all patients need to be provided with clear dietary advice and emergency contact details. A timely discharge summary with full clinical details must also be delivered.

Major Complications of Airway Management in the UK: NAP4

The combined 4th National Audit Project (NAP4) between The Royal College of Anaesthetists and The Difficult Airway Society was published in March 2011. The project was based on the report of 184 major airway-related events occurring in the UK over a 1-year period from a nationwide sample. An expert panel that identified themes reviewed each of these cases and combining this with previous knowledge, extracted lessons that might guide improvements in care.

Key Findings Related to Obesity

- The proportion of obese adults reported to NAP4 was twice that of the general population and for morbidly obese adults the rate was four times higher.
- Difficulty with mask ventilation was comparatively higher in obese individuals (5.7%) compared to the non-obese (1.3%).

- The use of supraglottic airway devices was associated with a significantly higher complication rate in obese patients (9.4%) as compared to the non-obese group (6.3%).
- Several reports demonstrated adverse events in obese patients under general anaesthesia with a spontaneous breathing technique in either the trendelenburg or lithotomy position.
- Airway issues occurred more commonly on emergence and in recovery.
- Senior involvement and planning were encountered less in obese patients with a number of cases presenting on the day of surgery.

Key Recommendations

1. Hospital management need to be aware of the additional time and resources needed to safely anaesthetise obese patients.

2. Provision must be made for anaesthetic pre-assessment of all obese patients without time constraint.

3. Part of the pre-operative evaluation must include a search for co-morbidities with the potential to promote airway issues. Notably sleep disordered breathing.

4. Airway assessment must include an evaluation of possible rescue techniques should adverse events arise.

5. Awake fibreoptic intubation should be considered in patients where it would be difficult to establish rescue oxygenation or an emergency surgical airway.

6. If awake fibreoptic intubation is chosen, extreme care is required in titration of sedatives and monitoring, in order to avoid airway obstruction and periods of apnoea.

7. A rescue airway strategy should be planned in case of failed regional anaesthesia. All theatre staff must be aware of the hazards posed by intra-operative conversion from regional to general anaesthesia.

8. Pre-oxygenation, performed to high standards, should be used for all obese patients prior to induction of general anaesthesia.

9. Healthcare providers should ensure appropriate equipment and techniques are embraced to meet the specific needs of obese patients.

10. At the end of anaesthesia, pre-oxygenation should be a standard of care prior to extubation and transfer to the recovery room. The possible need

for re-intubation should be anticipated and planned for.

11. Anaesthetic training should emphasise the importance of obesity as a risk factor for complications of airway management.

Accidental Awareness during General Anaesthesia (AAGA) in the United Kingdom and Ireland 5th National Audit Project: NAP5

This combined audit project led by the two biggest UK anaesthetic organisations, the Royal College of Anaesthetists (RCOA) and the Association of Anaesthetists of Great Britain and Ireland (AAGBI) looked at the incidence of accidental awareness under general anaesthesia (AAGA). Over a calendar year, a nationwide network of local health service coordinators anonymously reported all records of accidental awareness under general anaesthesia to a central, secure online database. The data detailed information about the event, anaesthetic and surgical techniques and any sequelae. Four hunderd cases were reported. After expert panel review, 300 were included for in-depth review. Of these 141 were certain AAGA, with others due to residual muscle paralysis, intensive unit (ITU) therapy-related awareness and sedation-related awareness.

Key Findings and Recommendations in Obesity

1. AAGA occurred in 35% of obese patients, mainly at induction of general anaesthesia.
2. The obese patient has an increased fat load, with associated increased cardiac output. This results in a rapid redistribution of fat-soluble drugs, with the potential to reduce their action on target organs.
3. Dosing of drugs with lean body weight may result in underdosing, while total body weight may result in cardiovascular instability.
4. Induction of general anaesthesia in obese individuals is associated with a higher risk of AAGA. It is essential to give titrated doses of induction agent in the obese population, with further incremental doses in cases of airway difficulty.
5. Eliminating induction of general anaesthesia in anaesthetic rooms for obese patients will reduce

the 'gap time' between intravenous drug concentrations and vapour levels.

6. Routine use of depth of anaesthesia (DOA) monitoring is not supported by NAP5 data, but obesity being one of the risk factor for developing AAGA, it is advisable to consider DOA monitoring, especially alongside neuromuscular blockade.

Maternal Obesity in the UK: Findings from a National Project Report by the Centre for Maternal and Child Enquiries 2010

In 2008, the Confidential Enquiry into Maternal and Child Health (CEMACH), now known as the Centre for Maternal and Child Enquiries (CMACE), commenced a 3-year UK-wide obesity in pregnancy project.

Key Findings

- The UK prevalence of women with a known BMI ≥35 at any point in pregnancy, who give birth ≥ 24+0 weeks' gestation, was 4.99%, which translates into approximately 38 478 pregnancies each year. The prevalence of women with a pregnancy BMI ≥40 in the UK is 2.01%, while BMI ≥50 affects 0.19% of all women giving birth.
- 38% of women within the obese category had a minimum one obesity co-morbidity diagnosed prior to and/or during pregnancy. The most frequently reported conditions were pregnancy-induced hypertension and gestational diabetes.
- Among women with a BMI ≥35 who laboured prior to delivery, each unit increase in BMI was associated with a 3% increased risk for the need for induction of labour.
- The caesarean sections rate for BMI >35 accounted for 37% of all singleton deliveries, which is substantially higher than the caesarean rate of 25% in the general maternity population in England.
- The incidence of primary post-partum haemorrhage (PPH) was 38% for women with a BMI ≥35, which was four times higher than the rate in the general obstetric population.
- Among women with a BMI ≥35, each unit increase in BMI was associated with a 7% increased risk of stillbirth.

- Babies born to mothers with a BMI ≥50 were almost twice as likely to be admitted to the neonatal unit as babies born to mothers with a BMI 35–39.9, even after adjusting for maternal age, parity, maternal diabetes and gestation at delivery.

Key Recommendations

1. Pregnant women with obesity should receive routine obstetric care supplemented by specialist services that are specific to their needs, including specialist midwives, senior anaesthetic expertise and senior obstetric reviews.
2. Maternal weight should be re-measured in the third trimester to allow appropriate plans to be made for equipment and personnel required during labour and delivery.
3. All pregnant women with a booking BMI ≥30 should be provided with accurate and accessible information about the risks associated with obesity in pregnancy and how these risks may be minimised.
4. Women with a booking BMI ≥35 who also have at least one additional risk factor for pre-eclampsia should have referral early in pregnancy for specialist input to care.
5. Pregnant women with a booking BMI ≥40 should have an antenatal anaesthetic consultation with an obstetric anaesthetist, which would allow potential difficulties with venous access, regional or general anaesthesia to be identified and anticipated.
6. All women with a BMI ≥40 should be offered post-natal thromboprophylaxis regardless of their mode of delivery.
7. To minimise the risk of complications, venous access should be established early in labour. In addition, an obstetrician and anaesthetist at Speciality Trainee Year 6 or above, should be informed and available for the care of women with a BMI ≥40 during labour and delivery.

Measuring Up: The Medical Profession's Prescription for the Nation's Obesity Crisis

The Obesity Steering Group was formed in early 2012, representing over 220 000 UK doctors from differing specialist fields. Over a period of 6 months, this inquiry received more than 100 submissions to its call for written evidence, from organisations and individuals representing the food and drink industry, weight management groups, charities, the UK government, the sports industry, educators, dieticians and healthcare professionals. The steering group came up with 10 key recommendations that fall into the following three groups:

Action by Healthcare Professions

1. Education and training programmes for healthcare professionals in both primary and secondary care to ensure that 'making every contact counts' becomes a reality.
2. Weight management services: the Departments of Health in the four nations should together invest at least £100 m in each of the next three financial years to extend and increase provision of weight management services across the country. This should include both programmes for early interventions and greater provision for severe and complicated obesity, including bariatric surgery.
3. Nutritional standards for food in hospitals: food-based standards in line with those put in place for schools in England in 2006 should be introduced in all UK hospitals in the next 18 months.
4. Increase support for new parents: give more support to deliver basic food preparation skills, to guide appropriate food choices, which will ensure nutritionally balanced meals, and continue to encourage breastfeeding.

The Obesogenic Environment

5. Nutritional standards in schools: a new statutory requirement on all schools to provide food skills, including cooking and growing, alongside a sound theoretical understanding of the long-term effects of food on health and the environment.
6. Fast food outlets near schools: Public Health England should develop formal recommendations on reducing the proximity of fast food outlets to schools, colleges, leisure centres and other places where children gather.
7. Junk food advertising: a ban on advertising of foods high in saturated fats, sugar and salt before 9pm, and an agreement from commercial broadcasters that they will not allow these foods to be advertised on internet 'on-demand' services.

Making the Healthy Choice the Easy Choice

8. Sugary drinks tax: for an initial period of 1 year, a duty should be levied on all sugary soft drinks, increasing the price by at least 20%.

9. Food labelling: improved food labelling (to be based on percentage of calories for men, women, children and adolescents) and visible calorie indicators for restaurants, especially fast food outlets.

10. The built environment: Public Health England should provide guidance to directors of public health in working with local authorities to encourage active travel and protect or increase green spaces to make the healthy option the easy option.

Further Reading

Cook TM, Woodall N, Frerk C, on behalf of the Fourth National Audit Project. Major complications of airway management in the UK: results of the Fourth National Audit Project of the Royal College of Anaesthetists and the Difficult Airway Society. Part 1: Anaesthesia. *Br J Anaesth.* 2011;**106**:617–31.

Fitzsomons K, Sullivan A. Maternal Obesity in the UK: Findings from a National Project. 2010. www.publichealth .hscni.net/publications/maternal-obesity-uk-findings-national-project (accessed April 2018).

Health and Social Care Information Centre. Statistics on Obesity, Physical Activity and Diet: England 2015. 2015. www.gov.uk/government/statistics/statistics-on-obesity-physical-activity-and-diet-england-2015 (accessed April 2018).

National Confidential Enquiry Into Patient Outcome and Deaths (NCEPOD). Too Lean a Service? A Review of the Care of Patients who Underwent Bariatric Surgery. 2012. www.ncepod.org.uk/2012report2/downloads/BS_fullreport .pdf (accessed April 2018).

Pandit JJ, Andrade J, Bogod DG, et al. The 5th National Audit Project (NAP5) on accidental awareness during general anaesthesia: protocol, methods and analysis of data. *Anaesthesia* 2014;**69**:1078–88.

Joch BYA, By P, Forrest S. Measuring Up: The Medical Profession's Prescription for the Nation's Obesity Crisis. 2007. www.aomrc.org.uk/publications/reports-guidance/m easuring-up-0213/ (accessed April 2018).

Education and Training in Peri-operative Care

Chris Carey

Introduction

Bariatric surgery is a relatively new and rapidly developing area of care. As such there is an essential requirement to train a healthcare workforce that is suitably skilled to support evolving services. Peri-operative care encompasses the pre-operative, intra-operative and post-operative periods and requires a multiprofessional team-based approach to ensure safe and effective patient care at all stages of treatment. There is very little in the way of historical basis on which to base the training of medical and non-medical healthcare staff in peri-operative medicine, especially when it comes to services specifically tailored to the requirements of bariatric patients. The knowledge, skills and professional values required of all members of the workforce providing peri-operative care for bariatric patients must be established and a suitable infrastructure needs to be in place to ensure that staff can be trained to an appropriate level to provide high-quality care in both existing and developing services.

The breadth of training for different professions working within different healthcare systems is enormous. This chapter focuses mainly on postgraduate anaesthetic training within the UK. There is considerable international variation in training configuration, and the organisation and staffing of services. Many of the essential principles of adult learning are generic and apply across all healthcare groups.

The Scope of Peri-operative Medicine

The aim of peri-operative medicine is to deliver the best possible care for patients before, during and after major surgery. The exact requirements for any individual relates to both the management of pre-existing medical and surgical conditions, and also the prevention and management of any medical complications that may arise during treatment. Given the potential for medical co-morbidity seen in obese patients presenting for surgery, the peri-operative care delivered represents a fundamentally important part of a patient's overall management.

Conditions such as diabetes mellitus, hypertension and ischaemic heart disease are all more prevalent in obese individuals undergoing surgery. There is also a greater incidence of many significant complications, such as respiratory failure, wound infection and venous thromboembolism witnessed in this group. Comprehensive skilled peri-operative care is essential to ensure the best possible outcomes from surgery and improvements in anaesthetic and peri-operative care have been credited with improving mortality rates in obese individuals undergoing bariatric surgery.

The complexity of care required by this group of patients necessitates the requirement for appropriately trained specialist healthcare staff to be involved at every stage of the peri-operative pathway. Successful services demand a multiprofessional approach with hospital medical and nursing staff, therapists and the patient's primary care team each fulfilling an important role. Consideration must be given to ensuring that every member of the team has the requisite skills and experience to perform their role successfully.

Peri-operative anaesthetic management of bariatric patients requires a considerable degree of specific training and experience in order to become expert. This is best achieved through a specific period of time spent working within a bariatric unit and there are many opportunities for training in such establishments. However, an understanding of the principles of management of bariatric patients is essential for all anaesthetists and many of the required skills can be gained through the care of obese patients presenting for other forms of surgery.

The Organisation and Structure of Anaesthetic Training

Management of Training

Anaesthetic training in the UK is provided through schools of anaesthesia which are managed by 17 deaneries across the country, each led by a Postgraduate Dean. At a national level responsibility for all postgraduate healthcare training rests with Health Education England and its equivalent bodies in Scotland, Wales and Northern Ireland. Schools of anaesthesia also work in close collaboration with the Royal College of Anaesthetists. Each school has a head of school and training programme directors who are responsible for the management of training rotations. Locally, each anaesthetic department has one or more college tutors who are responsible for the management of training in that particular organisation.

The Curriculum

In the UK, the requirements for post-graduate medical training are set out in specialty curricula that are set by the medical Royal Colleges. These set out the rules and regulations of training in a particular medical specialty, outlining both the specific knowledge and skills required to complete each stage of training and also the values and behaviours that are attributed to professional practice within each specialty, much of which are generic across the entire medical profession.

The anaesthetic curriculum is set by the Royal College of Anaesthetists and is divided into four stages: basic, intermediate, higher and advanced training. These stages each contain a number of units of training which encompass different areas of anaesthetic practice. Each unit of training has learning outcomes attached which must be achieved to complete that particular area of training. There are also a series of competencies within each unit which set out the specific areas of knowledge and skills that are associated with that particular unit.

In the early stages, each unit of training is mandatory and must be completed successfully. However, in the later stages of training some higher and advanced units of training are optional and allow trainees to develop specific areas of interest within anaesthesia. Bariatric anaesthesia is not a formally recognised area of sub-specialist practice in anaesthesia and in terms

of the scope of consultant practice comes under the broad umbrella of the term 'generalism'. However, most specialist bariatric surgical units offer dedicated training attachments and experience in such a post would be a pre-requisite for those wishing to practice in this field as a consultant.

Bariatric Anaesthesia and the Anaesthetic Training Programme

Anaesthesia for bariatric surgery is not currently recognised as a stand-alone unit of the training in the UK. However, gaining some form of experience in anaesthesia and peri-operative management of bariatric patients is highly valuable for all anaesthetists and essential for those who intend to specialise in this area of practice. It supports the development of understanding of the issues associated with management of obese patients in general and development of the skills required to deal with many of the specific clinical and technical challenges involved. Unfortunately access to such training may be limited, but should be encouraged whenever possible. The increasing levels of obesity seen in the general population presenting for all forms of surgery mean that the experience gained is invaluable for trainees wishing to specialise in all areas of anaesthetic practice.

When training in anaesthesia for bariatric surgery is undertaken within a UK training programme, the learning outcomes must be mapped to a specific unit of training. The most appropriate unit for this purpose is the 'General Surgery, Urology and Gynaecology Surgery' module. In the basic and intermediate levels of training some exposure to anaesthesia for bariatric surgery will support the development of many of the competences described in these modules.

For those anaesthetists who wish to undertake specialist practice in bariatric anaesthesia, training may be undertaken either within the training programme or as an out of programme attachment (OOP). OOP may be undertaken at appropriate stages of the training programme, usually towards the end, in agreement with the local training programme director. It may be undertaken as additional time (out of programme for experience or OOPE) or take the place of a part of a training programme (out of programme for training or OOPT). The regulations are set out in the Gold Guide, the reference guide for post-graduate specialty training in the UK.

It is also possible to undertake an attachment to a bariatric surgery unit within the training programme as part of advanced anaesthetic training. In order to gain recognition for training, such a placement needs to provide suitable training experience to allow the completion of each of the learning outcomes for the advanced unit of training in general surgery, urology and gynaecology surgery. These are relatively broad based and as such are easily mapped to a more specialised area of practice. They are set out below.

Learning outcomes for advanced training in general surgery, urology and gynaecology surgery (reproduced by kind permission from the Royal College of Anaesthetists):

- Gain mastery in the delivery of safe and effective peri-operative anaesthetic care to patients undergoing complex intra-abdominal surgical procedures, including those where pleural breach is anticipated.
- Gain mastery in the management of major abdominal surgery and in doing so demonstrate the necessary multidisciplinary leadership, communication and team-working skills necessary to ensure the care delivered benefits both the patient and the organisation.
- Gain maturity in understanding the importance of utilising the time allocated to clinical sessions effectively, optimizing throughput, whilst not compromising patient safety.
- Gain the necessary maturity to guide the choice of audit cycles/quality improvement projects in developing practice.
- Become familiar with recent developments in peri-operative anaesthetic care to this area of practice, to evaluate these developments and to advise colleagues of useful changes in practice.
- To be capable of undertaking the peri-operative anaesthetic care for a wide variety of complex abdominal surgical cases independently; this implies an ability to:
  - Provide peri-operative anaesthetic care to a wide range of surgical cases performed (including those where pleural breach may occur), demonstrating a fundamental understanding of the problems encountered.
  - Show the decision-making and organisational skills required of an anaesthetist to manage

busy operating sessions that involve patients having major abdominal surgery and ensuring that the care delivered is safe and timely, benefiting both the patient and the organisation.
  - Assist colleagues in decisions about the suitability of surgery in difficult situations.
  - Provide teaching to less experienced colleagues of all grades.

Training and Assessment

Competency-based Training

Historically, post-graduate medical training worked on an apprentice-type model, with trainees working in a particular unit gaining experience of the various aspects of clinical medicine, with post-graduate exams seen as the specific test of knowledge in each specialty. Progression through training was largely time-based, with separate points of entry for each grade of training. There was little in the way of formal assessment in the workplace and recording of progression in training was based on a combination of time served and a suitable reference that would allow promotion.

Over the past two decades there has been a shift towards competency-based training for doctors in training programmes in the UK. Competency-based training is commonly employed for many areas of vocational learning. It places the emphasis on the knowledge and skills that a trainee develops and demonstrates in the workplace to achieve the required outcomes rather than the time spent in a particular attachment. This in theory allows progression through training to take place at an appropriate pace for an individual trainee. Thus, those who demonstrate knowledge and skills at an early stage are at least in theory able to progress more quickly than those who take longer to demonstrate such competencies. This emphasis on the particular abilities demonstrated by an individual rather than the duration of a training attachment can be described as learner-centeredness and is considered to be a valuable approach to training.

Knowledge and skills are broken into individual areas defined as competencies for each unit of training, which are set out in appendices to specialty curricula for each level of the programme. In most cases there are numerous individual competencies set out within a single unit and trainees are expected to demonstrate competency in each of these areas in order to complete that particular unit of training.

Competencies gained in training are considered to be transferrable; for instance, intravenous cannulation skills learnt by medical students and foundation doctors are transferable to anaesthetic practice and advanced airway skills learnt in anaesthetic attachments are transferable to emergency medicine or pre-hospital care. This provides flexibility within the medical workforce and helps to ensure that there are sufficient numbers of appropriately trained medical staff to provide care for patients in a wide range of settings. In this way, many of the skills learnt in bariatric anaesthesia attachments are transferable and highly useful in other areas of anaesthesia.

Ensuring the successful attainment of standard competencies within a training programme also allows a consistent and reproducible standard of clinical practice. This promotes high standards in patient care and is of particular value to healthcare regulators such as the General Medical Council (GMC) in the UK, who are able to define the required knowledge and skills of the senior medical workforce through the competencies which must be achieved in training.

Controversies in Competency-based Training

The concept of competency-based training in medicine has been the subject of much debate over the years, not least because medical training remains largely time-based due to the logistical challenges of managing doctors in training rotations that are often complex, with numerous units of training requiring completion in a wide range of clinical areas. It can also be argued that consultant practice requires 'expertise' as opposed to 'competence' and that there is more to demonstrating expertise in medical practice than merely being proficient at a range of individual tasks. Indeed, competencies feature far less prominently in the advanced unit of training in anaesthesia, where the mandatory learning outcomes tend to specify the demonstration of expertise in a range of areas.

Many trainees and trainers have found that the complexity and time required to complete and record numerous assessments detracts from the clinical learning within the training programme. Whilst trainees will be expected to achieve all competencies within each unit of training, only a sample need to be specifically assessed to achieve successful completion. It must also be borne in mind that competencies achieved at a specific point in time will not be maintained without regular clinical exposure. They may also become out of date or obsolete over a period of time, given the rapid developments in many areas of clinical medicine; bariatric anaesthesia is a good example of such a rapidly changing field.

Spiral Learning

The anaesthetic training programme uses the concept of 'spiral learning', whereby trainees rotate through a range of specific clinical areas multiple times. As they return to each area, their previous learning is developed further with increasing levels of difficulty resulting in a higher level of competence and understanding being gained. This concept was first described in 1960 and its use is long established in both undergraduate and post-graduate medical education. An example of this in its simplest form could relate to the expected levels of supervision for clinical work afforded to trainees of different seniority. A junior trainee may require direct supervision for a given case, whilst a trainee near the end of the programme may only require indirect or distant supervision for the same case.

There are some specific considerations pertinent to training in bariatric anaesthesia. Firstly, the knowledge and skills required are challenging and most training in this area is likely to occur towards the end of a training programme. Secondly, the specialist, relatively low volume nature of this work means that trainees are unlikely to spend time working in bariatric centres on multiple occasions within a training programme.

The concept of spiral learning fits well with another widely adopted educational concept: Bloom's Taxonomy of Educational Objectives. This concept, first described in 1956, uses a series of descriptors to define levels of expertise. There are in fact three separate taxonomies describing the areas of knowledge-based goals, skills-based goals and affective goals. These set out levels of expertise in increasing complexity, providing a description of each level of expertise and verbs that describe that particular level. These may be ascribed to competencies associated with each level. The taxonomy for knowledge-based goals is set out in Figure 5.1.

It can be seen that the descriptors used for each level of expertise may be used to form competencies used within units of training at each level. Thus, units of

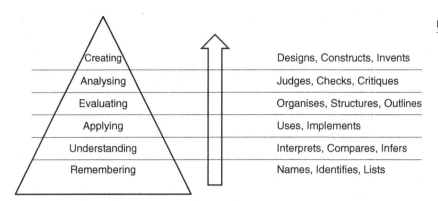

Figure 5.1 Modified Bloom's Taxonomy of knowledge-based goals.

training in the formative years of the training programme may feature competencies which relate to 'remembering' and 'understanding' a subject, whereas towards the end of training competencies could relate to higher-level understanding, such as 'evaluating' and 'analysing' a particular area of knowledge. In practice, this is often not clear cut, but it is useful to bear in mind when considering the level of understanding that senior trainees in attachments to bariatric surgery units should be achieving in order to meet the required learning outcomes.

Assessment

Types of Assessments

Assessments may be defined as 'formative' or 'summative'. Formative assessments are used to monitor learning in a particular area. They provide ongoing feedback that can be used by trainees to target areas of weakness and improve their performance. An example of a formative assessment would be a driving lesson where the teacher is providing feedback for the pupil to improve their skills. In contrast, summative assessments are used to evaluate performance or learning by comparing with a benchmark. This may have a binary 'pass/fail' outcome or be graded. An example of a summative assessment would be a driving test where the candidate either passes or fails. Post-graduate medical exams are also obvious examples of summative assessments.

Workplace-based Assessments in Anaesthetic Training

One of the key considerations of a competency-based training programme is how the attainment of individual competencies is measured. Workplace-based assessments (WBAs) were introduced to UK training

by the General Medical Council in 2010 to allow the assessment of competencies in a consistent and reliable manner. These assessments have become embedded in the anaesthesia training programme and are recorded in an educational portfolio to demonstrate completion of units of training.

Case-Based Discussion (CBD)

CBDs are based around the discussion of one or more aspects of a clinical case carried out by the trainee undertaking the assessment. This may be any aspect of knowledge associated with that particular case, such as discussion of the management of any aspect of pre-operative medical co-morbidity, assessment and consideration of anaesthetic technique, conduct of anaesthesia ·or post-operative care. CBDs are the mainstay of the workplace assessment of knowledge in everyday clinical practice.

Direct Observation of Procedural Skill (DOPS)

DOPSs are used to assess attainment of clinical skills and may be used for any practical technique, such as central venous cannulation or epidural catheter placement. Although by nature their scope is rather more limited than that of a CBD, they are nonetheless a central part of the assessment process. Successful completion of DOPSs ensures that trainees have the requisite skills to practice safely and they are especially valuable at the early stages of training.

Anaesthetic List Management Assessment Tool (ALMAT)

ALMATs are used to assess the ability of trainees to run an entire theatre list. As well as encompassing safe planning and conduct of anaesthesia they also encompass skills such as communication, teamwork and other aspects of non-clinical skills which are collectively known as 'human factors'. These skills are immensely important in ensuring safe and effective clinical practice, especially given the team-based approach required in the management of bariatric patients.

Multi-Source Feedback (MSF)

MSFs are completed annually by all trainees and allow trainees to gather feedback from trainers and colleagues at work, with typically around 15 individuals contributing to each assessment. They cover a number of individual areas which are grouped into the four areas of the GMC's Good Medical Practice: knowledge, skills and performance; safety and quality; communication, partnership and teamwork; maintaining trust. Responses in each area are graded with further space for comments.

These assessment tools are all intended to be formative in nature and provide trainees with guidance on how they can continue to develop their practice. For each unit of training they contribute to a completion of unit of training (CUT) form, which is a summative assessment of whether the trainee has passed that particular unit. The decision to complete a 'sign-off' should draw on a range of evidence, including WBAs, confirmation of having achieved learning outcomes and feedback from trainers within the department.

The FRCA Exam

The Fellow of the Royal College of Anaesthetists (FRCA) exam is the post-graduate examination that must be passed by anaesthetists in the UK in order to complete their training, gain a place on the GMC Specialist Register and take up a consultant post. The exam is a summative assessment and is divided into two parts, the Primary FRCA and Final FRCA. The exam syllabus encompasses a wide variety of areas relative to anaesthetic practice, including physiology, pharmacology, physics and clinical measurement, clinical anaesthesia and peri-operative medicine. Knowledge of the effects of obesity relevant to these areas and specific considerations for bariatric anaesthesia fall within the remit of the exam.

Annual Review of Competency Progression

ARCPs are conducted yearly for all doctors in training programmes. Evidence is reviewed from trainees' portfolios, including assessments, unit of training sign-offs, multi-source feedback and the results of any exams taken. Satisfactory completion of all required areas allows that particular year of training to be signed off and the trainee can progress to the next year of the training programme. Details of ARCP process and outcomes are set out in the Gold Guide.

Supervision of Training

Training in any area of clinical medicine requires appropriate workplace supervision and the support of longer-term career development. This is particularly important in an area such as bariatric anaesthesia where trainees undertake work which is frequently complex and challenging. Levels of day-to-day supervision of trainees in clinical attachments in bariatric anaesthesia depend on the seniority of a particular trainee and the competencies which they have demonstrated. In complex areas of anaesthetic practice such as this, it is generally accepted that services will be covered by consultants, with trainees adopting a supernumerary role. However, a degree of indirect supervision is advantageous for senior trainees in preparation for independent consultant practice. The exact requirements for supervision will be unique for each situation and should be based on the professional judgement of trainers rather than any particular service requirements.

The GMC has formally defined the roles of 'clinical supervisor' (CS) and 'educational supervisor' (ES) in post-graduate medical training and all training establishments are required to have trainers in these roles. Not all consultants are required to undertake such roles, but participation in training is a requirement of the GMC's Good Medical Practice for all doctors. The role of a CS is to lead day-to-day training, undertaking assessments and signing off units of training as appropriate, in liaison with colleagues and under the leadership of the departmental College Tutor. ES's are required to provide close supervision for individual trainees, being responsible for supporting career planning and professional development and contributing to an educational supervisor's structured report for use in ARCP. From 2016 a register has also been established of all trainers in these roles in the UK. Trainers will be required to undertake specific training and maintain continuing professional development in order to maintain registration.

Conclusion

Developing an appropriately trained medical work-force is of considerable importance to all bariatric surgical units. The processes and pathways involved in post-graduate medical education are complex, with a multitude of requirements for both trainees and trainers. Ensuring a robust and high-quality training environment has considerable benefits for the trainees who may rotate through a particular department. Furthermore, high standards in training have been shown to support excellence in patient care. The provision of high-quality training in bariatric anaesthesia will serve to ensure that the future consultant workforce has the clinical and professional skills to provide excellent patient care and further develop services in this area of practice.

Further Reading

Bloom, BS, Engelhart MD, Furst EJ, Hill WH, Krathwohl DR. *Taxonomy of Educational Objectives: The Classification of Educational Goals. Handbook I: Cognitive Domain.* New York: David McKay Company; 1956.

Brunner J. *The Process of Education.* Cambridge, MA: Harvard University Press; 1960.

COPMeD. A Reference Guide for Postgraduate Specialty Training in the UK (sixth edition). 2016. https://www.copmed.org.uk/publications/the-gold-guide (accessed April 2018).

Frank, J, Snell LS, Cate OT, et al. Competency-based medical education: theory to practice. *Med Educ.* 2010;32: 638–45.

Harden RM, Stamper N. What is a spiral curriculum? *Medical Teacher.* 1999;21:141–3.

Poirier P, Cornier M-A, Mazzone T, et al. Bariatric surgery and cardiovascular risk factors: a scientific statement from the American Heart Association. *Circulation.* 2011;123: 1683–701.

The General Medical Council. Good Medical Practice. 2013. www.gmc-uk.org/ethical-guidance/ethical-guidance-for-doctors/good-medical-practice (accessed April 2018).

The General Medical Council. Promoting Excellence: Standards for Medical Education and Training. 2016. www.gmc-uk.org/Promoting_excellence_standards_for_medical_education_and_training_0715.pdf_61939165.pdf (accessed April 2018).

The Royal College of Anaesthetists. CCT in Anaesthetics: Assessment Guidance. 2015. www.rcoa.ac.uk/document-store/cct-anaesthetics-assessment-guidance (accessed April 2018).

The Royal College of Anaesthetists. Perioperative Medicine: The Pathway to Better Surgical Care. 2015. www.rcoa.ac.uk/sites/default/files/PERIOP-2014.pdf (accessed April 2018).

The Royal College of Anaesthetists. CCT in Anaesthetic Annex E- Advanced Level Training. 2016. www.rcoa.ac.uk/system/files/TRG-CCT-ANNEXE.pdf (accessed April 2018).

The Royal College of Anaesthetists. Curriculum for a CCT in Anaesthetics. 2016. www.rcoa.ac.uk/system/files/TRG-CU-CCT-ANAES2010.pdf (accessed April 2018).

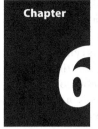

Chapter

6 Cardiovascular System Pathophysiology in Obesity

Peter Gregory

Introduction

According to the World Health Organization cardiovascular disease (CVD) is the leading cause of death. In 2012, 17.5 million people worldwide died as a consequence of CVD, which equates to 31% of all deaths. In Europe, CVD accounts for over a third of deaths in those less than 75 years of age, whilst in the UK 42 000 people die prematurely each year from its complications. The clinical care of CVD is expensive and places a huge burden on health services. The yearly cost to NHS England for the treatment of CVD is £6.8 billion, whilst the estimated annual cost to the UK economy is £15 billion.

Cardiovascular Pathophysiology in Obesity

Obesity, defined by body mass index (BMI) of >30 kg/m^2, is an independent risk factor for the development of CVD. Coronary artery disease, hypertension, cardiac dysrhythmias, sudden cardiac death, cardiomyopathy, pulmonary hypertension, heart failure, thromboembolism and stroke are all more common in the obese. There are three primary reasons for this. Firstly, the presence of obesity, particularly central obesity, predisposes to those conditions that also cause CVD in non-obese people. Hypertension, dyslipidaemia, diabetes mellitus, obstructive sleep apnoea and the metabolic syndrome all have an increased prevalence. Secondly, obesity is an inflammatory state and inflammatory mediators released from adipose tissue damage vascular endothelium, affecting arterial pressure regulation and accelerating atheroma formation. Thirdly, the increased burden of metabolically active adipose tissue in the obese requires compensatory changes to the function of the cardiovascular system to meet this demand, which over time and with increasing obesity become maladaptive and ultimately pathological.

This chapter will focus on the role of adipose tissue in the pathogenesis of CVD and the cardiovascular adaption to obesity. Finally, the impact of obesity on cardiomyopathy and heart failure, hypertension, cardiac dysrhythmias, sudden cardiac death and coronary artery disease (CAD) will be reviewed.

Adipose Tissue

Fat is not just an inert storage system for triglycerides. It is becoming increasingly clear that adipose tissue is highly metabolically active and plays an important role in many homeostatic mechanisms (Table 6.1). It secretes over 50 known mediators to regulate these processes and is considered to be a major endocrine tissue. In the pathogenesis of CVD, the interplay of three of these mediators; leptin, interleukin-6 (IL-6) and C-reactive peptide (CRP) is noteworthy.

Leptin, IL-6 and CRP

Leptin, also known as the 'satiety hormone', is a protein secreted into the circulation by adipose tissue. It crosses the blood–brain barrier and acts on the hypothalamus to inhibit hunger and stimulate satiety, or fullness. Given its mechanism of action on the hypothalamus it is not unreasonable to presume that obese individuals would have a deficiency of circulating leptin, resulting in increased hunger and reduced satiety; however, this is not the case. Instead, there is hyperleptinaemia reflecting not only the increased adipose tissue mass secreting more of this protein, but also the effects of increased leptin resistance, a situation analogous to insulin resistance in type 2 diabetes mellitus. Leptin has many complex peripheral interactions, including roles in insulin signalling pathways and in the modulation of arterial pressure by a direct effect on the vasculature. Leptin also stimulates release of the atherogenic agent tissue necrosis factor alpha (TNF-α) and, consequently, hyperleptinaemia has been implicated as an

Table 6.1. Homeostatic functions of adipose tissue

Lipid metabolism

Glucose homeostasis

Inflammation

Blood pressure regulation

Angiogenesis

Thrombogenesis

metabolically more active and is associated with an increased cardiovascular risk, whilst peripheral adipose tissue is more quiescent and may even have a protective cardiovascular effect. This central adipose tissue has a rich capillary network, reflecting its high metabolic activity. Adipose tissue blood flow (ATBF) is keenly regulated according to changes in nutritional state and to the metabolic activity of the adipose tissue. The physiological regulation of ATBF is com-

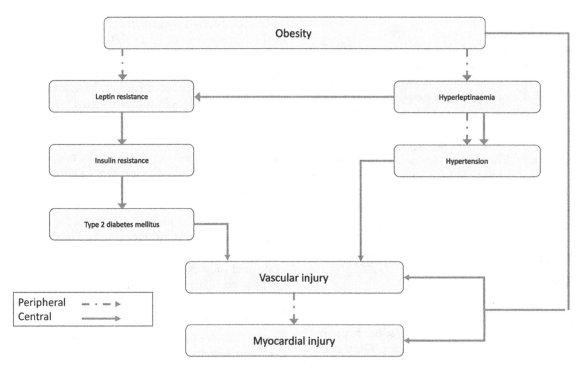

Figure 6.1 Mechanism of vascular injury by hyperleptinaemia.

independent risk factor for the development of atherosclerosis, ischaemic heart disease and stroke.

IL-6, also secreted by adipose tissue, is a proinflammatory cytokine that stimulates the release of CRP from the liver and from the vascular endothelium. CRP binds to leptin, reducing its efficacy by allosteric modulation, thus increasing leptin resistance.

Haemodynamic Adaptation to Obesity

The adaptive changes of the cardiovascular system to obesity arise as a consequence of both the increase in adipose tissue bulk and the increase in lean muscle required to carry the excess mass. Adipose tissue can be categorised into central (abdominal) and peripheral (hips, buttocks) stores. Central adipose tissue is

plex and not completely understood, although β and α_2 adrenergic receptor-mediated effects are known to predominate. Nitrous oxide, insulin, angiotensin II and prostacyclin are also implicated. Interestingly, compared with healthy, non-obese individuals, the resting and post-prandial rise in ATBF is lower in the obese. In the 1960s, Larson demonstrated with xenon clearance studies that resting ATBF in non-obese individuals is 2.6 ml/100 g tissue, increasing up to 10-fold following eating. This resting ATBF falls to 1.8 ml/100 g tissue in individuals with body fat content greater than 36% compared to individuals with 15% and 26% body fat. This down-regulation in obese states is thought to be an adaptation to the increased fat mass. Although ATBF per 100 g of tissue falls in obese individuals, more total blood is

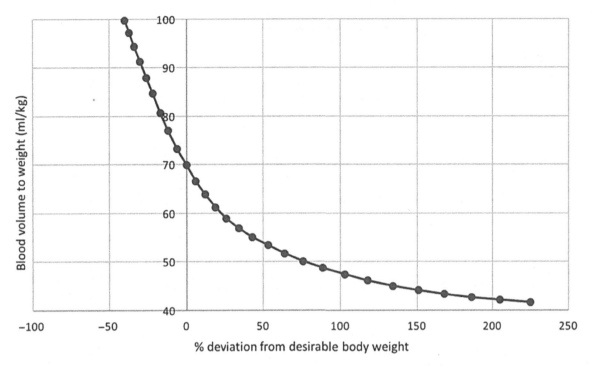

Figure 6.2 Change in blood volume by deviation from desirable body weight.

delivered, due to the large increase in adipose tissue bulk resulting in an overall increase in cardiac output.

Blood Volume

Until the late 1970s there was a commonly held belief that the ratio between an individual's blood volume and body weight or body surface area was constant, e.g. if a 50 kg person put on 50 kg of weight, their blood volume would double. Investigation of this, by measuring plasma volume with a radio-iodine marker and haematocrit to measure red cell mass in individuals of varying body weights, demonstrated this ratio is not constant. In the extremely underweight, a blood volume of 100 ml/kg was revealed. As body weight increases this falls, with the severely overweight having a volume 40 ml/kg. Although the ratio of blood volume to body weight or body surface area falls in obesity, overall total blood volume is increased compared to non-obese individuals with adverse consequences for the cardiovascular system.

Cardiac Output

Increased blood volume leads to increased cardiac filling pressures, increased pre-load and increased myocardial stretch, resulting in an increased stroke volume (SV). Usually there is little or no change in heart rate (HR). Cardiac output (CO) is primarily increased by increased stroke volume. Additionally, due to the inflammatory nature of obesity, which has been likened to early sepsis, there is a drop in systemic vascular resistance (SVR). As blood pressure is the product of CO and SVR, there is a higher CO and lower SVR for any given blood pressure compared to non-obese individuals. These changes result in a hyperdynamic state comparable to persistent exercise or the physiological changes seen in pregnancy. Accumulated evidence reveals that each unit increase in BMI is associated with a 1.35 ml increase in SV and a 0.08 l/min increase in CO. Increased lean muscle mass may also play a role. The North American Strong Heart Study links the increase in CO and SV to fat free mass suggesting that blood supply to other non-fatty tissues may also be of significance.

Progression to Obesity Cardiomyopathy and Heart Failure

Obesity is an independent risk factor for left ventricular hypertrophy (LVH) and other cardiac structural

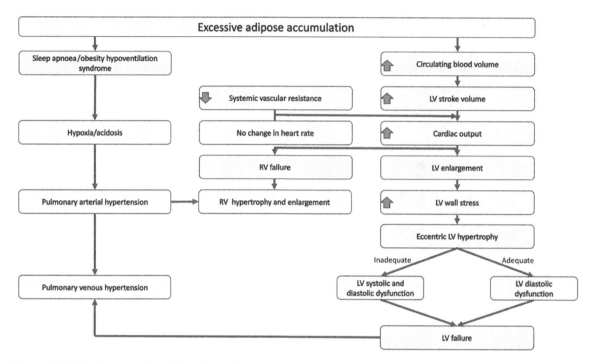

Figure 6.3 Pathophysiology of heart failure in the obese.

abnormalities. Echocardiograms of asymptomatic obese patients prior to bariatric surgery demonstrated 50% had eccentric dilatation of the ventricle and 55% had diastolic dysfunction. This could be predicted, as the hyperdynamic state, increased cardiac filling pressures and volumes shift the Frank–Starling curve to the left, resulting in a higher cardiac workload at any given level of activity for obese individuals. Over time, the increased wall stress in the left ventricle (LV) causes hypertrophy, making the ventricle bulkier, stiffer and increasing its oxygen demand. This hypertrophy is typically the eccentric type where the ventricular wall thickens and dilates with preservation of the size of the LV cavity. With progression, diastolic and systolic function decline, resulting in LV failure. The failed LV causes backpressure to build in the left atrium (with atrial dilatation and predisposing to atrial fibrillation) and then in the pulmonary circulation. Pulmonary hypertension, right ventricular hypertrophy and right ventricular (RV) failure follow. Progressive dyspnoea, ankle oedema, symptoms of LV failure and RV failure may then manifest. This obesity cardiomyopathy is prevalent in 10% of patients with BMI >40 kg/m^2 and in those who have been obese for >10 years. Heart failure is the leading cause of death in these patients.

Pathological States

Hypertension

Obesity, and particularly central obesity, has long been associated with increased cardiovascular mortality. Overweight individuals with hypertension are twice as likely to die from a cardiac cause, whilst those who are overweight but not hypertensive do not demonstrate an increased risk. This suggests it is the presence of hypertension that provides the link between obesity and CVD.

Hypertension is three times more likely to occur in obese individuals, with prevalence and severity increasing with increasing BMI. The National Health and Nutrition Examination Survey (NHANES) III study revealed that men with a BMI >30 kg/m^2 had a 42% risk compared with a 15% risk for lean men for developing hypertension. This risk was similar in women, i.e. 38% risk BMI >30 kg/m^2 compared to 15% lean.

Hypertension in obesity has a complex and multifactorial aetiology and is likely to be determined by interplay between genetic and environmental factors. An illustration of this is provided by the Framingham study that found that normal weight, hypertensive individuals were more likely to gain excessive weight than normal weight, normotensive individuals

Table 6.2 Aetiology of hypertension in the obese

Activation of Sympathetic nervous system (SNS)

Activation of renin–angiotensin system (RAS)

Endothelial dysfunction

Insulin resistance

Decreased atrial natriuritic peptide (ANP)

Leptin resistance

Obesity hypoventilation syndrome

Sub-clinical inflammation

Procoagulability

suggesting either individual susceptibility or shared environmental triggers between hypertension and obesity. Implicated mechanisms of the pathogenesis of hypertension in obesity are given in Table 6.2. The LVH typically associated with essential hypertension is concentric, i.e. LV wall thickening with diminution of the LV cavity. When present in obesity where eccentric hypertrophy is present, a dimorphic eccentric/concentric hypertrophy results.

Conduction Abnormalities

Obesity cardiomyopathy is characterised by cardiomegaly, LV dilatation and myocyte hypertrophy, with the absence of interstitial fibrosis. In the obese state, there is increased fat deposition, not only in predictable peri-organ sites such as the pericardium but also in non-adipose tissue sites. The presence of fat cells in these areas causes lipotoxicity resulting in dysfunction and death of nearby native organ cells. In the myocardium, cords of myocytes trap fat cells between them causing apoptosis of cardiac cells, with the cells of the sinoatrial and atrioventricular nodes particularly vulnerable. Damage to the cardiac conducting system predisposes obese patients to increased electrical irritability that can lead to significant dysrhythmias, even in the absence of LV dysfunction or heart failure. Electrocardiogram studies of obese patients have demonstrated that the PR interval, QRS duration and QTc interval are commonly prolonged and the cardiac axis is directed more leftward than in the non-obese. Other prevalent findings include left atrial abnormalities, flattened T waves in inferior and posterior leads and low-voltage QRS complexes.

Sudden Cardiac Death

Sudden death is more common in those who are naturally fat than in the lean.
Hippocrates (460–370 B.C.)

The Framingham study reported that sudden cardiac death (SCD) is 40 times more likely to occur in obese than non-obese patients. SCD occurs in both the 'healthy', asymptomatic obese and in those with obesity cardiomyopathy, although the risk is greatest in those patients with eccentric LV hypertrophy. The incidence of premature ventricular complexes was observed to be 30 times higher in obese patients with eccentric LVH and 10 times higher in obese patients without eccentric LVH compared to lean. In addition, bigeminy, quadrigenminy and ventricular tachycardia were observed to be present in those with obesity cardiomyopathy, but absent in the other two groups. The propensity of ventricular ectopic beats in the obese may make SCD in this population more likely. Obesity is also associated with abnormalities of autonomic balance, leading to higher heart rates and reduced heart rate variability, factors known to increase the risk of SCD.

Atrial Fibrillation

There are a number of large studies that identify obesity as an independent risk factor for the development of atrial fibrillation (AF). Known risk factors such as sleep disordered breathing, left atrial dilatation, left ventricular diastolic dysfunction and increased p-wave dispersion, i.e. the difference between minimal and maximal p-wave duration, are all more common in the obese. It is the structural changes that occur to the atria as a consequence of obesity that forms the basis of this predisposition. Hearts of obese patients are typically heavier and larger than non-obese hearts. Post mortem examinations demonstrate that the hearts of obese patients are on average 40% heavier than lean hearts, mainly due to an increase in peri-cardial fat. Wang et al. observed over 5000 patients without AF over a 13.7-year period. Echocardiography demonstrated larger atrial diameters in obese men (4.4 cm) compared to overweight men (4.1 cm) and non-obese men (3.8 cm). Findings were similar in the female group. This study also found that after adjusting for age, blood pressure, use of anti-hypertensive medications, cigarette smoking, diabetes mellitus, LVH and previous myocardial infarction, the risk of developing AF increases by 4% for every BMI unit increase for both men ($p = 0.2$) and women (p = 0.1). Interestingly, when atrial diameter was removed from the calculation this increased risk disappeared, supporting the hypothesis it is structural change to the atria that is the common pathway to AF in obesity.

Coronary Artery Disease

Although seemingly intuitive, an independent causal relationship between obesity and CAD is unproven and continues to be a subject of dispute. Early studies such as the 'Seven Countries Trial' in 1984 and 'The Geographic Pathology of Atherosclerosis' by HC McGill Jr in 1986 failed to show any significant correlation. Although the Framingham Heart Study has consistently demonstrated an increased incidence of CAD with increasing BMI, multivariate analysis of this data reveals this is most likely due to an indirect effect of obesity increasing the prevalence of known CAD risk factors, such as hypertension, dyslipidaemia and insulin resistance. One possible explanation for the lack of a clear link is that recently identified or emerging risk factors may be playing a role. Atherogenic dyslipidaemia, insulin resistance and pro-inflammatory and pro-thrombotic states common in obesity are recent concepts that have been implicated, but are not yet fully understood. In spite of the paucity of strong evidence of a direct effect of obesity on atherogenesis the observation it directly promotes other conditions associated with CAD means it is considered a primary modifiable risk factor for CAD by both the American Heart Association and the British Heart Foundation.

Obesity Paradox

That which does not kill us makes us stronger.
Freidrich Nietzsche (1844–1900)

This chapter has demonstrated that obesity is an established independent risk factor for mortality and morbidity from CVD in the general population, largely due to the presence of the metabolic syndrome and other associated pathophysiological changes. However, there is a growing body of evidence suggesting there are certain overweight and obese patient populations with CVD that do not have a worse outcome than comparable, non-obese groups and, in fact, may actually have more favourable outcomes. This 'reverse epidemiology' is known as the obesity paradox. In medical populations, obese patients with known CAD undergoing percutaneous coronary

intervention with either known heart failure, hypertension or CAD all had a lower incidence of mortality compared to normal and underweight patients. In one surgical study, a prospective, multicentre cohort study of 118 707 patients undergoing non-bariatric, general surgery, demonstrated the lowest rates of crude and risk-adjusted mortality in the overweight and moderately obese groups (BMI 30–34.9 kg/m^2) compared to normal weight. The highest rates of mortality were seen in the underweight and in those patients with BMI >40 kg/m^2.

Several pathophysiological and methodological mechanisms for this phenomenon have been postulated, including alterations in circulating cytokines, inflammatory pre-conditioning, endotoxin–lipoprotein interactions, reverse causality, survival bias and time discrepancies among critical risk factors, but more studies are needed to conclusively prove the existence of this paradox and its basis in medicine.

Further Reading

Alpert MA, Terry BE, Cohen MV, et al. The electrocardiogram in morbid obesity. *Am J Cardiol.* 2000;**85**(7):908–10.

Anand RG, Peters RW, Donahue TP. Obesity and dysrhythmias. *J Cardiometab Syndr.* 2008;**3**:149–54.

Bernick S, Davis CB. The Economic Cost of Cardiovascular Disease from 2014–2020 in Six European Countries. London: Centre for Economic and Business Research; 2014.

Cole VW, Alexander JK. Clinical effects of extreme obesity on cardiopulmonary function. *South Med J.* 1959;**52**(4): 435–8.

Curtis JP, Selter JG, Wang Y, et al. The obesity paradox: body mass index and outcomes in patients with heart failure. *Arch Intern Med.* 2005;**165**:55–61.

Duflou J, Virmani R, Rabin I, et al. Sudden death as a result of heart disease in morbid obesity. *Am Heart J.* 1995;**130**(2): 306–13.

Frank S, Colliver JA, Frank A. The electrocardiogram in obesity: statistical analysis of 1,029 patients. *J Am Coll Cardiol.* 1996;**7**(2):295–9.

Goncalves IE, Rocha M, et al. Echocardiography evaluations for asymptomatic patients with severe obesity. *Arq Bras Cardiol.* 2007;**88**(1):48–53.

Gruberg L, Weissman NJ, Waksman R, et al. The impact of obesity on the short-term and long-term outcomes after percutaneous coronary interven- tion: the obesity paradox? *J Am Coll Cardiol.* 2002;**39**:578–84.

Larsen OA, Lassen NA, Quaade F. Blood flow through human adipose tissue determined with radioactive xenon. *Acta Physiol Scand.* 1996;**66**(3):337–45.

Martin SS, Qasim A, Reilly MP. Leptin resistance a possible interface of inflammation and metabolism in obesity-related cardiovascular disease. *J Am Coll Cardiol*. 2008;**52**:1201–10.

Messerli FH, Nunez BD, Ventura HO, et al. Overweight and sudden death. Increased ventricular ectopy in cardiopathy of obesity. *Arch Intern Med*. 1987;**147**(10): 1725–8.

Mullen J, Moorman D, Davenport D. The obesity paradox: body mass index and outcomes in patients undergoing non-bariatric general surgery. *Ann Surg*. 2009;**250**(1): 166–72.

Rimm EB, Stampfer MJ, Giovannucci E, et al. Body size and fat distribution as predictors of coronary heart disease among middle-aged and older US men. *Am J Epidemiol*. 1995;**141**:1117–27.

Seyfeli E, Duru M, Kuvandick G, et al. Effect of obesity on P-wave dispersion and QT dispersion in women. *Int J Obes*. 2006;**30**(6):957–61.

Smith HL, Willius FA. Adiposity of the heart: a clinical and pathologic study of 136 obese patients. *Arch Intern Med*. 1933;**52**:910–39.

Stelfox HT, Ahmed SB, Ribeiro RA, et al. Haemodynamic monitoring in obese patients: the impact of body mass index on cardiac output and stroke volume. *Crit Care Med*. 2006;**34**(4):1243–6.

Thomas F, Bean K, Pannier B, et al. Cardiovascular mortality in overweight subjects: the key role of associated risk factors. *Hypertension*. 2005;**46**:654–9.

Townsend N, Williams J, Bhatnagar P, et al. *Cardiovascular Disease Statistics*. London: British Heart Foundation; 2014.

Uretsky S, Messerli FH, Bangalore S, et al. Obesity paradox in patients with hypertension and coronary artery disease. *Am J Med*. 2007;**120**:863–870.

Wang TJ, Parise H, Levy D, et al. Obesity and the risk of new-onset atrial fibrillation. *J Am Med Assoc*. 2004;**292**(20): 2471–7.

The Respiratory System and Airway Pathophysiology in Obesity

Nathan Ware and Christopher Bouch

Introduction

The influences of obesity on physiological functions are wide ranging and multiorgan in nature. Deposition of truncal adipose tissue has direct and indirect affects on the airway and lower respiratory tract. There is a clear relationship demonstrating airway and respiratory dysfunction as BMI increases. These changes affect the upper airway with anatomical changes and the lower airway with changes in compliance, lung volumes, work of breathing and gas exchange. This chapter will review these changes in relation to obesity. Differences exist between obese patients with and without the obesity hypoventilation syndrome (OHS) and will be discussed.

Upper Airway

The upper airway consists of the oral cavity, the nasal cavity and the pharynx (nasopharynx, oropharynx and laryngopharynx). The oral cavity is divided in to the oral vestibule, extending externally from the lips and cheek mucosa to the alveolar processes of the teeth. The oral cavity proper is bound by the hard palate superiorly, the floor of the mouth and mandible inferiorly and the pharynx posteriorly. The tongue occupies the majority of the space in the oral cavity.

Nasal structures are formed from bone and cartilage, with a muscosal lining. Where the nasal and laryngeal airways are supported by bone and cartilaginous structures, the pharyngeal airway is not.

The pharynx is a U-shaped fibro-muscular tube extending from the base of the skull to the cricoid cartilage. The nasopharynx portion extends from the posterior nasal cavity and lies superior to the soft palate. The base of the tongue down to the valleucula and epiglottis borders the oropharynx anteriorly. Superiorly is the soft palate and posteriorly the cervical spine. Laterally are found the palatoglossal and palatopharyngeal arches. The laryngopharynx sits inferior to the pharynx, running from the epiglottis to the inferior border of the cricoid cartilage.

Over 20 pairs of muscles form the pharynx. Whilst they are used for swallowing, for example, they also play a vital role in maintaining pharyngeal patency; allowing the passage of air during respiration. The muscles (particularly genioglossus, geniohyoid, sternohyoid, sternothyroid and thyrohyoid) are under neural control and have phasic inspiratory activity. They act to maintain a patent airway in response to both chemoreceptors and negative pressure in the nose and pharynx.

In health, a careful balance between constriction and dilatation exists in the pharynx. This tension control across the muscles maintains patency of this muscular tube. Neural control is reduced during sleep and anaesthesia, potentially precipitating a loss of a patent airway. In its simplest form, the pharynx can be considered as a cylindrical tube connecting the oral and nasal cavities to the trachea and lungs.

Several forces act across and along this tube (Figure 7.1). When these forces are balanced the tube remains patent. These forces include:

- the intra-luminal pressure, where a decrease in pressure may precipitate collapse;
- the external (tissue) pressure, which may be increased in obesity due to fat deposition in the upper airway soft tissues;
- longitudinal tension, where stress along the length of the tube increases the stability and therefore patency of the tube;
- surface tension, which will increase as the airway size reduces.

Posterior movement of the mandible may collapse the anatomically normal airway during sleep, flexion of the head and neck, pressure over the hyoid bone or compression of soft tissue around the mandible. Any increase in resistance in the nasal passages or pharynx will increase the likelihood of collapse with inspiratory effort and consequent generation of negative pressure.

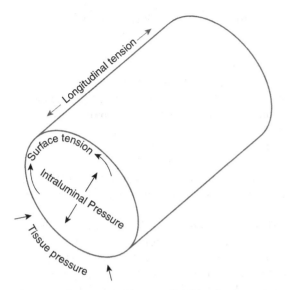

Figure 7.1 Forces acting about a collapsible tube

This pharyngeal tube is contained within the bone structure of the maxilla and mandible. This is not a sealed box, but may remain closed during periods of sleep and anaesthesia. Considering the stresses across and along the tube, we can surmise that a proportional increase in soft tissue volume, a decrease in the size of the bone housing or a decrease in the length of the tube will all promote a tendency to collapse. In addition, any anatomical abnormality will facilitate pharyngeal collapse.

Once closure of the tube has occurred, the body must overcome the adherence of the tissue from mucosal surface tensions before opening. In addition, as the pharyngeal airway becomes comparatively smaller with increasing soft tissue volume, the surface tension around the tube increases, which will favour collapse.

In obesity, an increase in fat deposition is seen throughout the upper airway. Pharyngeal airway collapse in obesity occurs predominately in the retropalatal region owing to fat deposition in the tongue (where fat deposition is predominantly in the posterior portion) and the lateral pharyngeal walls. Obese patients with sleep disordered breathing have both increased tongue and lateral pharyngeal wall volume, which have been identified as independent risk factors for airway collapse.

The excessive tissue deposition seen in obesity may displace outside the enclosure of the mandible into the submandibular space, seen as a double chin or reduced cricomental distance.

During the respiratory cycle there is tracheal tug as the lungs move caudally with inhalation. This tracheal tug helps to increase the tension along the pharyngeal tube, increasing stability and patency. However, lung volumes are altered in the obese patient during anaesthesia and in the supine patient. This reduction in volume decreases the caudal movement of the trachea, decreasing the tug and therefore the tension along the tube within the pharynx, leading to a reduction in stability.

Although not within the airway, the increased deposition of fatty tissue over the upper thorax, across the upper back and around the neck can lead to difficulty when managing the patient's airway. Pressure over excess soft tissues surrounding the neck easily compresses the airway; the increased tissue deposition may cause difficulty when holding and maintaining position for facemask ventilation. Fat deposition over the upper back can reduce atlantoaxial movement leading to difficulty manipulating the neck and head. The size of the upper thorax can obstruct access to the airway when intubating. Careful patient positioning is paramount.

The Lower Respiratory Tract

Compliance

Compliance is defined as the volume change per unit pressure change; it is a measure of distensibility. In health, it is reduced when supine due to a decrease in functional residual capacity (FRC). Total thoracic compliance measures both lung and chest wall compliance. Lung compliance is influenced by connective tissue within the lung (elasticity) and alveoli surfactant (surface tensions at air–water interfaces). In obesity, total respiratory compliance has been shown to decrease by as much as two-thirds compared to normal values, reflecting a threefold increase in resistance. The fall in lung compliance results from an increase in truncal fat, reducing total lung volumes, leading to closure of dependant airways and increased surface tension in the alveoli due to a reduced FRC. This reduction in lung volume is furthered by an increase in pulmonary blood volume. In addition, it has been observed in spontaneously breathing individuals that a decrease in chest wall compliance occurs owing to the increased deposition of fat amongst the ribs and diaphragm.

Changes in Lung Volumes and Spiromtery

Obesity is associated with a number of changes in measured lung volumes (Table 7.1). There is associated loss of FRC and expiratory reserve volume (ERV). With increasing BMI, FRC has been observed to decrease exponentially. FRC and ERV decrease approximately 3% and 5%, respectively, for each unit increase in BMI from 20 to 30 kg/m². Above this point, both the FRC and ERV decrease approximately 1% for each unit increase in BMI, such that severe obesity can result in patients breathing near their residual volume. A decrease in ERV may lead to an increase in areas of atelecstasis, disrupting ventilation/perfusion mismatch. Total lung capacity (TLC), vital capacity (VC) and residual volume (RV) are all affected once BMI >30 kg/m², but the impact is relatively small; on the lower end of normal, even in severe obesity. Studies observe an approximate decrease of 0.5% in VC, TLC and RV with each unit increase in BMI, the decrease continues proportionately with an increasing BMI. As the obese patients FRC encroaches on their RV, closing capacity may exceed the FRC and airway closure can occur with tidal volume breathing.

Breathing at tidal volume during rest in mild-moderate obesity shows little variation from the lean population; however, in severe obesity a reduced tidal volume with an increased respiratory rate is observed. This is believed to be a physiological response to lung volume reduction, a similar respiratory pattern can be observed in patients with restrictive lung conditions.

Contrary to dependant regional ventilation patterns in the healthy lean patient, regional ventilation is seen to be the opposite in the severely obese population with ventilation occurring predominantly in the upper (noted particularly when ERV is markedly reduced) non-dependant zones with associated air trapping in the lower zones. With perfusion still predominately in dependant zones, there is significant potential for ventilation perfusion mismatch.

There is an increased incidence of asthma in the obese population. Debate continues as to the association and pathophysiology of this. Spirometry in the obese patient demonstrates a decreasing forced vital capacity (FVC) and FEV_1 (forced expiratory volume in 1 second), with a normal or slightly increased FEV_1/FVC ratio, suggesting a decrease in lung volume, as opposed to bronchial obstruction. Breathlessness on exertion has been reported in a high proportion of the obese population. Dyspnoea in these patients may well be multifactorial. It is considered that even in the healthy obese patient, the sensation of breathlessness may be brought about due to the increased work of breathing overcoming decreased lung compliance and increases in resistance. The increased airway resistance with increasing BMI is due to the decreased and/or an intrinsic narrowing of the airways, thought to occur with reduced lung volumes. Compared to a patient with a BMI of 20, airway resistance increases by approximately 33%, 49% and 62% for people with BMI values of 30, 35 and 40, respectively.

As well as a reduction in lung volume, other causes of increased airway resistance have been investigated and postulated, owing to biological and functional mechanisms within the parenchyma. With a lower operating lung volume, the airways and associated smooth muscle may accommodate to smaller dimensions. Over time its contractile elements adjust accordingly to maintain the appropriate dimensions. As a result, there is further contraction when stimulated, but a decrease in the ability to distend on stretching. Fatty tissue in the obese patient is capable of expressing pro-inflammatory substances, many of which are implicated in asthma and associated with inflammation of small airways, which are then prone to collapse.

Table 7.1 Respiratory physiological changes in obesity

Respiratory parameter	Change compared to standard values
FRC	Decreased
ERV	Decreased
TLC	Normal
VC	Normal
RV	Normal
FEV_1/FVC	Normal
FEV_1	Normal or decreased
FVC	Normal or decreased
Airways resistance	Increased
Diffusing capacity	Slight increase
Work of breathing	Increased

Although they have been shown to exaggerate airway responsiveness in obese animal studies, there is little evidence to suggest that a link between asthma and obesity exist as a result of the inflammatory effects of obesity.

The Work of Breathing

The respiratory muscles of the obese patient have a greater load, compared to their lean counterparts, owing to the need to overcome the decreased compliance and increased airway resistance. There is much conflict between studies, regarding both respiratory muscle strength and muscle endurance. Several have demonstrated no gross difference between muscle strength and the ability to generate pressure. However, others have shown that the obese population generates lower pressures and has weaker respiratory muscles, for example maximal voluntary ventilation can be reduced by up to 20% in the healthy obese and as much as 45% in OHS patients. Severely obese patients have a higher work of breathing, using up to 15% of their total oxygen consumption versus 3% in the lean population.

Gas Exchange

Gas exchange as measured by carbon monoxide diffusion capacity (DL_{CO}) has been shown to increase in the healthy obese patient. The increase in DL_{CO} is due to an increase in pulmonary blood volume. DL_{CO} is estimated to increase by approximately 0.3% for each unit increase in BMI. Owing to the ventilation perfusion mismatch associated with obesity, there is an increased alveolar–arterial oxygen tension gradient and a reduced partial pressure of arterial oxygen (PaO_2). The majority of obese patients maintain a normal partial pressure of arterial carbon dioxide ($PaCO_2$), owing to an increase in minute ventilation. OHS patients will be discussed elsewhere.

Key Points

- Fat deposition outside and within the respiratory system leads to changes in respiratory physiology.
- An appreciation of factors affecting airway patency may help in its management.
- Compliance is decreased.
- FRC decreases exponentially with increasing BMI and explains the rapid desaturation seen in obese patients.
- Work of breathing is increased; however, there is ongoing debate regarding respiratory muscle strength and fatigue.

Further Reading

Behazin N, Jones SB, Cohen RI, et al. Respiratory restriction and elevated pleural and esophageal pressures in morbid obesity. *J Appl Physiol*. 2010;**108**(1):212–18.

Holley HS, Milic-Emili J, Becklake MR, et al. Regional distribution of pulmonary ventilation and perfusion in obesity. *J Clin Invest*. 1967;**46**:475–81.

Jones Rl, Nzekwu MM. The effects of body mass index on lung volumes. *Chest*. 2006;**130**(3):827–33.

Naimark A, Cherniack RM. Compliance of the respiratory system and its components in health and obesity. *J Appl Physiol*. 1960;**15**(3):377–82.

Nicolacakis K, Skowronski ME, Coreno AJ, et al. Observations on the physiological interactions between obesity and asthma. *J Appl Physiol*. 2008;**105**(5):1533–41.

Pelosi P, Croci M, Ravagnan I, et al. The effects of body mass on lung volumes, respiratory mechanics and gas exchange during general anaesthesia. *Anaesth Analg*. 1998;**87**(3):654–60.

Salome CM, King GG, Berend N. Physiology of obesity and effects on lung function. *J Appl Physiol*. 2010;**108**(1):206–11.

Stanchina ML, Malhotra A, Fogel RB, et al. The influence of lung volume on pharyngeal mechanics, collapsibility, and genioglossus muscle activation during sleep. *Sleep*. 2003;**26**(7):851–6.

Sutherland TJ, Cowan JO, Young S, et al. The association between obesity and asthma: interactions between systemic and airway inflammation. *Am J Respir Crit Care Med*. 2008;**1789**(5):469–75.

Tagaito Y, Isono S, Remmers JE, et al. Lung volume and collapsibility of the passive pharynx in patients with sleep-disordered breathing. *J Appl Physiol*. 2007;**103**(4):1379–85.

The Pathophysiology of Sleep Disordered Breathing in the Morbidly Obese

Pei Kee Poh and Andrew Hall

Introduction

The constellation of signs and symptoms associated with sleep disordered breathing (SDB) has been known for millennia. As early as the fourth century BC, Dionysius, 2nd tyrant of Heraclea, who became extremely obese due to his gluttony, lived in constant fear of 'drowning in his own fat during sleep'. To counteract this, he ordered his physicians to stick needles into his abdomen every time he fell asleep to enable him to breathe.

In 1836, Charles Dickens published his first novel *The Pickwick Papers*, in which he characterised 'Joe the fat boy' from his childhood experiences of being bullied. Dickens described Joe as a (130 kg) boy who could fall asleep at any time of the day. Joe 'snored so loud it could be heard from the distant kitchen'. He had a 'ruddy complexion' and suffered from the dropsy. These were probably symptoms of polycythaemia, and oedema resulting from right heart failure – features we now recognise in end-stage obstructive sleep apnoea (OSA) and obesity hypoventilation syndrome (OHS).

Medical descriptions of OSA lagged behind their literary contemporaries; case reports only began emerging in the nineteenth century. It was in 1956 when sleep disordered breathing became a formal medical entity. A 51-year-old businessman attended hospital, having become angry at himself for missing a 'full house' during a game of poker when he fell asleep. He weighed 120 kg, had polycythaemia, hypoventilation whilst awake, apnoeic spells during sleep and suffered from right heart failure. He lost 18 kg and the problems of hypersomnolence and 'periodic respiration' went away. His attending physician, Burwell, termed the condition 'Pickwickian syndrome' having noticed the resemblance to Dickens' Joe.

Whilst the term 'Pickwickian syndrome' is now used more for OHS, Dickens and Burwell may have described co-existent OSA and OHS. In fact, 90% of patients with OHS suffer from OSA, and the two probably form part of a continuum of disease process that in its mildest form is represented by uncomplicated simple snoring. For the purposes of this article, we will be concentrating on OSA.

Epidemiology

OSA is becoming more prevalent due to the increasing burden of obesity. Most texts quote an incidence of 4% and 2% in middle-aged men and women, respectively. The British Lung Foundation estimates 2.9% of the adult UK population have OSA, with 85% of these undiagnosed.

Risk Factors

Males with an androgenic fat distribution are at highest risk. Women have a fourfold risk increase after the menopause. Conversely, women on hormonr replacement therapy (HRT) have this risk halved, likely due to the effect of oestrogen on upper airway muscles.

In adulthood, the risk of OSA doubles every 10 years to 65, at which point it reaches a plateau. Reasons suggested for this include under-reporting, as sleepiness becomes less of an issue in the elderly along with increased mortality after this age.

OSA runs in families; the risk doubles if an immediate family member has OSA. It is thought that genetics influence facial structure (retrognathia being more common) and increased distribution of fat in the airways. Obesity may be hereditary, but it is also more likely in families due to common eating and social habits.

Africans, Asians, Hispanics and Polynesians have an increased risk of OSA. Asians in particular have a crowded airway and increased retrognathia compared to Caucasians. Therefore, obesity predisposes to OSA more so in whites than Chinese, who are more affected by craniofacial features.

Other risk factors include alcohol, smoking (mucositis), sedatives, sleeping supine, Down's

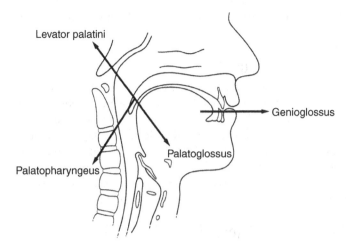

Levator palatini

Genioglossus

Palatoglossus

Palatopharyngeus

Figure 8.1 Actions of upper airway dilator muscles. (Adapted from Douglas N. *Clinician's Guide to Sleep Medicine*. Fig 2.3, Page 29. Arnold Publishers; 2002.)

syndrome, acromegaly, hypothyroidism, Cushing's syndrome and diabetes mellitus.

Pathophysiology

The pharynx is a complex structure, serving three distinct functions – breathing, swallowing and talking. The airway needs to be rigid to prevent collapse on inspiration from the generated negative pressure; conversely, swallowing tubes need to be compliant for peristalsis, while speech requires fine-tuning of airway diameter. Remarkably, the pharynx achieves all these requirements despite these conflicts.

In the awake state, the palatal muscles and tongue work together to maintain airway patency. Palatopharyngeus and palatoglossus contract, while levator palatini relaxes to increase nasal airflow. Genioglossus, the main tongue muscle, expands the oropharynx by protruding the tongue forward. Interestingly, genioglossus weakens with age.

During sleep, these muscles assume a more relaxed state, as the reflexes that regulate muscle tone become blunted. This is not normally a problem, but with increased fat deposition in the pharynx or posterior displacement of the tongue from retrognathia, this can cause airway obstruction, giving rise to OSA. Localised oedema then occurs due to vibration trauma between the pharyngeal walls and soft palate, exacerbating the problem.

A common misconception is that hypoxaemia causes arousal as the brain becomes oxygen-deprived. This is not entirely true. A decrease in intra-pleural pressure leads to electroencephalogram (EEG) arousal and termination of the apnoea. Hypoxaemia and

hypercapnia indirectly stimulate the respiratory centres to increase the force of inspiratory muscle contraction, thereby decreasing intra-pleural pressure.

At the point of arousal, the patient emerges from a deeper to a lighter stage of sleep. The palatal muscles and genioglossus regain their muscle tone. The airway opens with the patient producing the classic sudden, loud snorting sound.

Consequences of SDB

Neuropsychological Impairment

It is unsurprising that many patients complain of daytime somnolence, due to sleep fragmentation. Studies demonstrate a decrease in global cognitive function affecting concentration, memory and judgement. Productivity at work falls and work-related accidents are more common. Marriages can become strained from unemployment and snoring, with some partners sleeping in another bedroom. Mood swings and depression may develop as a result. Many studies have shown improvements in these areas of life after treatment.

Accidents

Many patients with OSA will admit to having fallen asleep at the wheel. More than one-third will have experienced an accident or near-accident because of sleep driving. Patients with OSA have a 2.5 times increased risk of having a road traffic accident (RTA). One study revealed that inebriated subjects performed better on a driving simulator than sober

OSA counterparts. NICE estimates that one RTA could be prevented for every 8.5 patients treated with continuous positive airway pressure (CPAP). If all patients with moderate-severe OSA were treated, this would mean 40 000 fewer RTAs per year in the UK.

Cardiovascular

At the start of an apnoeic spell, inspiratory effort against a closed airway stimulates a parasympathetic response. As hypoxia ensues, sympathetic activity builds up, peaking at the point of arousal before returning to baseline. This is associated with alternating bradycardic and tachycardic episodes, which have been mistaken for tachy-brady syndromes and pacemakers fitted unnecessarily. Ectopics, atrial fibrillation, ventricular tachycardia, and first- and second-degree heart blocks may also occur.

The surge in sympathetic activity leads to a rise in blood pressure. This may be sustained during the daytime if the hypoxic spells are prolonged and frequent. The Wisconsin Sleep Cohort Study found a 2.9-fold increase in the risk of developing hypertension. OSA-induced hypertension may be resistant to medications, but is potentially reversible with CPAP, which can reduce 24-hour diastolic blood pressure by 5 mmHg. This fall may be small, but over a 5–10 year period, translates to a 20% reduction in cardiovascular risk and 40% decrease in strokes.

OSA is associated with myocardial infarction. The Wisconsin Study demonstrated OSA patients were 1.9 times more likely to develop coronary heart disease or heart failure. Those with severe OSA had their risks increased to 2.6-fold.

Respiratory

Hypercapnia is a well-recognised but infrequent finding in OSA patients. It is more common in OHS and the morbidly obese due to mass loading of the chest wall, reducing compliance and tidal volume. OSA also increases the risk of type 2 respiratory failure in those with chronic obstructive airway and neuromuscular disease.

Daytime hypoxaemia is also more common in the above patient groups, and is integral to the development of pulmonary hypertension from prolonged pulmonary vasoconstriction. Right ventricular hypertrophy may then ensue with development of right heart failure. CPAP has the potential to reduce pulmonary artery pressures and improve ventricular function.

Neurological

There appears to be an association between OSA and strokes, possibly due to common risks between the two conditions, e.g. alcohol, age, diabetes mellitus, hypertension and obesity. Sustained daytime hypertension from OSA is likely the most important cause, although sympathetic surges during apnoeic spells may play a role. Studies reveal an increased risk of stroke in snorers. The reason is unknown.

Haematological

Most OSA patients have normal erythropoietin levels and do not suffer from polycythaemia; those who do usually have a concurrent disease causing daytime hypoxaemia. Polycythaemia increases blood viscosity, predisposing to thrombosis. Prolonged hypoxaemia may also elevate fibrinogen levels, as it is an acute phase protein.

OSA induces a pro-inflammatory state because of hypoxia. CRP, TNF-α, IL-6 and oxygen free radical production increases (due to re-oxygenation after apnoea), while nitric oxide levels fall, causing platelet aggregation and increased atheroma formation. This promotes the increased risks of cardiovascular disease and stroke.

Endocrine

Sleep is required for growth hormone and IGF-1 (insulin-like growth factor 1) production; these fall in OSA patients who have reduced deep (slow wave) sleep, leading to loss of muscle, but increased fat deposition. Increased sympathetic activity stimulates pancreatic β-cells. This increases insulin production, fat storage and eventually, insulin resistance develops. OSA is associated with decreased testosterone levels, reduced libido and causes erectile dysfunction.

Anaesthetic Risks

OSA patients may have a tendency to increased risk of difficult intubations compared to the non-OSA group. OSA is associated with an increased risk of cardiorespiratory complications, delirium, increased length of stay, unplanned intensive care unit (ICU) admissions and death in the peri-operative setting.

Cost-benefit

Just under half of patients with moderate-severe OSA in the UK are currently receiving treatment. The Office of Health Economics estimates that if all were to receive treatment, a potential saving to the NHS of £28 million could be realised.

Obesity Hypoventilation Syndrome

When 'Pickwickian syndrome' and OHS was first described, these patients had features of obesity, hypersomnolence, polycythaemia and right heart failure. Nocturnal observations in this patient group led to the first descriptions of OSA; however, not all patients with OHS had OSA. Many of those with OSA also did not have daytime hypoxaemia. This led to considerable variation in the diagnosis of these patients, leading the American Academy of Sleep Medicine (AASM) to define them as two separate entities. OHS is now diagnosed when a patient has:

- a BMI of ≥30;
- daytime alveolar hypoventilation defined as P_aCO_2 >45mmHg (6.0kPa) ± P_aO_2 >70mmHg (9.3kPa);
- associated sleep-related breathing disorder (90% have OSA, while the others have sleep hypoventilation that is not due to airway obstruction);
- absence of other known causes of hypoventilation.

The main differences between OHS and OSA are that the former has:

- daytime hypercapnia;
- longer and more continuous episodes of hypoventilation overnight (may or may not be secondary to upper airway obstruction).

OHS is much less common than OSA; it is estimated to occur in 0.3% of the population. Most patients have a BMI >40 and severe OSA. The pathophysiology of OHS is complex; it can be thought of as a disease process at the upper end of the spectrum where sleep disordered breathing is complicated by lung mechanics, obesity-related excessive production of CO_2, depressed respiratory drive and leptin resistance (impairs brainstem response to hypercapnia) due to morbid obesity. This leads to longer and continuous episodes of hypoventilation, causing hypoxaemia and hypercapnia not just at night time, but during the day as well. Hence, these patients are much more likely to develop pulmonary hypertension and right heart failure from pulmonary vasoconstriction. Treatment is the same as for OSA; mortality is high without it.

Peri-operative Management of OSA

General anaesthesia commonly includes administration of sedatives, muscle relaxants and respiratory depressants. When given to an obese patient with OSA, who may have low saturations, adverse events are frequently encountered. In 2014, the American Society of Anesthesiologists Task Force published guidelines for the peri-operative care of these patients.

Pre-operative

Assessment should include a review of the patient's medical notes, and patient assessment for potential difficult airway, previous anaesthetic issues, hypertension and evidence of cardiovascular disease. Snoring, apnoeic episodes and daytime somnolence should alert one to the possibility of OSA; these patients should be evaluated with an appropriate screening tool, such as the STOP-BANG questionnaire (Table 18.2 and see Chapter 14). If a patient has been diagnosed with OSA previously, compliance with treatment and residual symptoms should be explored. Physical examination should include an airway assessment, neck circumference, tongue and tonsil size.

Undiagnosed moderate-high risk patients should be referred for formal sleep studies. The decision to postpone a patient for further investigations and treatment should be based on:

- severity of OSA (especially those with signs of hypoxaemia, OHS and right heart failure);
- nature and urgency of surgery;
- proposed anaesthetic technique;
- need for post-operative analgesia.

Intra-operative

For superficial and peripheral procedures, local and regional anaesthesia is ideal, which avoids administration of sedative agents.

Where general anaesthesia is used, difficult intubation should be anticipated. A secure airway with an endotracheal tube utilising controlled ventilation is preferable to a spontaneous ventilation technique and supraglottic airway device. Quick-offset agents, e.g. desflurane will be of patient benefit.

Neuromuscular blockade should be fully reversed with tracheal extubation awake and full recovery of airway reflexes.

Post-operative

A multimodal analgesic regime involving simple analgesia and regional techniques should be used to avoid opioid use. The use of patient-controlled opioid delivery systems should be avoided in this patient group.

CPAP should be re-instituted to maintain airway patency as soon as possible. Supplemental oxygen is recommended for high-risk patients to maintain oxygen levels, though they run the risk of increasing apnoea duration and hypercapnia. Supplementary oxygen can be introduced into the normal CPAP circuit. These patients should be nursed in a monitored environment with continuous pulse oximetry until they can maintain oxygen saturations on room air and apnoeas are non-existent.

Key Points

- OSA is common in obese patients.
- There is an association with peri-operative adverse events and practitioners must be prepared for this.
- OSA is associated with numerous morbidities.
- A simple approach to peri-operative care facilitates a smooth patient journey.

Further reading

American Society of Anesthesiologists. Practice guidelines for the perioperative management of patients with obstructive sleep apnea. *Anesthesiology*. 2014;**120**(2):268–86.

Douglas N. *Clinician's Guide To Sleep Medicine*. London: Arnold; 2002.

Downey R. Obstructive sleep apnea. 2017. http://emedicine.medscape.com/article/295807-overview (accessed April 2018).

Mokhlesi B. Obesity hypoventilation syndrome: a state-of-the-art review. *Respir Care*. 2010;**55**(10):1347–65.

Shneerson J. *Sleep Medicine*. Malden: Blackwell Publishing; 2005.

Drug Compartments and Body Systems

Christopher Hebbes and Jonathan Thompson

Pharmacokinetics

Body Composition in the Obese

Total body weight (TBW) comprises fat mass and lean mass (cell mass, extracellular water and non-fat connective tissue). In the non-obese adult, TBW is approximately 80% lean mass and 20% fat. The relative proportion of fat mass increases with obesity (Figure 9.1). Lean body weight (LBW) plateaus at around 100 kg. Therefore the overall LBW/TBW ratio is reduced due to the preferential increase in fat in the obese. At extremes of weight, LBW only accounts for 20–40% of the TBW. The high extracellular water content of fatty tissue leads to an overall increase in extracellular fluid volume, and therefore increased drug volume of distribution (V_D) as fatty mass increases, for both fat and water soluble drugs.

Increases in LBW correspond to increases in rates of drug metabolism, elimination, clearance and cardiac output. Increased cardiac output and tissue blood flow deliver greater amounts of drug to the liver and kidneys for metabolism and clearance.

The main values used for expressing weight (Table 9.1) are explained below. TBW is the mass as measured and can be divided into fat-free mass (or LBW) and fat mass. Subtracting the fat mass from TBW leaves mass due to lean tissues, the LBW. Ideal body weight (IBW) is the maximum weight for a given height and sex associated with the longest lifespan (based on insurance tables).

X-ray absorptiometry is the gold standard technique for measurement of lean mass, but is neither practical nor economical, and therefore calculated LBW is used in clinical practice. The relationships between lean mass, fat mass and water are often non-linear, and whilst TBW approximates LBW in the non-obese this is not true in the obese, requiring a surrogate variable for drug dosing (Table 9.1). Furthermore, most clinical and basic pharmacokinetic studies have studied non-obese patients; hence the calculations used to derive drug doses (such as LBW) are often invalid and inaccurate in the obese.

Adiposity is determined by individual characteristics and genetic variables. However, TBW, IBW and LBW are all derived from weight, height and sex. The use of derived measures based either on a correction factor applied to TBW, or values based on 'normal' population characteristics may therefore lead to inaccuracies in the obese. Allometric models, which account for body shape, size, metabolic rate and composition may reduce the inaccuracies of conventional variables such as TBW at extremes of weight. However, these models are complex and difficult to apply clinically.

Total Body Weight

TBW is readily obtainable, traditionally used to calculate drug dosage and straightforward to use. However, it does not take into account the pharmacokinetic effects of differences in lean and fat mass as TBW changes (Figure 9.1). Therefore, using TBW for drug dosing becomes inaccurate at high TBW, where TBW, IBW and LBW diverge (Figure 9.1). In those with a normal BMI, TBW approximates to LBW, although dosing by TBW may result in overdosing in the obese, particularly during repeated administration or infusion. In general, the use of TBW assumes equal drug distribution across all body compartments, which may be appropriate for a highly lipid soluble drug with a large volume of distribution, or where the clearance, metabolism or elimination are enhanced in obesity (such as for suxamethonium). However, the increase in body mass and particularly fat mass is offset by relatively poor perfusion to adipose tissue, therefore distribution is not always equal.

Lean Body Weight

LBW is TBW excluding fat mass. In clinical practice, it is calculated using a correction factor for TBW, as it is impractical to measure clinically. James' formula (Table 9.1) is a simple and straightforward calculation to derive LBW based on TBW, height and sex.

Table 9.1 Measures used in drug dosing

Marker	Derivation	Notes
Total body weight (TBW) (kg)	Measured weight, including lean and fatty tissues	Accurate, but does not take into account body composition. No correction for drug properties.
Ideal body weight (IBW) (kg)	Derived from height using formulae below Lemmens $IBW = 22 \times H_M^2$ Devine $IBW_{MALE} = 50 + (2.3 \times H_{I>60})$ $IBW_{FEMALE} = 45.5 + (2.3 \times H_{I>60})$ Robinson $IBW_{MALE} = 52 + (1.9 \times H_{I>60})$ $IBW_{FEMALE} = 49 + (1.7 \times H_{I>60})$ Miller $IBW_{MALE} = 56.2 + (1.41 \times H_{I>60})$ $IBW_{FEMALE} = 53.1 + (1.36 \times H_{I>60})$	Based on assumptions of an ideal weight for a given height, but does not take body composition into account. Therefore, as the obese patient, by definition, is of high body mass relative to their height, using IBW will underdose. No correction for drug properties.
Lean body weight (LBW)	Closely correlated with FFM, TBW − mass of adipose tissue. Derived based on TBW, sex and height James $LBW_{MALE} = (1.1 \times TBW) - 128 \times \left(\dfrac{TBW}{H_{CM}}\right)^2$ $LBW_{FEMALE} = (1.07 \times TBW) - 148 \times \left(\dfrac{TBW}{H_{CM}}\right)^2$ Janmahasatian $LBW_{MALE} = \dfrac{9270 \times TBW}{6680 + (216 \times BMI)}$ $LBW_{FEMALE} = \dfrac{9270 \times TBW}{8780 + (244 \times BMI)}$	Based on assumptions about changes in body composition; accurate at low mass (where LBM equates to TBW), inaccurate at extremes of weight. Linearly correlated with drug clearance and metabolism. Makes no correction for drug composition.
Adjusted body weight (ABW) (kg)	Based on TBW, fat composition and a drug-specific correction factor based on lipid solubility Servin's formula ABW = IBW + 0.4 × (TBW −IBW)	Adjusted body weight corrects the IBW for the additional fat weight, assuming a 40% increase in IBW. This is a recognised correction used in the dosing of propofol infusions.
Body mass index (BMI) (kg m^{-2})	Quetelet index $BMI = \dfrac{TBW}{H_M^2}$	Does not take body composition into account. An 'ideal' recommended BMI for men and women is 18.5–25
Body surface area (BSA) (m^2)	Mosteller $BSA = \sqrt{\dfrac{H_{CM} \times TBW}{3600}}$ DuBois $BSA = 0.007184 \times H_M^{0.725} \times TBW^{0.425}$	Used for the dosing of cytotoxic agents in chemotherapy. Does not take the role of sex in body composition into account.

Abbreviations: H_M – Height (m), H_{CM} – Height (cm), $H_{I>60}$ – Height (inches) over 60 inches, TBW – Total body weight (kg)

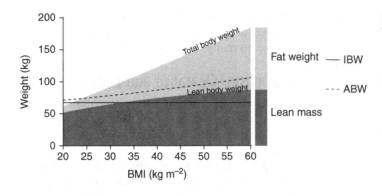

Figure 9.1 Relationship between BMI, LBW and TBW, based on a man 1.75 m tall.

Table 9.2 Changes in body composition in obesity

Variable	Changes in obesity	Significance
Extracellular fluid volume	Increased	Increased V_D for hydrophilic drugs
Cardiac output	Increased	Rapid distribution
Lean body mass	Increased	Increased metabolism relative to the non-obese
Fat mass	Increased	Increased compartmentalisation of lipophilic drugs

However, this has been shown to underestimate LBW in the obese. The Janmahasatian formula is more complex, but more accurate in obesity. LBW has traditionally been advocated for drug dosing in the obese, due to its close correlation with physiological properties such as cardiac output, and pharmacokinetic properties such as drug clearance.

Ideal Body Weight

IBW uses equations, initially derived from insurance company data relating life expectancy to height and sex. The formulae of Lemmens, Robinson, Miller and Devine (Table 9.1) are based on different datasets, although all are approximately equivalent and can be used interchangeably. As these calculations are based around a theoretical 'optimal' body composition for a given height and sex, they do not take into account individualised body composition, and may therefore underestimate TBW and LBW in the obese, leading to underdosing.

Adjusted Body Weight

ABW is used in drug dosing for the obese patient, and expands on IBW to include a metabolic contribution by fatty tissue (the product of TBW – IBW and a dose weight correction factor). The disadvantages of this approach are that it is drug-specific and requires individual pharmacokinetic studies of each drug in order to determine the appropriate correction factor to be used.

Body Surface Area

BSA is traditionally used in the dosing of chemotherapeutic agents. However, BSA does not correlate with pharmacokinetic variables, can be complicated to calculate, and is not widely used outside oncology.

In summary, a variety of measures are used in clinical practice for drug dosing by weight; LBW gives a measure of the metabolically active lean mass which correlates with drug clearance and may be useful for giving single boluses of drugs. However, it is difficult to calculate and the formulae can be inaccurate in obesity. The only clear recommendations are that there is no single perfect measure for dosing in the obese, and that drugs with a narrow therapeutic range should be monitored for toxicity, particularly for repeat dosing or infusions.

Compartment Models

Drug distribution is described using compartment models; with a central vascular compartment and several peripheral compartments comprising other body tissues responsible for metabolism, storage, distribution and elimination of drugs. Movement between compartments depends on the chemical properties of the drug (lipid solubility, pK_a, degree of ionisation, molecular mass and concentration gradient), as well as the compartment (vascularity, membrane surface area, membrane integrity and protein binding). These properties are affected by both obesity and its complications (see Table 9.2).

In obesity, there is an overall increase in TBW with a disproportionate increase in fatty mass. Total body water and particularly extracellular water increases representing greater circulating volume and interstitial fluid. In general, these changes promote an increased volume of distribution, clearance and a rapid offset due to drug redistribution.

Absorption and Bioavailability

Gastrointestinal absorption is unchanged in obesity. The limited data on bioavailability in obesity are conflicting, with both an increase and no significant change in bioavailability being reported. Any difference is likely to be insignificant – as exemplified by propanolol (bioavailability 35% (obese), 27% (non-obese)), and midazolam (bioavailability 42% (obese), 40% (non-obese)). Whilst gastric capacity is increased in obese patients, rapid gastric emptying times render this unimportant in practice.

Distribution

In general, the V_D of all drugs is increased to some degree in obesity, more significantly for lipophilic drugs. However, dosing based on TBW to account for this can result in overdosing, particularly if a drug is confined to the vascular compartment, as in the case of neuromuscular blocking drugs, which show increased duration of action when dosed by TBW. Therefore, for boluses, drugs should be dosed according to LBW, with the expectation that offset may be more rapid due to redistribution. Toxicity and accumulation may become significant for drugs given by intravenous infusion, or where repeat dosing is required. Continuous drug administration results in a relative increase in the reservoir of drug 'trapped' in a poorly perfused area, giving delayed clearance, and prolonged offset of effect, especially for lipid-soluble drugs. In general, drugs requiring repeat doses or infusions should be prescribed on the basis of LBW.

Drugs in the central compartment are in equilibrium between the free and protein-bound states. Protein binding and therefore free drug fraction itself is affected by obesity because total plasma protein content is increased. Drugs bound to albumin display similar kinetics in the obese and normal-weight individual. However, binding to α_1-acid glycoprotein is increased in the obese, although the effects of this are

unpredictable; studies have demonstrated a reduced free fraction of propranolol, increased free fraction of diazepam and no change in the free fraction of phenytoin.

Metabolism, Clearance and Elimination

Drug metabolism, clearance, and elimination are consistently increased in the obese because of increased cardiac output, splanchnic blood flow, renal filtration and LBW.

Hepatic metabolism is affected by obesity to a variable degree. The overall increased cardiac output increases hepatic blood flow. However, where obesity causes heart failure, or fatty liver, the effects of hepatic congestion reduce flow, reducing the metabolism of drugs with a flow-restricted metabolism. Studies of Phase 1 and Phase 2 metabolic pathways show conflicting results in the obese patient. Phase 1 reactions are responsible for the removal of functional groups, and may increase, decrease or show no change in obesity. Phase 2 reactions modify groups to enhance water solubility for elimination, and are increased in obesity. Non-alcoholic steatohepatitis (NASH) and non-alcoholic fatty liver disease (NAFLD) are common in obesity, and may also affect liver function.

There is conflicting evidence regarding renal clearance in obesity, which may increase, decrease, or remain unchanged.

Drug Handling in the Obese

Anaesthetic Induction Agents (and Target Controlled Infusions)

The drugs commonly used for induction of anaesthesia (propofol, sodium thiopentone, etomidate and ketamine) are all highly lipid soluble with a large V_D. The effects of obesity on the pharmacokinetics of these drugs are all similar. Onset of action depends on equilibration between ionised and unionised forms (pK_a), effect site and plasma (K_{eo}) and the V_D, lipid solubility and drug dose. The effects of obesity include increased V_D, cardiac output and renal clearance, and these combine to predict a higher dose in order to achieve a given effect site concentration, and therefore clinical effect.

Offset of effect of these agents is by redistribution of drug from the effect site, with subsequent renal or hepatic clearance from the central compartment. In the case of drug infusions, offset relates to context-sensitive half time and is dependent on duration of infusion and peripheral V_D. The increase in cardiac output seen in obese patients may lead to more rapid distribution and offset of action, and therefore rapid awakening (and concomitant risk of anaesthetic awareness).

Both propofol and thiopentone have a reduced duration of clinical effect in the obese following a bolus dose for induction of anaesthesia. However, the risk of cardiovascular compromise precipitated by TBW dosing favours the use of LBW for an initial dose with cautious titration to mitigate against this.

There are no specific pharmacokinetic data available for ketamine or etomidate in the obese. However, guided by the principles above, both risk accumulation with prolonged infusion (and rapid offset of a bolus dose due to redistribution) and should be dosed according to LBW and titrated to effect.

Target controlled infusions (TCI) use computer modelling to predict the distribution of a drug between body compartments. Drug-specific models are used, using TBW to estimate compartment size and therefore distribution. This approach can be inaccurate in obesity because of weight-related differences in compartments and the inability to measure and validate compartment concentrations *in vivo*.

Propofol may be delivered via TCI using the Marsh or Schnider models. The Marsh model estimates a larger central compartment than the Schnider model, delivering a higher bolus dose in order to achieve a given effect site concentration for a given TBW. For induction, in order to avoid the haemodynamic instability associated with large initial bolus drug doses, and as offset is largely governed by cardiac output and redistribution, LBW or ABW is preferred for dosing. Allometric models, based on body shape and size, correct for the proportion of fatty tissue and LBW, and may therefore be more accurate, although such models are not in current usage pending clinical validation. The Schnider model calculates LBW from input data, although this model will not permit a greater BMI than 42 for men or 37 for women, and is therefore not useful in the morbidly obese. This model is only recommended in effect site targeting mode, as the calculated drug boluses are small and have inadequate effect, which predisposes to awareness.

These challenges in anaesthetic dosing have led to recommendations that depth of anaesthesia monitoring is used for all patients undergoing TIVA. This is even more important in obesity.

Volatile Anaesthetic Agents

The volatile agents are lipophilic substances acting centrally for induction and maintenance of anaesthesia. They are sequestered in fat, requiring higher inhaled concentrations to maintain a constant minimum alveolar concentration (MAC). This can cause delayed recovery of consciousness in the obese, more markedly for longer exposures and more lipid-soluble agents. Therefore isoflurane and sevoflurane both take longer for recovery than desflurane. The inverse correlation between solubility and onset results in a rapid onset for nitrous oxide, as well as a slow on/offset for halothane and enflurane.

Specific Examples: Opioids

Most opioids in clinical use have relatively high lipid solubility and therefore high V_D, which is increased significantly in obesity. Combined with the pathophysiological changes in obesity, the risk of opioid sensitivity and obstructive sleep apnoea, these patients may require increased monitoring following opioid administration. In general, opioid doses are guided by LBW and titrated carefully.

Codeine and morphine can be associated with an increased incidence of adverse effects such as nausea, vomiting and respiratory depression in the obese. Codeine is metabolised to morphine by acetylation, a process unaffected by obesity. However, the pharmacodynamic concerns raised by the adverse effects of morphine and increased sensitivity have led to cautious prescribing in this population. As morphine has intermediate lipid solubility and V_D, its effects may be prolonged in the obese, but no specific pharmacokinetic data are available. However, it is reasonable to administer opioids in conventional doses according to LBW. Studies demonstrate no deleterious effects when PCA (patient-controlled analgesia) morphine is given in standard doses. There are significant inter-individual differences in opioid requirements, related to pharmacogenetics, drug tolerance, pain intensity, and psychological and physiological differences between individuals; these are probably more important than the effects of obesity per se. In the absence of more detailed studies, obese patients should be regularly assessed and their analgesia titrated with appropriate respiratory and cardiovascular monitoring.

Fentanyl has similar kinetic properties to propofol; the initial offset is governed by cardiac output and it has a high lipid solubility. There are limited

Table 9.3 Recommendations for dosing of drugs used in anaesthesia in the obese

Drug	Class	Dosing recommendations
Propofol (Bolus)	Induction agent	LBW
Propofol (TCI)	Induction agent	TBW
Thiopentone	Induction agent	LBW
Ketamine	Induction agent	LBW (no data – based on likely pharmacokinetics)
Etomidate	Induction agent	LBW (no data – based on likely pharmacokinetics)
Morphine	Opioid	LBW
Remifentanil TCI	Opioid	LBW
Suxamethonium	Neuromuscular blocker	TBW
Atracurium	Neuromuscular blocker	IBW
Rocuronium	Neuromuscular blocker	IBW
Sugammadex	Cyclodextran	TBW/ABW
Neostigmine/Glycopyrrolate	Reversal of neuromuscular blockade	TBW/ABW

pharmacokinetic studies of fentanyl in the obese; however, given its properties are related to clearance and cardiac output, both of which increase in line with LBW, this is recommended for use in single bolus dosing. None of the available pharmacokinetic models for fentanyl have been validated for use in morbid obesity, and may inaccurately predict plasma concentrations. Due to its high lipid solubility and large V_D, fentanyl accumulates after infusion or repeated bolus dosing, leading to a prolonged context-sensitive half time and delayed offset; this is expected to be greater in the obese, leading to delayed recovery.

Remifentanil has a small V_D and rapid clearance which are both unchanged in obesity, requiring dosing by LBW for bolus, and TCI (Minto) administration. However, the Minto equation used may underestimate LBW, causing underdosing.

Neuromuscular Blocking Drugs

Neuromuscular blocking drugs are highly polar, charged hydrophilic molecules, typically distributing to extracellular water. They have a characteristically small volume of distribution and are rapidly cleared. Aminosteroid drugs also undergo hepatic metabolism. The increased circulating volume and body water in the obese patient require an increased dose in order to achieve an effective clinical effect. Conventionally, these drugs are dosed according to LBW or IBW; studies have demonstrated a prolonged duration of effect when TBW is used.

Suxamethonium is a rapidly acting depolarising neuromuscular blocker with a fast onset and offset of action. Onset is governed by peak concentration, and offset by rapid metabolism by plasma cholinesterase, the concentrations of which are increased in obesity. Therefore, suxamethonium is dosed according to TBW to negate these changes, and provide optimal neuromuscular blockade without significant adverse effects.

Rocuronium is increasingly used for rapid sequence induction and situations where there may be airway difficulties, such as morbid obesity, because of its rapid onset of action, excellent intubation conditions, avoidance of the adverse effects of suxamethonium and the availability of sugammadex as a reversal agent. In patients with a significant incidence of obstructive apnoea, the availability of an agent to provide complete reversal and avoid postoperative narcosis from residual paralysis is attractive. Rocuronium is dosed based on LBW or IBW, as dosing based on ABW or TBW increases recovery times without any significant differences in onset. Rocuronium is metabolised in the liver, and this may explain the relatively prolonged duration when TBW is used in the obese.

Sugammadex is a cyclodextrin with a moderate volume of distribution used for reversal of rocuronium. When dosed using TBW, there is no clinically significant difference in time to recovery between obese and non-obese patients, suggesting that TBW should be used for dosing. The distribution profile of sugammadex includes the central vascular compartment and relatively little of the peripheral compartments. This profile would usually favour dosing based on LBW, supported by a lack of residual paralysis when IBW is used. However, where the risks of inadequate reversal outweigh those of sugammadex overdose, TBW is the most appropriate guide to dosing of sugammadex and other reversal agents such as neostigmine.

Conclusions

The pharmacokinetic changes in obesity are complex and varied, but follow general principles. A knowledge of the underlying pharmacokinetic principles enables safe and effective prescribing, but an individualised approach is required to dosing of drugs used in anaesthesia and critical care (Table 9.3). Drugs with a narrow therapeutic range pose a particular problem, as do target controlled infusions. Further research and validation of existing models in this patient group is required in order to tailor recommendations. However, for the majority of drugs, clearance and metabolism correlate to LBW, a general recommendation is that (with the exception of a few drugs discussed above), this should be used for dosing, and titrated to effect with cautious monitoring.

Further Reading

Andreasen PB, Dano P, Kirk H, Greisen G. Drug absorption and hepatic drug metabolism in patients with different types of intestinal shunt operation for obesity: a study with phenazone *Scand J Gastroenterol.* 1977;**5**:531–5.

Benedek IH, Blouin RA, McNamara PJ. Serum protein binding and the role of increased alpha 1-acid glycoprotein in moderately obese male subjects. *Br J Clin Pharmacol.* 1984;**6**:941–6.

Benedek IH, Fiske WD 3rd, Griffen WO, et al. Serum alpha 1-acid glycoprotein and the binding of drugs in obesity. *Br J Clin Pharmacol.* 1983;**6**:751–4.

Blouin RA, Warren GW. Pharmacokinetic considerations in obesity. *J Pharm Sci.* 1999;**1**:1–7.

Bowman SL, Hudson SA, Simpson G, Munro JF, Clements, JA. A comparison of the pharmacokinetics of propranolol in obese and normal volunteers *Br J Clin Pharmacol.* 1986;**5**:529–32.

Brill MJ, Diepstraten J, van Rongen A, et al. Impact of obesity on drug metabolism and elimination in adults and children *Clin Pharmacokinet.* 2012;**5**:277–304.

Brodsky JB, Lemmens HJ. *Anesthetic Management of the Obese Surgical Patient.* Cambridge: Cambridge University Press; 2011.

Carron M, Freo U, Parotto E, Ori C. The correct dosing regimen for sugammadex in morbidly obese patients. *Anaesthesia.* 2012;**3**:298–9.

Cortinez LI, Anderson BJ, Penna A, et al. Influence of obesity on propofol pharmacokinetics: derivation of a pharmacokinetic model. *Br J Anaesth.* 2010;**4**:448–56.

Cortinez LI, De la Fuente N, Eleveld DJ, et al. Performance of propofol target-controlled infusion models in the obese: pharmacokinetic and pharmacodynamic analysis. *Anesth Analg.* 2014;**2**:302–10.

Das SK, Roberts SB, McCrory MA, et al. Long-term changes in energy expenditure and body composition after massive weight loss induced by gastric bypass surgery. *Am J Clin Nutr.* 2003;**1**:22–30.

Ducharme MP, Slaughter RL, Edwards DJ. Vancomycin pharmacokinetics in a patient population: effect of age, gender, and body weight. *Ther Drug Monit.* 1994;**5**: 513–18.

DuBois D, DuBois EF. A formula to estimate the approximate surface area if height and weight be known. *Arch Int Med.* 1916;**17**:863–71.

Egan TD, Huizinga B, Gupta SK, et al. Remifentanil pharmacokinetics in obese versus lean patients. *Anesthesiology.* 1998;**3**:562–73.

Erstad BL, Patanwala AE. Ketamine for analgosedation in critically ill patients. J Crit Care. 2016:145–149.

Graves DA, Batenhorst RL, Bennett RL, et al. Morphine requirements using patient-controlled analgesia: influence of diurnal variation and morbid obesity. *Clin Pharm.* 1983;**1**:49–53.

Green B, Duffull SB. What is the best size descriptor to use for pharmacokinetic studies in the obese? *Br J Clin Pharmacol.* 2004;**2**:119–33.

Greenblatt DJ, Abernethy DR, Locniskar A, et al. Effect of age, gender, and obesity on midazolam kinetics. *Anesthesiology.* 1984;**1**:27–35.

Gurney H. Dose calculation of anticancer drugs: a review of the current practice and introduction of an alternative. *J Clin Oncol.* 1996;**9**:2590–611.

Han PY, Duffull SB, Kirkpatrick CM, Green B. Dosing in obesity: a simple solution to a big problem. *Clin Pharmacol Ther.* 2007;**5**:505–8.

Ingrande J, Brodsky JB, Lemmens HJ. Lean body weight scalar for the anesthetic induction dose of propofol in morbidly obese subjects. *Anesth Analg.* 2011;**1**:57–62.

Ingrande J, Lemmens HJ. Dose adjustment of anaesthetics in the morbidly obese. *Br J Anaesth.* 2010:i16–23.

James W. *Research on Obesity.* London: Her Majesty's Stationery Office; 1976.

Janmahasatian S, Duffull SB, Ash S et al. Quantification of lean bodyweight. *Clin Pharmacokinet.* 2005;**44**:1051–65

Juvin P, Vadam C, Malek L, et al. Postoperative recovery after desflurane, propofol, or isoflurane anesthesia among morbidly obese patients: a prospective, randomized study. *Anesth Analg*. 2000;3:714–19.

Keys A, Fidanza F, Karvonen MJ, Kimura N, Taylor HL. Indices of relative weight and obesity. *J Chronic Dis*. 1972;**25** (6–7):329–43.

Kirkegaard-Nielsen H, Helbo-Hansen HS, Lindholm P, Severinsen IK, Pedersen HS. Anthropometric variables as predictors for duration of action of atracurium-induced neuromuscular block. *Anesth Analg*. 1996;5:1076–80.

Kyle UG, Piccoli A, Pichard C. Body composition measurements: interpretation finally made easy for clinical use. *Curr Opin Clin Nutr Metab Care*. 2003;4:387–93.

La Colla L, Albertin A, La Colla G, et al. Predictive performance of the 'Minto' remifentanil pharmacokinetic parameter set in morbidly obese patients ensuing from a new method for calculating lean body mass. *Clin Pharmacokinet*. 2010;2:131–9.

Lemmens HJ, Brodsky JB. The dose of succinylcholine in morbid obesity. *Anesth Analg*. 2006;2:438–42.

Lemmens HJ, Brodsky JB, Bernstein DP. Estimating ideal body weight–a new formula. *Obes Surg*. 2005;5(7):1082–3.

Lemmens HJ, Saidman LJ, Eger EI, 2nd, Laster MJ. Obesity modestly affects inhaled anesthetic kinetics in humans. *Anesth Analg*.2008;6:1864–70.

Leykin Y, Pellis T, Lucca M, et al. The pharmacodynamic effects of rocuronium when dosed according to real body weight or ideal body weight in morbidly obese patients. *Anesth Analg*. 2004;4:1086–9.

Linares CL, Decleves X, Oppert JM, et al. Pharmacology of morphine in obese patients. *Clin Pharmacokinet*. 2009;10: 635–51.

Martinoli R, Mohamed EI, Maiolo C, et al. Total body water estimation using bioelectrical impedance: a meta-analysis of the data available in the literature. *Acta Diabetol*. 2003: S203–6.

McCarron MM, Devine BJ. Clinical pharmacy: case studies case number 25 gentamicin therapy. *Ann Pharmacother*. 1974;11:650–5.

McLeay SC, Morrish GA, Kirkpatrick CM, Green B. The relationship between drug clearance and body size: systematic review and meta-analysis of the literature published from 2000 to 2007. *Clin Pharmacokinet*. 2012;5:319–30.

Miller D, Carlson J, Loyd B, Day B. Determining ideal body weight (letter). *Am J Hosp Pharm*. 1983:1622.

Monk TG, Rietbergen H, Woo T, Fennema H. Use of sugammadex in patients with obesity: a pooled analysis. *Am J Thera*. 2015;24(5):e507–16.

Moore FD. Energy and the maintenance of the body cell mass. *J Parent Ent Nutr*. 1980;3:228–60.

Moretto M, Kupski C, Mottin CC, et al. Hepatic steatosis in patients undergoing bariatric surgery and its relationship to body mass index and co-morbidities. *Obes Surg*. 2003;4: 622–4.

Mosteller RD. Simplified calculation of body-surface area. *N Engl J Med*. 1987;17:1098.

Nightingale CE, Margarson MP, Shearer E, et al. Peri-operative management of the obese surgical patient 2015. *Anaesthesia*. 2015;7:859–76.

Pai MP, Paloucek FP. The origin of the 'ideal' body weight equations. *Ann Pharmacother*. 2000:1066–9.

Reiss RA, Haas CE, Karki SD, et al. Lithium pharmacokinetics in the obese. *Clin Pharmacol Ther*. 1994;4:392–8.

Robinson JD, Lupkiewicz SM, Palenik L, Lopez LM, Ariet M. Determination of ideal body weight for drug dosage calculations. *Am J Hosp Pharm*. 1983;6: 1016–19.

Rose DK, Cohen MM, Wigglesworth DF, DeBoer DP. Critical respiratory events in the postanesthesia care unit: patient, surgical, and anesthetic factors. *Anesthesiology*. 1994;2:410–18.

Sakizci-Uyar B, Celik S, Postaci A, et al. Comparison of the effect of rocuronium dosing based on corrected or lean body weight on rapid sequence induction and neuromuscular blockade duration in obese female patients *Saudi Med J*. 2016;1:60–5.

Schwartz AE, Matteo RS, Ornstein E, Halevy JD, Diaz J. Pharmacokinetics and pharmacodynamics of vecuronium in the obese surgical patient. *Anesth Analg*. 1992;4:515–18.

Servin F, Farinotti R, Haberer JP, Desmonts JM. Propofol infusion for maintenance of anesthesia in morbidly obese patients receiving nitrous oxide: a clinical and pharmacokinetic study. *Anesthesiology*. 1993;4:657–65.

Sharma V, McNeill JH. To scale or not to scale: the principles of dose extrapolation *Br J Pharmacol*. 2009;6: 907–21.

Shibutani K, Inchiosa MA, Jr, Sawada K, Bairamian M. Pharmacokinetic mass of fentanyl for postoperative analgesia in lean and obese patients. *Br J Anaesth*. 2005;3: 377–83.

Stokholm KH, Brochner-Mortensen J, Hoilund-Carlsen PF. Increased glomerular filtration rate and adrenocortical function in obese women. *Int J Obes*. 1980;1:57–63.

Strum EM, Szenohradszki J, Kaufman WA, et al. Emergence and recovery characteristics of desflurane versus sevoflurane in morbidly obese adult surgical patients: a prospective, randomized study. *Anesth Analg*. 2004;6: 1848–53.

Van Lancker P, Dillemans B, Bogaert T, et al. Ideal versus corrected body weight for dosage of sugammadex in morbidly obese patients. *Anaesthesia*. 2011;8:721–5.

WHO Expert Consultation. Appropriate body-mass index for Asian populations and its implications for policy and intervention strategies. *Lancet*. 2004;9403:157–63.

Chapter 10

Diabetes Mellitus and the Metabolic Syndrome

Hsiu L. Yap and Harvinder Chahal

Introduction

There has been a staggering rise worldwide in the number of people diagnosed with diabetes, especially type 2 diabetes mellitus (T2DM). In most instances, the diagnosis is related to obesity, which is in turn, connected to lifestyle factors such as diet and decreased activity levels. The 'obesity epidemic' is an immense problem on multiple levels, and essentially clarifies the extraordinary increase in the incidence and prevalence of type 2 diabetes over the past two decades. In England, the prevalence of obese adults has increased significantly between 1993 to 2012 from 13% to 24% for males, and 16% to 25% for females. Globally, it is also a mounting problem with tremendous socio-economic consequences. In 2008, the World Health Organization (WHO) estimated that 35% of the adult population worldwide was overweight and 12% obese. This equates to more than 1.4 billion overweight and approximately 500 million obese adults.

Obesity and Type 2 Diabetes Mellitus

Type 2 diabetes mellitus (T2DM) is typified by peripheral insulin resistance with or without atypical insulin production. T2DM usually presents later in adulthood, although it is currently presenting earlier in life due to increasing rates of obesity in the young. It can have devastating effects on other body systems, resulting in morbidity and mortality from cardiovascular and cerebrovascular events, diabetic retinopathy, nephropathy and neuropathy.

In obesity, genetic and lifestyle factors combine to form a state of surplus energy thereby producing additional adipose tissue. An individual is defined as overweight if their body mass index (BMI) ranges between 25 and 30 kg/m^2, and obese if their BMI is greater than 30 kg/m^2. Lower cut-off points for BMI apply to certain ethnic groups. The vast majority of patients with type 2 diabetes are overweight; however,

obese people largely do not acquire T2DM. There have been multiple studies recognising the complex relationships between T2DM and obesity. These include insulin resistance resulting from:

1. the release of non-esterified fatty acids creating a lipotoxic state;
2. adipokine or cytokine production causing an inflammatory reaction;
3. impairment in mitochondrial function;
4. ectopic fat deposition.

Adipose Tissue as an Endocrine Organ

Adipose tissue plays a large role in insulin sensitivity and is involved in endocrine, inflammatory, immune and neuronal pathways. Fat cells, or adipocytes collectively make up the largest endocrine organ in the body. They release various bioactive peptides (also known as adipokines), growth factors and proteohormones, which control energy homeostasis via complex interactions and pathways.

Visceral fat, which is fat padding the main organs in the intra-abdominal cavity, is dissimilar to the subcutaneous fat found underneath the skin and intramuscular fat. Although subcutaneous fat makes up more than 80% of body fat, visceral fat carries more metabolic significance, and is associated with a greater risk of insulin resistance, type 2 diabetes, metabolic syndrome and cardiovascular disease. Consequently, adipose tissue may be viewed as an organ with different endocrine and metabolic functions, depending on its type and/or location in the body.

Adipose tissue is also the location of glucocorticoid regulation. Biologically inactive cortisone is converted to active cortisol by the action of 11-beta-hydroxysteroid dehydrogenase type 1 (11βHSD-1) enzyme, which is expressed in fundamental metabolic organs like adipose tissue (particularly visceral fat) and the liver. Preventing 11βHSD-1 enzyme action has been shown to improve insulin sensitivity, paving

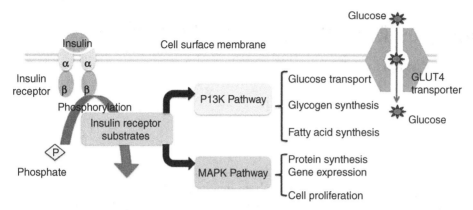

Figure 10.1 Insulin receptor signalling and effects on glucose metabolism.

the way for further work into developing therapeutic interventions for insulin resistance and obesity.

The Insulin Receptor and its Signalling Pathways

To understand insulin resistance in obesity, we should have a basic appreciation of how the insulin receptor works (Figure 10.1). The insulin receptor is a tyrosine kinase receptor, which, when activated, phosphorylates (addition of a phosphate group) insulin receptor substrates 1 and 2 (IRS-1, IRS-2). Consequently, this triggers the activation of the mitogen-activated protein kinase (MAPK) and phosphatidylinositol-3′-kinase (PI3 K) signalling pathways. The MAPK pathway regulates cell proliferation and gene expression, and the PI3 K pathway is responsible for glucose metabolism, as well as glycogen, fatty acid and protein synthesis. Through the phosphorylation cascades in the PI3 K pathway, the glucose transporter GLUT-4 migrates to the cell surface membrane and mediates influx of glucose into cells.

Fatty Acids and Lipotoxicity

Circulating triglycerides derived from diet and very low-density lipoproteins (VLDL) are converted by lipoprotein lipase (secreted by adipocytes) into fatty acids. Fatty acids are stored as triacylglycerol deposits within fat cells.

Constant overload of nutrients and a state of surplus energy raises triglyceride levels. Excess adipose tissue induces intra-cellular lipolysis and release of more fatty acids into the bloodstream, which are then oxidised and utilised by the liver and muscle

for energy and gluconeogenesis. Fatty acid metabolites impede insulin receptor signalling by blocking phosphorylation of insulin receptor substrates and activation of the PI3 K pathway, subsequently enhancing gluconeogenesis. Meanwhile, lipogenesis is inhibited as the extra free fatty acids obstruct breakdown of serum triacylglycerol concentrations. These dysfunctional changes in the fatty acid cycle ultimately result in insulin resistance and elevated glucose levels (Figure 10.2).

The increase in free fatty acid and metabolite levels in the circulation provokes cell oxidative stress and a lipotoxic state. The endoplasmic reticulum and mitochondria are mainly affected, in various organs throughout the body. Lipotoxicity hinders the action of GLUT-4 glucose transporters, reducing glucose movement into the cell. Lipotoxicity also affects the secretion of insulin from the beta-cells of the pancreas, leading to cell fatigue and insulin insuffiency.

Adipokines in Inflammation and Insulin Resistance

It is now understood that obesity is a chronic state of inflammation (Figure 10.3). Enlarging adipose tissue releases inflammatory cytokines, namely interleukin-6 (IL-6) and tumour necrosis factor alpha (TNF-α). TNF-α hinders phosphorylation of the insulin receptor and its substrate IRS-1, in turn hampering post-receptor signalling. This ultimately results in insulin resistance. TNF-α and IL-6 decrease the action of lipoprotein lipase (LPL), stimulates lipolysis within the cell, and leads to higher levels of fatty acids in the circulation.

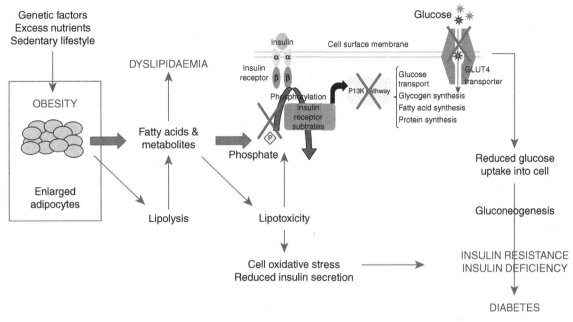

Figure 10.2 Increase in fatty acids leading to a lipotoxic state and insulin resistance.

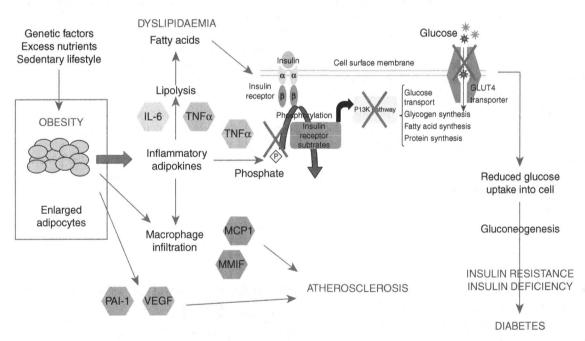

Figure 10.3 Inflammatory adipokines and their role in insulin resistance.

Adipocytes promote secretion of monocyte chemoattractant protein (MCP-1), as well as macrophage migration inhibiting factor (MMIF) from macrophages, which contributes to ongoing inflammation. The MAPK pathway is also activated, subsequently impeding glucose transporter action and causing insulin resistance and hyperglycaemia. In addition, there is upregulation of other pro-inflammatory and acute phase markers such as CRP and alpha-1 acid glycoprotein.

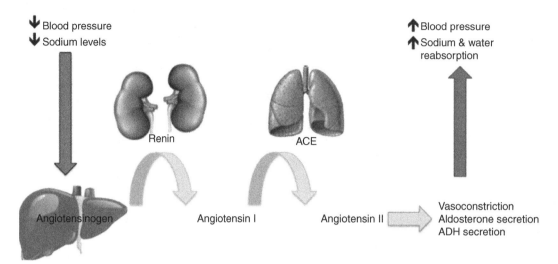

Figure 10.4 The renin–angiotensin system.

This state of inflammation also enables atherosclerosis. Fat cells produce vasoactive endothelial growth factor (VEGF), plasminogen activator inhibitor 1 (PAI-1) and metalloproteinases, leading to endothelial damage, collagen remodelling and plaque formation. As the damage develops, macrophages add to atherogenesis through release of MCP-1, MMIF and endothelin-1. Inflammatory adipokines (IL-6) that inhibit lipolysis further exacerbate hypertriglyceridaemia, and procoagulant adipokines (IL-6, PAI-1, TNFα, tumour growth factor β) contribute to ongoing plaque formation and eventual rupture.

Adipocytes also release anti-inflammatory adipokines (adiponectin, leptin, visfatin) to protect against continuing inflammation and improve insulin sensitivity. However, levels of adiponectin decline with advancing obesity and is likely a factor in growing insulin resistance.

Other Relevant Adipokines

Fat cells also produce a whole variety of other adipokines such as retinol binding protein 4 (RBP4), leptin, and adiponectin.

RBP4 is responsible for the transport of retinol, or vitamin A. Higher concentrations of the binding protein are seen in obesity, with hyperglycaemia resulting from reduced glucose uptake in muscle and accelerated hepatic gluconeogenesis via a retinol-dependent pathway.

Leptin is chiefly produced by adipose tissue, but also produced elsewhere in the body (stomach, bone marrow). It is thought to activate adenosine monophosphate kinase (AMPK) pathways to heighten insulin sensitivity, but conversely has inflammatory effects elsewhere. It also has a role in the oxidation of fatty acids. Its endocrine effects include central regulation of appetite by inducing satiety. Even though higher levels of circulating leptin are found in obese people, there is leptin resistance and subsequent inability to curb hunger and weight gain.

Adiponectin receptors are found in the pancreatic islet cells, muscle and liver, and participate in insulin signalling, fatty acid oxidation and glucose uptake. As stated previously, adiponectin has anti-inflammatory actions, but it also protects against atherosclerosis by increasing nitric oxide levels and enhancing vasodilation.

Mitochondrial Function and Increased Oxidative Stress

Metabolism of glucose and lipids relies on cell mitochondria to produce energy, with adenosine triphosphate (ATP) being the main energy 'currency'. Studies have shown mitochondrial dysfunction in type 2 diabetes, insulin resistance and obesity. Elevated concentrations of fatty acids and glucose leads to generation of reactive oxygen species (ROS) and diminishing ATP production. ROS cause lower

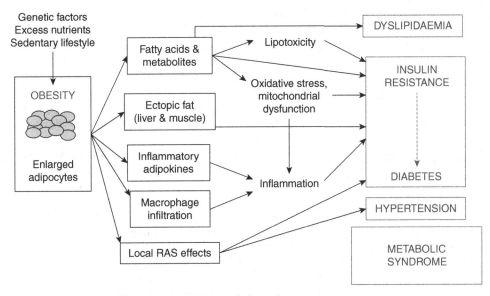

Figure 10.5 Obesity, insulin resistance and the metabolic syndrome.

quantities and smaller-sized mitochondria, which therefore possess reduced mitochondrial oxidative capacity. These disturbances in mitochondrial form and function lead to build-up of fatty acid metabolites, stimulation of inflammatory adipokines and generation of more ROS, creating a vicious cycle.

ROS is understood to encourage phosphorylation of IRS-1 and IRS-2, and reduce the activity of the PI3 K insulin signalling pathway, thereby interfering with intra-cellular glucose uptake and reducing insulin sensitivity. In summary, impairment in mitochondrial function is frequently correlated with insulin resistance, and the pathogenesis of obesity, type 2 diabetes and fatty liver disease.

Adipokines and the Renin–Angiotensin System in Obesity

The renin–angiotensin system (RAS) has a chief role in the regulation of systemic arterial blood pressure, as well as salt and water balance (Figure 10.4). Changes in blood volume or blood pressure are detected by baroreceptors in the carotid sinus, which triggers conversion of angiotensinogen to angiotensin I by the enzyme renin. Angiotensin I is then converted to angiotensin II by angiotensin-converting enzyme (ACE). Angiotensin II is the major mediator of arteriole vasoconstriction, aldosterone secretion from the adrenal glands, anti-diuretic hormone (ADH) secretion from the posterior pituitary gland, and sodium

reabsorption and water retention in the kidneys. With regards to metabolic effects, angiotensin II also increases gluconeogenesis in the liver, reduces lipolysis and has effects on adipocyte development. The RAS influences insulin signalling pathways and endothelial function, leading to cardiovascular disease.

It is also known that RAS has local effects on organs such as the myocardium, kidneys and adrenals. There is growing evidence that adipose tissue also has a local RAS. Adipose tissue has been found to secrete angiotensinogen, angiotensin I and II, and ACE. Adipose tissue expresses angiotensin receptors, particularly in visceral fat versus subcutaneous fat. Activity of RAS components is higher in obese people and mice models have demonstrated that overexpression of angiotensinogen in fat is linked to hypertension and obesity. Thus, local RAS elements in fat tissue may have important roles in the pathophysiology of insulin resistance, diabetes and obesity in humans, although further research is ongoing.

Ectopic Fat Deposition

Ectopic fat found in the liver, skeletal muscle and the beta cells of the pancreas has been significantly linked to insulin resistance. The degree of ectopic fat in these areas has a positive correlation with the extent of insulin resistance. Patients with lipodystrophy have abnormal lipid accumulation in the liver, muscle and pancreatic beta cells, leading to insulin resistance and diabetes. Obese patients share this feature, having enlarged adipocytes that predispose to ectopic fat deposition.

Reversal of ectopic fat deposition in muscle and liver through weight loss interventions has been shown to normalize triglyceride and glucose levels, subsequently stabilising insulin sensitivity.

Metabolic Syndrome and Obesity

To fulfil the criteria of having metabolic syndrome, the individual should possess three of five risk factors – central adiposity, hypertension, elevated triglyceride, low high-density lipoprotein (HDL) levels and raised fasting glucose. Central obesity is measured by waist circumference, with the WHO advising cut off points of more than 102 cm in men and more than 88 cm in women. These thresholds are lower for the Asian population, being more than 90 cm and 80 cm, respectively. Indeed, waist circumference measurements should be adjusted for different ethnic populations.

You will have noticed that the concepts discussed earlier regarding obesity and its links to insulin resistance are essentially the components making up the metabolic syndrome (Figure 10.5). Besides local RAS in adipose tissue in obese patients contributing to hypertension, other likely mechanisms are increased sympathetic activity and ROS reducing nitric oxide levels leading to elevated vascular tone. This is a syndrome that merits greater awareness, as patients have double the risk of cardiovascular disease and an astonishing fivefold increase of developing type 2 diabetes. It is very much a disease of our modern times, but fundamentally reversible with lifestyle interventions.

Conclusion

There are several mechanisms linking obesity to the development of insulin resistance and diabetes. The production of fatty acids and metabolites, an inflammatory state created by adipokines and macrophages, oxidative stress and changes in mitochondrial function, and local RAS effects from adipose tissue all combine to form a potent mix of dyslipidaemia, insulin insensitivity and hypertension – all features of metabolic syndrome.

Further Reading

Alberti KG, Eckel RH, Grundy SM, et al. Harmonizing the metabolic syndrome: a joint interim statement. *Circulation*. 2009;**120**(16):1640–5.

Berg AH, Scherer PE. Adipose tissue, inflammation, and cardiovascular disease. *Circul Res*. 2005;**96**(9):939–49.

Brownlee M. The pathobiology of diabetic complications: a unifying mechanism. *Diabetes*. 2005;**54**(6):1615–25.

Cooper SA, Whaley-Connell A, Habibi J, et al. Renin-angiotensin-aldosterone system and oxidative stress in cardiovascular insulin resistance. *Am J Physiol Heart Circul Physiol*. 2007;**293**(4):2009–23.

Dandona P, Aljada A, Chaudhuri A, Mohanty P, Garg R. Metabolic syndrome: a comprehensive perspective based on interactions between obesity, diabetes, and inflammation. *Circulation*. 2005;**111**(11):1448–54.

Day C, Bailey CJ. Obesity in the pathogenesis of type 2 diabetes. *Br J Diabetes Vasc Dis*. 2011;**11**(2):55–61.

Després JP, Lemieux I. Abdominal obesity and metabolic syndrome. *Nature*. 2006;**444**(7121):881–7.

Hajer GR, van Haeften TW, Visseren FL. Adipose tissue dysfunction in obesity, diabetes, and vascular diseases. *Eur Heart J*. 2008;**29**(24):2959–71.

Kahn SE, Hull RL, Utzschneider KM. Mechanisms linking obesity to insulin resistance and type 2 diabetes. *Nature*. 2006;**444**(7121):840–6.

Kershaw EE, Flier JS. Adipose tissue as an endocrine organ. *J Clin Endocrinol Metab*. 2004;**89**(6):2548–56.

Petersen KF, Shulman GI. Etiology of insulin resistance. *Am J Med*. 2006;**119**(5 Suppl 1): S10–S16.

Qatanani M, Lazar MA. Mechanisms of obesity-associated insulin resistance: many choices on the menu. *Genes Develop*. 2007;**21**(12):1443–55.

Redinger RN. The pathophysiology of obesity and its clinical manifestations. *Gastroenterol Hepatol*. 2007;**3**(11): 856–63.

Shoelson SE, Lee J, Goldfine AB. Inflammation and insulin resistance. *J Clin Invest*. 2006;**116**(7):1793–801.

Unger RH. Lipotoxicity in the pathogenesis of obesity-dependent NIDDM: genetic and clinical implications. *Diabetes*. 1995;**44**(8):863–70.

Airway Assessment in Obesity

Naveen Eipe and Adele S. Budiansky

Introduction

In the general population, morbid obesity (MO) has been frequently identified as a risk factor for challenges in airway management. The increasing global prevalence of obesity coupled with the widespread use of weight loss (bariatric) surgery as a treatment option has given investigators the opportunity to study large cohorts of patients with MO undergoing elective surgery. These and other studies have identified clinical features that would more accurately predict difficult airways (DAs) and develop appropriate management strategies.

The dual emphasis in anaesthetic management in MO was to secure the potentially DA while minimising patient oxyhaemoglobin desaturation. Traditionally, these goals were facilitated by either a technique of rapid sequence induction-intubation (RSII) or awake fibreoptic intubations (AFOI). Over the past decade, the introduction of innovative drugs and the use of video laryngoscopy have resulted in a paradigm shift to many conventional DA practices and algorithms.

While the circumstances and needs of airway management will vary widely, depending on the patient, practitioner and procedure, this chapter will focus mainly on assessment for tracheal intubation as the primary goal of airway management of patients with MO.

Predicting Difficult Airways in Morbid Obesity

BMI and Distribution

The UK 4th National Audit Project (NAP4) report stated that though the proportion of primary airway problems related to tracheal intubation was similar in MO and non-obese patients, patients with MO represented 42% of the major airway management complication cases. These findings suggest that either the airway management of patients with MO did not

follow established DA guidelines or that more MO-specific DA guidelines are needed. Prior to the NAP4 report, it was well established that MO was a risk factor for DA. Indeed, multiple previous studies have reported that when compared to lean patients, facemask ventilation and tracheal intubation are both significantly more difficult in MO and the difficulty encountered increases with increasing BMI. Contradicting these are other studies reporting that BMI itself is a weak predictor for difficulty in airway management. These conflicting findings must also be taken in the context that widely variable and often inconsistent definitions of DA were used.

Clearly, BMI alone cannot predict DA and other MO-related factors should be sought. Looking beyond BMI, bariatric anaesthesia experts have emphasised the importance of distribution of the excessive body mass as a predictor of peri-operative outcomes in MO. It is recommended that the pattern of distribution of the excessive weight in MO is objectively measured by comparing the waist circumference (WC) to the height of the patient. When the WC exceeds half the height, the distribution is more 'central' or 'android'. This distribution is already well described to be associated with difficulty in securing the airway, ventilation, metabolic syndrome, OSA and increased peri-operative morbidity. The opposite 'peripheral' or 'gynaecoid' pattern of MO (where the WC is less than half the height) is much less likely to be associated with DA and other negative peri-operative outcomes. In patients with MO, it is therefore important for future research to address the pattern of excessive fat distribution, as this may well explain the previous studies failure of BMI alone in predicting DA.

Age

As patients with MO get older, apart from age-related changes to their airway anatomy, their co-morbidity burden increases and their cardiorespiratory reserve diminishes. These age-related anatomical and physiological changes may also be disproportionately accelerated in patients with MO when compared to their non-obese counterparts. Almost in conflict with increasing weight, increasing age decreases the pharmacological choices and the doses that can be safely administered during anesthetic induction. All these implicate age as an almost greater peri-operative risk factor that MO (measured by BMI). Nevertheless, in this population with MO, age, even over a modest 40 years, has been identified as a significant independent risk factor for DA. This is further supported by the observation of significant difference in the age of patients with MO having uneventful intubation, difficult intubation and those planned for fiberoptic intubation. Other studies have also confirmed that with increasing age both difficulty with face mask ventilation and worse direct laryngoscopy views will be encountered. Indeed, as described elsewhere in this book, age and BMI (either or both >50) are the major diagnostic criteria for OSA and other peri-operative MO risk scores. In our opinion (unpublished observation), when the sum of the age and BMI exceeds 100, difficulty in airway management and other peri-operative risk increases considerably.

Gender

As described in the preceding section, the distribution of excessive fat, expectedly so, causes the central pattern of obesity in male patients with MO to be an independent predictor of difficult facemask ventilation. This difficulty can be up to 8.5 times higher in males compared to females. Attributed also to the deposition of fat tissue in the upper airway, men undergoing bariatric surgery are also more likely to present with difficulty in both laryngoscopy and tracheal intubation. It is also reasonable to advise men with MO who sport large beards (itself an independent risk factor for difficult face mask ventilation) to become clean shaven before elective surgery, as is advised in many bariatric surgery programmes. Despite these, the male gender remains an important risk factor for DA that needs to be taken into consideration together with the BMI, distribution and age of the patient with MO.

Obstructive Sleep Apnea

OSA is an important co-morbidity seen in patients with MO. Interestingly, OSA has also been previously identified as a risk factor for both difficult facemask ventilation and difficult intubation. MO patients with a confirmed diagnosis of OSA and patients with high screening test scores are also known to be significantly more difficult to ventilate with a facemask when compared to non-OSA patients, irrespective of the administration of neuromuscular blockade. The presence of OSA is also an independent predictor of difficult intubation in MO, both in the operating theatre and in the ICU. As is the case for BMI, studies of OSA as an independent DA predictor have produced conflicting results – some studies fail to find an association. It is therefore likely that in patients with MO who have OSA, additional factors are needed to predict DA. These include severity, treatment with positive pressure therapy (CPAP or BiPAP (bilevel positive airway pressure)) adequacy and compliance with prescribed treatment. In our opinion and experience, difficulty in facemask ventilation frequently observed in patients with MO who have OSA can be correlated with the positive pressure settings. Though this has been previously suggested, further investigation is required. Additionally, it is also important to note that the 'obstructive' component in OSA is not always overcome or bypassed by oropharyngeal or nasopharyngeal airways, as the deposition of soft tissues can extend into the peri-laryngeal space.

Mallampati Score

Amongst the specific airway examination findings, the Mallampati score is a well-established measure of available space in the upper airway relative to the MO-related oropharyngeal soft tissue mass. This explains why it is the most consistent DA test reported in multiple studies of patients with MO. Mallampati scores >2 have been identified as independent predictors of difficult face mask ventilation and intubation.

Neck Circumference

With its origins in the contributory pathophysiology of OSA, increasing neck circumference (of greater than 40 cm) has been described as a significant predictor of difficult facemask ventilation. Neck circumference has also been proposed as a predictor of difficult tracheal intubation due to increased anterior neck soft tissue. However, more recent use of ultrasound imaging of the neck in MO suggests that increased neck circumference does not necessarily predict soft tissue deposition at the level of the

Table 11.1 List of predictors of difficult airway in patients with morbid obesity

	0	1	2
Age	<40	40–60	>60
Sex		Women	Men
Habitus		Waist <½ height	Waist >½ height
OSA	Absent	CPAP 5–15 cmH$_2$0	CPAP>15 cmH$_2$0
BMI	<40	40–60	>60
Neck circumference (cm)	<40	40–60	>60
Mallampati score		I, II	III, IV
ULBT		I	II, III

The sum of scores (0–2) from each predictor suggested here can be used to create a range of scores with increasing difficulty. Total scores predict increasing difficulty (<5 = low, 5–10 = moderate to serious difficulty and >10 = considerably serious difficulty) and can be used to direct appropriate management strategies.

vocal cords. Nevertheless, there is a clear association between increased neck circumference, worse laryngoscopy views and difficult intubation in patients with MO. In their landmark study, Brodsky and colleagues found that neck circumference was the only significant predictor of difficult intubation. They also suggest that the probability of difficult intubation progressively increased with neck circumference at or beyond 60 cm. It is also probably worthwhile to note that increased neck circumference is also one of the diagnostic criteria for OSA.

Upper Lip Bite Test

The upper lip bite test (ULBT) is a simple test that provides an objective assessment of the anatomy of the lower jaw, its mobility and protrusion, and also assesses the submandibular space. In patients with MO, this test may offer important information with regards to space available for the caudad displacement of the tongue, which improves laryngeal visualisation on direct laryngoscopy. Even though the role of ULBT has not been specifically tested in patients with MO, restricted jaw mobility was found to be an independent predictor of difficult tracheal intubation in patients undergoing bariatric surgery.

We have summarised the predictors of DA in patients with MO based on the available evidence discussed in Table 11.1. Taking into consideration the multifactorial aetiology of predicting DA in patients with MO, further investigation and validation will be required.

Conclusion

As obesity continues to increase globally, patients with morbid obesity will continue to frequently present for elective and emergency procedures where they require airway management. We need to carefully predict DAs in these patients and manage them appropriately.

Further Reading

Brodsky JB, Lemmens HJ, Brock-Utne JG, et al. Morbid obesity and tracheal intubation. *Anesth Analg.* 2002;**94**: 732–6.

Cook TM, Woodall N, Frerk C, et al.; Fourth National Audit Project. Major complications of airway management in the UK: results of the Fourth National Audit Project of the Royal College of Anaesthetists and the Difficult Airway Society. Part 1: anaesthesia. *Br J Anaesth.* 2011;**106**:617–31.

De Jong A, Molinari N, Pouzeratte Y, et al. Difficult intubation in obese patients: incidence, risk factors, and complications in the operating theatre and in intensive care units. *Br J Anaesth.* 2015;**114**:297–306.

Kheterpal S, Healy D, Aziz MF, et al. Incidence, predictors, and outcome of difficult mask ventilation combined with difficult laryngoscopy: a report from the multicenter perioperative outcomes group. *Anesthesiology.* 2013;**119**: 1360–9.

Kim WH, Ahn HJ, Lee CJ, et al. Neck circumference to thyromental distance ratio: a new predictor of difficult intubation in obese patients. *Br J Anaesth.* 2011;**106**:743–8.

Lavi R, Segal D, Ziser A. Predicting difficult airways using the intubation difficulty scale: a study comparing obese and non-obese patients. *J Clin Anesth.* 2009;**21**:264–7.

Law JA, Broemling N, Cooper RM, et al. The difficult airway with recommendations for management–part 2–the anticipated difficult airway. *Can J Anaesth*. 2013;**60**:1119–38.

Leoni A, Arlati S, Ghisi D, et al. Difficult mask ventilation in obese patients: analysis of predictive factors. *Minerva Anestesiol*. 2014;**80**:149–57.

Lundstrom LH, Møller AM, Rosenstock C, et al. High body mass index is a weak predictor for difficult and failed tracheal intubation: a cohort study of 91,332 consecutive patients scheduled for direct laryngoscopy registered in the Danish Anesthesia Database. *Anesthesiology*. 2009;**110**:266–74.

Gonzalez H, Minville V, Delanoue K, et al. The importance of increased neck circumference to intubation difficulties in obese patients. *Anesth Analg*. 2008;**106**:1132–6.

Shailaja S, Nichelle SM, Shetty AK, Hegde BR. Comparing ease of intubation in obese and lean patients using intubation difficulty scale. *Anesth Essays Res*. 2014;**8**:168–74.

Riad W, Vaez MN, Raveendran R, et al. Neck circumference as a predictor of difficult intubation and difficult mask ventilation in morbidly obese patients: a prospective observational study. *Eur J Anaesthesiol*. 2016;**33**:244–9.

Sheff SR, May MC, Carlisle SE, et al. Predictors of a difficult intubation in the bariatric patient: does preoperative body mass index matter? *Surg Obes Related Dis*. 2013;**9**:344–9.

Siriussawakul A, Limpawattana P. A validation study of the intubation difficulty scale for obese patients. *J Clin Anesth*. 2016;**33**: 86–91.

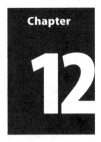

Respiratory Assessment in Obesity

Nick Reynolds and Christopher Bouch

Introduction

The majority of morbidly obese patients presenting for surgery will complain of breathlessness. This may be associated with a level of activity considered normal for a lean individual to the other end of the spectrum; breathlessness at rest or with very minimal exertion. The difficulty in assessment lies in delineating the extent of the symptoms, the degree of contributing co-morbid disease and from this provide an indication of how to optimise or improve the symptoms and function.

Respiratory system assessment of the obese is important. Sleep disordered breathing is common but so are asthma and chronic obstructive pulmonary disease (COPD). One must remember that the cardiovascular system is intimately associated with the respiratory system and disorders such as cardiac failure and pulmonary hypertension will have respiratory effects.

Dyspnoea is not a diagnosis but a symptom with a myriad of potential aetiologies and no fixed definition. There is rarely a neat relationship of a single contributing factor causing symptoms in a patient. Contributors to perception of breathlessness may be physiological or pathophysiological, and related to the excess fat deposition and/or associated pathology. Classically, obese patients are considered to have much higher risk and prevalence of cardiac and respiratory disease compared to ideal weight counterparts.

For any obese patient, a full history and examination should be undertaken prior to investigation. Should this reveal disease then referral to a respiratory physician is essential.

Epidemiological Risk and Prevalence of Respiratory Conditions

Sleep disordered breathing is by far the commonest respiratory condition present in obese individuals. Up to 70% of obese individuals may have this disorder, the majority undiagnosed when presenting to medical care.

Asthma and COPD are also frequently diagnosed. It is accepted that there is an overlap in the diagnostic spectrums of these conditions. The pathophysiological effects of obesity can mimic and amplify underlying symptoms and cloud diagnostic clarity. Animal models and human laboratory trials of respiratory disease suggest that dysregulated adipose tissue with release of adipokines produces a pro-inflammatory milieu for exaggerated airway inflammation and hyper-reactivity. Literature demonstrates that this airway narrowing and resultant symptoms worsen with increasing BMI.

An obese patient is around 1.5 to 3.5 times more likely to have a diagnosis of asthma compared with a normal weight individual, with a much stronger association in females.

Unfortunately, many investigations of asthma do not use consistent definitions. Reliance of self-reported symptoms may result in this increased incidence being observed.

The relationship between COPD and obesity is even less clear. Studies suggest that there is a higher prevalence in higher BMI patients and when waist measurement criteria, not BMI, are used, the incidence of diagnosed chronic respiratory disease doubles in the obese group. COPD associated with obesity is more likely to present as chronic bronchitis rather than emphysema.

Clinical Assessment

History

About 40% of bariatric patients will report breathlessness on questioning, with symptoms known to increase with increasing adipocyte load. It is essential to expand on the associations of breathlessness; is this cardiac in origin, functional limitations and progression over time.

Table 12.1 Medical Research Council (MRC) dyspnoea scale

Grade	Degree of breathlessness related to activities
1	Not troubled by breathlessness except on strenuous exercise
2	Short of breath when hurrying or walking up a slight hill
3	Walks slower than contemporaries on level ground because of breathlessness, or has to stop for breath when walking at own pace
4	Stops for breath after walking about 100 m or after a few minutes on level ground
5	Too breathless to leave the house, or breathless when dressing or undressing

Used with the permission of the Medical Research Council.

Table 12.2 Metabolic equivalent

MET	Activity
1	Can take care of self (e.g. eat, dress, use toilet)
4	Can walk up a flight of steps or a hill or a hill or walk on level ground at 3–4 miles/hour
4–10	Can do heavy work around the house (e.g. scrubbing floors, or moving heavy furniture)
>10	Can participate in strenuous sports such (e.g. swimming, singles tennis, football, basketball, skiing)

The MRC dyspnea scale (Table 12.1) is a five-point scale that quantifies the clinical grade of breathlessness, originally devised for research in COPD patients. However, it is a useful tool to document dyspnoea as part of pre-assessment.

Assessment of functional capacity via metabolic equivalents (METs) (Table 12.2), is of value. Inability to climb a flight of stairs (4 METs) implies significant impairment of cardiorespiratory functional status and increased post-operative complications. One MET is equivalent to 3.5 ml oxygen uptake/kg/min at rest. It is important to be aware of the limitation to MET. It was devised from physiological measurements obtained in a healthy, ideal body weight individual. Increased fat and fat-free mass will impact on the oxygen consumption. However, as an easy assessment tool it is useful.

Cigarette smoking is a major contributor to development of both cardiovascular and respiratory disease. There is overwhelming evidence of an increased incidence of post-operative complications in smokers. In obesity, cigarette smoking is an easily identifiable risk factor and direct questioning must take place. A minimum of 8 weeks smoking cessation must be enforced prior to any surgical procedure to facilitate a reduction in respiratory complications.

It is vital to screen for the presence of sleep disordered breathing using the STOP-BANG questionnaire.

Clinical Examination

The presence of oedema, cyanosis, inability to speak in sentences and use of accessory muscles should be noted. Auscultation and percussion can be faint and indistinct. This also applies to both cardiac and blood pressure auscultation through increased subcutaneous tissue depth due to fat.

Increased tissue depth may not always represent adiposity. Lymphoedema is a very common finding; occurring in up to 75% of individuals with a BMI of 40 or more, compared with around 1 in 10 of normal weight individuals.

Sarcopenic obesity is an important risk factor for development of post-operative complications and mortality. Defining the presence of this condition, which is increasingly recognised, is vital. However, that is easier said than done. With increasing obesity and age there is loss of muscle mass. Although BMI as a simple measure of obesity may remain constant, lean mass reduces. This is due to the complex interplay of adipokines and the inflammatory state produced by obesity. The result is an older individual with poor exercise tolerance and reduced muscle mass. CT scans and complex X-ray imagery can identify this condition. However, assessment of handgrip strength, knee flexion and extension, combined with slow gait and poor performance will assist identification.

Investigations

There are many ways in which to investigate the respiratory system. The decision on which test is best should be determined by signs and symptoms revealed as part of the history and examination. Routine investigation requests are never of benefit and not only are costly, but some may carry a degree of risk to the patient.

Arterial Blood Gas Analysis and Oxygen Saturations

Peripheral oxygen saturation measurement is a simple and non-invasive method of respiratory assessment. It should be undertaken on all patients pre-operatively as part of assessment. Resting oxygen saturations on air of less than 95% should result in an arterial blood gas being sampled and tested. Demonstration of $PaCO_2$ greater than 6 kPa suggests respiratory failure and further investigation is warranted to elucidate the cause.

In patients who smoke cigarettes it is useful to measure expired carbon monoxide levels. This investigation can also be of value in individuals suspected of smoking. Of the available tests, this is simple, cheap and provides an acceptable measure.

Spirometric Lung Function Testing

Spirometric measurement is a relatively quick and easy investigation to perform. Portable devices are available for use in the outpatient setting. These outpatient measurements may lack the precision and expertise of those taken in specialist clinical measurement departments, but, when taken in context, this immediate data can be very useful to screen and target subsequent investigations.

Obese subjects with abnormal pre-operative spirometry have a threefold risk of complications after laparoscopic bariatric surgery. When extrapolated to surgery in general for the obese patient this may provide a useful predictor of risk of complication development.

In general, results for a patient that reveal an FVC of less than 3 l or a FEV_1 of less than 1.5 l signal significant respiratory disease that requires further specialist investigation and management from a respiratory physician.

Radiological Imaging

Medical imaging techniques can be helpful for delineating pathological conditions. However, there are a number of practical aspects to consider when requesting and interpreting imaging requests. Routine performance of radiological investigations should not occur because of obesity. Selection should be based on clinical history and examination.

Physical Constraints

The radiology department needs to know about the obese patient. Even for a simple plain film, changes can be made to staff availability; the number of imaging cassettes used and following discussion may offer a better investigation.

Imaging techniques such as CT and MRI might require the use different imaging equipment, suites or even another hospital/location with larger-sized radiological imaging facilities. An example of this is the use of veterinary and zoo facilities where large animal resources are available. It is therefore important to be aware of the limitations of the range of equipment within a specific hospital.

Patient weight and body habitus will affect the nature of the imaging protocols used to optimise the quality of the images obtained. Changes such as a higher radiological dosing and scanning time may be required.

The general perceived rule for all imaging modalities is that increasing body mass leads to a degradation of image quality.

Plain Chest X-ray

Plain film images taken of obese patient chests require proportionately increased radiation doses and increased exposure time. This will impact on the utility of mobile systems in comparison to static departmental devices to obtain the best possible diagnostic image. On occasion, multiple cassettes may be necessary to obtain an adequate field of view.

Cross-sectional Imaging

The challenges of plain film imaging are compounded in tomographic cross-sectional imaging. This includes table weight limits and the orifice size of the scanner itself. It should also be remembered that most cross-sectional images are acquired when patients are in a supine position. This may be a recipe for poor patient tolerance due to dislike of lying flat and worsening of dyspnoea with resultant poor quality scans.

Analogous to plain films, tomographic images require increased radiation dose. However, fat deposition around organs can help to increase contrast between anatomic structures and actually improve organ image quality.

Some computing protocols can estimate abdominal fat proportions and weight, making corresponding changes to help improve image quality. This data can be useful when estimating the relative proportions of internal and external fat mass, organ infiltration, and muscle mass and lymphoedema fluid.

Objective Exercise Testing

The history, examination and investigations listed above take place with the patient more or less at rest. While useful, they do not assess respiratory function during exercise. This is a situation that will truly reveal lung function.

Six-minute Walk Test (6MWT) and Incremental Shuttle Walk Test (ISWT)

Both of these tests have been proposed as a screening test for cardiorespiratory fitness in the 'normal' population. These simple tests combined with activity status questionnaires may be quite sensitive to those with possible limitation.

Studies in the bariatric population have used populations with BMIs at the lower end of the spectrum. These groups are much less likely to have limiting musculoskeletal disease or cardiorespiratory comorbidity. In this group, a single test appears to be reliable and reproducible. However, the time-limited nature of the ISWT appears to be better at revealing limitation than allowing a patient to set his or her own pace in the 6MWT.

Cardiopulmonary Exercise Testing

Cardiopulmonary exercise testing (CPET) has the potential to offer a 'one stop' diagnostic differentiation of the contributing factors causing breathlessness whilst the patient exercises.

Simplistically, CPET testing has the ability to record pulmonary function, cardiac and gas exchange data. The data is collected initially at rest, then over a range of increasing exercise power output states. The exercise testing can be performed using either ambulatory protocols or through the use of static bicycles. To accommodate differing body habitus and disability, the bicycles may be leg driven in the normal erect posture, by a semi-recumbent posture standard bicycle or hand-cranked systems. However, it should be borne in mind that in the practical testing of pre-operative patients around 1 in 10 patients are unable to undertake the test, in particular the ability to achieve the required revolutions per minute to start the ramped protocol. These issues are particularly pertinent in the obese individual.

In the obese population, cardiopulmonary exercise testing can be used to quantify cardiorespiratory fitness and predict possible risk.

In bariatric surgery candidates, peak oxygen consumption below 15 ml/kg/min or anaerobic thresholds of less than 10 ml/kg is associated with post-operative complications and increased hospital length of stay.

Ultimately, any CPET test undertaken in an obese individual will need individual interpretation by an experienced physician to analyse results and quantify risk.

Summary

Obese patients are highly likely to report shortness of breath as a symptom. The context of these symptoms for that patient is important.

All obese patients presenting for surgery should have a full history and examination. Any concerns elicited from this in combination with low peripheral oxygen saturation (less than 95% on room air) should prompt further investigation, initially by arterial blood gas analysis.

Investigation beyond this point is determined by possible diagnosis and availability of investigations in the local healthcare facility.

Whilst difficult to undertake for the patient, CPET testing offers the better all-round assessment of respiratory function and offers a risk profile.

Ultimately, any abnormality revealed will require assessment and management by an experienced respiratory physician.

Further Reading

Böhmer A, Wappler F. Preoperative evaluation and prearation of the morbidly obese patient. *Curr Opin Anaesthesiol.* 2017;**30**(1):126–32.

Hodgson LE, Murphy PB, Hart N. Respiratory management of the obese patient undergoing surgery. *J Thoracic Dis.* 2015;**7**(5):943–52.

West AJ, Burton D. Effect of obesity on pulmonary function and its association with respiratory disease. *Can J Respir Ther.* 2009;**45**(1):25–30.

Donohoe CL, Feeney C, Carey MF, et al. Perioperative evaluation of the obese patient. *J Clin Anesth*. 2011;**23**:575–86.

Lorenzo S, Babb TG. Quantification of cardiorespiratory fitness in healthy nonobese and obese men and women. *Chest*. 2012;**141**(4):1031–9.

Hennis PJ, Meale PM, Grocott MP. Cardiopulmonary excercise testing for the evaluation of perioperative risk in non-cardiopulmonary surgery. *Postgrad Med J*. 2011;**87**:550–7.

Hennis PJ, Meale PM, Hurst RA, et al. Cardiopulmonary exercise testing predicts postoperative outcome in patients undergoing gastric bypass surgery. *Br J Anaesth*. 2012;**109**: 566–71.

Cullen A, Ferguson A. Perioperative management of the severely obese patient: a selective pathophysiological review. *Can J Anesth*. 2012;**59**:974–96.

Van Huisstede A, Biter LU, Luitwieler R, et al. Pulmonary function testing and complications of laparoscopic bariatric surgery. *Obes Surg*. 2013;**23**:1596–603.

Jubber AS. Respiratory complications of obesity. *Int J Clin Pract*. 2004;**58**(6):573–80.

Farina A, Crimi E, Accogli A, et al. Preoperative assessment of respiratory function in severely obese patients undergoing biliopancreatic diversion. *Eur Surg Res*. 2012;**48**:106–10.

Chapter 13

Cardiovascular Assessment in Obesity

Neil Ruparelia and Iqbal S. Malik

Introduction

Obesity is a leading preventable cause of death and disability and its worldwide incidence is rapidly increasing. In the developed world, the prevalence of obesity has doubled in the last 20 years, with approximately 70% of adults now classed as overweight or obese. Obesity leads to both cardiovascular and non-cardiovascular disease, including an increase in the risk of cancer. Consequently, clinicians are now frequently faced with overweight or obese patients requiring surgery. Obesity increases adverse cardiac events, and cardiovascular complications pose one of the most significant risks to any patient in the peri-operative period. Optimal pre-operative cardiac assessment is therefore important in optimising clinical outcomes. During the course of this chapter the impact of obesity upon the cardiovascular system, special considerations when clinically assessing the obese patient and finally the potential benefits of pre-surgical interventions upon cardiovascular outcomes in this patient population will be discussed.

Obesity and Cardiovascular Disease

Obesity has direct effects upon the cardiovascular system and is also associated with numerous co-morbidities that are independent risk factors of future events resulting in reduced overall survival (Table 13.1).

Table 13.1 Adverse effects of obesity

Type 2 diabetes mellitus

Hypertension (systemic and pulmonary)

Dyslipidaemia

Arrhythmias

Obstructive sleep apnoea

Cardiac failure

Coronary artery disease

Cardiomyopathy

Cancer

Systemic inflammation

Systemically, the presence of large volumes of adipose tissue results in the release of adipokines and inflammatory plasma proteins e.g. interleukin-6, tumour necrosis factor and insulin-like growth factor-1 that create a pro-inflammatory and pro-thrombotic state resulting in vascular endothelial damage increasing the likelihood of atherosclerotic disease, the formation of unstable plaque and plaque rupture.

Cardiac Failure

Physiologically, adipose tissue has a resting blood flow of 2–3 ml/100 g/min, but this can increase up to 10-fold, especially after food intake, with associated increase in total blood volume. This increased cardiac output is predominantly achieved through an increase in stroke volume. In the long-term, the left ventricle becomes volume loaded, dilated and commonly also develops eccentric hypertrophy. This is often initially associated with diastolic dysfunction, but with time systolic impairment also develops, resulting in congestive cardiac failure.

Cardiomyopathy

Cardiomyopathy of obesity (adipositas cordis) is caused by the direct effect of adipose tissue upon the heart. Early in the process the fat content of the heart is increased. With time, cardiac tissue is replaced by fat cells (e.g. sinus node, atrioventricular node) and can occasionally cause conductive defects. In the latter stages of the process, irregular bands of adipose tissue may separate and cause pressure-induced atrophy of the myocardial cells and result in cell dysfunction and cardiac failure.

Metabolic Syndrome

Obesity also negatively impacts the cardiovascular disease indirectly through the increased prevalence of concomitant cardiovascular risk factors, including type 2 diabetes mellitus, hypertension and obstructive sleep apnoea. Metabolic syndrome is associated with central or abdominal obesity, with increased values conferring additional cardiovascular risk.

Coronary Artery Disease

Obesity is an independent risk factor for coronary artery disease with an approximately twofold increase in comparison to lean individuals. The extent of coronary disease has been found to directly correlate with the extent of visceral fat.

Hypertension

Both systemic and pulmonary hypertension are more common in patients with obesity. Systemic hypertension is likely a result of a number of factors, including low-grade inflammation, endothelial dysfunction and increased cardiac output. Pulmonary hypertension is also more prevalent in this patient population and is elevated in more than 50% of individuals and is likely due to an increase in pulmonary vascular resistance secondary to combination of intrinsic pulmonary disease, thromboembolic disease or left ventricular dysfunction. The presence of elevated pulmonary artery pressures is an independent risk factor for adverse outcomes following surgery.

Arrhythmias

Obesity-associated cardiomyopathy, as discussed previously, may result in conduction disorders. Furthermore, due to physiological and haemodynamic changes in the heart associated with obesity, the atria may also dilate, predisposing to atrial arrhythmias. Obesity is also associated with ventricular arrhythmia, most commonly in the context of heart failure, but also possibly due to a higher prevalence of QT prolongation on resting ECG and abnormal late potentials.

Sleep Apneoa

Obesity is a cause of alveolar hypoventilation and obstructive sleep apnoea (OSA). OSA contributes to the pathogenesis of hypertension and is associated with a higher risk of heart failure, myocardial infarction, stroke and overall mortality.

Cardiac Pre-operative Assessment: General Considerations

The risk of the occurrence of cardiovascular events in the peri-operative period is related to both patient- and surgery-specific characteristics. Identification of increased risk provides both the patient and the clinical teams further information with regards to the risk-to-benefit ratio of any given procedure, and also affords the opportunity for interventions that may reduce that risk. As discussed above, patients classed as obese or overweight are at higher risk than lean individuals. Some general considerations for the assessment of pre-operative cardiac risk in any patient will be discussed first, followed by additional specific factors that should be taken into account in the obese patient.

Clinical Evaluation

The initial clinical evaluation and assessment of all patients begins with a thorough clinical history. The clinician should ask about symptoms such as angina, breathlessness, syncope and palpitations, in addition to ascertaining the presence (or absence) of other co-morbidities that increase cardiac risk, including hypertension, dyslipidaemia, diabetes mellitus, previous myocardial infarction, chronic kidney disease, and cerebrovascular and peripheral arterial disease. Cardiac functional status should also be determined. An important indication of poor functional status and predictor for post-operative cardiopulmonary complications is the inability to climb two flights of stairs. Function status is often expressed in metabolic equivalents (METs) and is defined as 3.5 ml oxygen uptake/kg/min that is the resting oxygen uptake in a sitting position (Table 13.2). Therefore patients unable to perform

Table 13.2 Metabolic equivalent

MET	Activity
1	Can take care of self (e.g. eat, dress, use toilet)
4	Can walk up a flight of steps or a hill or walk on level ground at 3–4 miles/hour
4–10	Can do heavy work around the house (e.g. scrubbing floors, or moving heavy furniture)
>10	Can participate in strenuous sports such (e.g. swimming, singles tennis, football, basketball, skiing)

activities >4 METs are regarded as having a poor functional state.

Physical examination should focus on the cardiovascular system and include blood pressure measurement, auscultation of the heart to exclude valvular pathology and determination of the presence of organ decompensation.

A resting electrocardiogram (ECG) can be useful to document a baseline reading and the presence of any arrhythmia (e.g. atrial fibrillation), evidence of previous myocardial infarction and any conduction abnormality (e.g. pre-excitation, bundle branch block). If the patient has no cardiovascular symptoms, no risk factors, and is under 50, not obese and having minor surgery, the ECG is often not performed.

Estimating Operative Cardiac Risk

The history, physical examination and ECG are used to identify patient-specific risk factors and together with the risk associated with the specific procedure (Table 13.3) are used in combination to predict cardiac risk. The estimated calculated risk will determine whether surgery should proceed without any further cardiac investigation, be postponed pending further tests (e.g. echocardiography, stress testing) and/or cardiac intervention (e.g. cardiac revascularisation or heart valve replacement) or be cancelled altogether.

There are a number of models that have been developed to aid in cardiac risk prediction. One that is most commonly used is the revised (Lee) cardiac risk index (RCRI) that is prospectively validated and predicts the risk of a cardiac event in patients undergoing non-cardiac surgery. It identifies six independent predictors:

1. high-risk surgery;
2. history of ischaemic heart surgery;
3. history of congestive cardiac failure;
4. history of cerebrovascular disease;
5. pre-operative treatment with insulin;
6. pre-operative serum creatinine (>2.0 mg/dl, >177 μmol/l).

The risk of major cardiac complications (cardiac death, non-fatal myocardial infarction, non-fatal cardiac arrest, post-operative cardiogenic pulmonary oedema, complete heart block) varies according to the number of risk factors present (Table 13.3).

The estimated cardiac risk is then used to categorise patients into low risk (<1%) or higher risk to guide further management.

Table 13.3 Revised cardiac risk index (Lee index)

Number of risk factors	Predicted risk
0	0.4%
1	1%
2	2.4%
3 or more	5.4%

Patients with an anticipated low cardiac risk following evaluation should proceed to surgery without delay. In this patient group it is unlikely that any risk-reduction strategies will further reduce peri-operative risk and/or improve outcomes.

Higher-risk patients are often individuals with known or suspected coronary or valvular disease and in these patients further cardiac testing may be indicated with the aim of determining the presence (and severity) of three cardiac risk markers: left ventricular dysfunction, myocardial ischaemia and heart valve abnormalities, all of which are major determinants of adverse post-operative outcomes. In general, any further cardiac testing (and resultant intervention) should only be performed if there is a clear indication regardless of proposed surgery and not just as a 'screening tool' due to the paucity of evidence demonstrating improved outcomes utilising this approach. These will be discussed further in the following section in the context of the obese patient.

Having said that, the local policy at Imperial College when it comes to renal transplant assessment is to perform coronary re-vascularisation due to the high cardiovascular event rates *after* surgery, and over the next few years. For major vascular surgery, pre-screening with stress echocardiography has been used when aortic cross-clamping is planned.

Specific Considerations for the Obese Patient

As discussed previously, obese patients are at higher risk of cardiac events when compared to lean individuals. Nonetheless, a similar approach should be applied to this patient group when performing cardiac assessment in the pre-operative period. However, there are a number of factors specific to this population that should be considered.

The clinical history will again be central to determining patient symptomology. However, it may be difficult to assess functional state due to immobility or concomitant orthopaedic limitations. In these instances, the use of bicycle or arm ergometry stress testing can be useful to evaluate functional status and is important to both cardiac risk assessment and post-procedural planning and rehabilitation.

Physical examination may also be limited due to patient habitus (e.g. auscultation of heart sounds), but evidence of cardiac decompensation, venous insufficiency and peripheral arterial disease may be present. The blood pressure should be taken with a large cuff to avoid misdiagnosis of hypertension.

Following clinical assessment, a proportion of patients with symptoms may be deemed to be at higher risk of cardiac events on the basis of co-morbidities and functional state and therefore further cardiac testing may be indicated. Again, due to patient habitus, conducting investigations and interpretation of their results may be challenging.

Electrocardiogram

Changes in cardiac morphology secondary to obesity can cause changes in the surface ECG with numerous patient series reporting that over 50% of obese patients have abnormal resting ECGs in the absence of any symptoms or evidence on further testing of any cardiac abnormality. Causes for the observed abnormalities include the increased distance of the heart to the surface electrodes, displacement of the heart and increased cardiac output. Resultant ECG abnormalities include, low voltages, leftward trend in the cardiac axis, non-specific T wave flattening and ST changes. It is therefore important to be aware of the significant false-positive rate of ECG abnormalities in this patient population; however, an abnormal ECG should not be ignored.

Echocardiography

The principal aims of performing resting echocardiography are to determine left ventricular ejection fraction and to determine the presence or absence of significant valvular pathology. Other information, including pulmonary arterial pressure assessment is also invaluable to peri-operative patient management. However, transthoracic echocardiography (TTE) can be technically challenging in obese patients, with limited views, poor resolution and difficulty in interpreting obtained images. Additional challenges with TTE in this patient group include the misinterpretation of pericardial fat for pericardial effusion and pronounced fat

deposition in the inter-atrial septum that may be confused for tumour. With regards to the assessment of left ventricular function, diastolic impairment is very common, although the increased intra-vascular volume in obesity may mask the Doppler-derived abnormalities of diastolic filling. Difficulty in adequately obtaining all of the views may make objective assessment of left ventricular systolic ejection fraction impossible.

Stress Testing

The aim of stress testing is to identify the presence (and extent) of cardiac ischaemia. It can also be used as an objective tool to quantify functional status. It should be noted again here that several studies have been unable to demonstrate the benefit of coronary revascularisation before non-cardiac surgery in the absence of symptoms or a clear indication for intervention and so suggest stress testing should only be performed if clinically indicated and not as a 'screening tool'. Since breathlessness and fatigue are common in the obese population, and exercise capacity an independent predictor of risk, 'screening' can guide risk assessment. A number of modalities are available and whilst each has limitations with regards to sensitivity and specificity in lean individuals, the presence of obesity further limits their efficacy, as discussed below.

Exercise testing using a bicycle or arm ergometer to provoke ischaemia (symptoms, ECG changes) may be limited in the obese patient due to immobility and related orthopaedic issues and also poor ECG traces due to patient habitus. Stress TTE may also be limited due to difficulty in obtaining adequate views to make an objective assessment of left ventricular function. Stress transoesophageal echo has been performed successfully to detect ischaemic burden, although this is too invasive for routine use. Nuclear imaging is limited due to attenuation artefacts and a higher incidence of false positives and may not practicably be possible due to weight limitations of the table. Perfusion and stress cardiac magnetic resonance imaging may also be limited due to size limits of the table and the bore, but when it can be carried out has been shown to be feasible, safe and efficacious.

A normal study or one demonstrating a small (<5%) volume of ischaemia is reassuring and in the absence of any other limiting condition should allow one to proceed to planned surgery without further delay, following the instigation of optimal medical therapy to address all concomitant risk factors.

In symptomatic patients that have been shown to have a large volume (>10%) of inducible ischaemia, cardiac revascularisation may be indicated in addition to medical therapy to improve cardiac outcomes.

Evaluation of Coronary Disease

Whilst initially the quality of the imaging of computed tomography angiography (CTA) was compromised in obese patients, newer protocols and improved technology have to a large extent overcome this and therefore this modality can be useful in excluding underlying coronary disease. However, the clinical significance of intermediate lesions is difficult to assess, and this supports the preferential use of functional testing.

In the presence of a positive stress test in a symptomatic patient, invasive coronary angiography is indicated, and is the 'gold standard' in coronary artery evaluation. It provides the option to perform coronary physiology studies (e.g. fractional flow reserve (FFR) or instantaneous wave free ratio (iFR)) to determine the presence of functionally important coronary lesions and the opportunity for percutaneous revascularisation at the same sitting. In the obese patient, radial arterial access is preferable to reduce the risk of access site vascular complications. Radiation doses to the patient will be inevitably higher than those for non-obese individuals.

Patient Management

On the basis of clinical evaluation and diagnostic tests, a management plan can be devised. The cornerstone of all patients is risk factor modification, which includes lifestyle changes and pharmacotherapy (e.g. aspirin, statins, angiotensin converting enzyme inhibitors and beta-blockers) that have been associated with both short- and longer-term outcomes. Additionally patients may also have medical treatments for long-standing conditions optimised, for example rate control medication for permanent atrial fibrillation or diuretics for peripheral oedema.

Weight loss prior to surgery can also play a role in the pre-operative period to reduce subsequent cardiac risk. Benefits include decreased blood pressure, decreased incidence of diabetes mellitus, improved lipid profile, decreased insulin resistance and improved endothelial function. However, achieving and then more importantly maintaining weight loss is a challenge. Furthermore, in the pre-operative period, any meaningful reduction in weight would inevitably cause a lengthy delay in any planned procedure.

There is now good evidence for the cardiovascular benefits of bariatric surgery, with reduction in blood pressure, improved glycaemic control and lipid levels. This type of surgery in particular requires not only cardiovascular optimisation, but psychological counselling to ensure the risk of surgery produces a long-term and sustained benefit.

Finally, in patients that are symptomatic with positive stress testing and a high volume of ischaemia, coronary revascularisation may improve prognosis. In common with all interventions, the benefits need to be weighed against the risk of both the procedure and also the resultant delay of the planned operation due to the need for recovery from open-heart surgery, or the use of dual anti-platelet therapy after the use of drug-eluting stents.

Conclusions

Obesity both directly and indirectly has negative effects upon the cardiovascular system, increasing morbidity and mortality. Due to the nature of obesity, clinical assessment can be very challenging, with interpretation of the clinical history, physical examination and diagnostic tests difficult. Appreciation and understanding of these limitations is critical to the optimal management of this patient group in the pre-operative period to improve outcomes.

Further Reading

Lavie CJ, Milani RV, Ventura HO. Obesity and cardiovascular disease. Risk factor, paradox and impact of weight loss. *J Am Coll Cardiol*. 2009;**53**(21):1925–32.

Poirier P, Alpert MA, Fleisher LA, et al. Cardiovascular evaluation and management of severely obese patient undergoing surgery: a science advisory from the American Heart Association. *Circulation*. 2009;**120**:86–95.

Poirier P, Giles TD, Bray GA et al. Obesity and cardiovascular disease: pathophysiology evaluation, and effect of weight loss. An update of the 1997 American Heart Association scientific statement on obesity and heart disease from the obesity committee of the Council on nutrition, physical activity, and metabolism. *Circulation*. 2006;**113**:898–918.

Sleep Disordered Breathing: Assessment and Management in Obesity

Brian Kent and Joerg Steier

Definitions and Diagnosis

The presence and severity of obstructive sleep apnoea (OSA) is quantified by the assessment of the number of apnoeas (cessation of airflow) and hypnonoeas (reductions of airflow) occurring per hour of sleep, the apnoea/hyponoea index (AHI). An AHI of <5 events per hour is considered normal, with an AHI of 5–15, 15–30 or >30 events per hour categorised as mild, moderate or severe sleep apnoea, respectively. Obstructive sleep apnoea syndrome (OSAS) is defined by the presence of OSA on a sleep study, accompanied by significant subjective daytime sleepiness. The gold-standard investigation for the diagnosis of OSA is inpatient, attended nocturnal polysomnography (PSG), incorporating measurement of oro-nasal air-flow, respiratory effort, pulse oximetry and ECG, alongside electroencephalography, electrooculography and electromyography of the chin and anterior tibialis. On PSG, an apnoea is defined as a reduction of airflow to ≤10% of baseline, lasting ≥10 seconds; an apnoeic event is classified as 'obstructive' if respiratory effort persists, or as 'central' if respiratory effort ceases.

How a hypopnoea should be best defined is rather controversial, with different hypopnoea definitions applied to the same sleep study leading to significant differences in AHI values. The most commonly used scoring rule defines a hypopnoea as a reduction in airflow of ≥30% from pre-event baseline, lasting ≥10 seconds, accompanied by a 3% arterial oxygen desaturation and/or a related arousal from sleep.

The recording of a PSG is a resource intensive and time-consuming test, and is rather inconvenient for the patient. Moreover, the prevalence of OSA is such that it is simply not feasible to perform PSG on all suspected cases within an acceptable time frame. Consequently, a number of ambulatory diagnostic methods, ranging from home PSG, to cardio-respiratory sleep studies and overnight home oximetry studies, have been assessed. Good evidence now exists to support ambulatory testing in subjects with a high pre-test clinical probability of OSA, with PSG reserved for more nuanced or complex cases.

Epidemiology

Sleep apnoea is the most common physical sleep disorder, and is probably also the most prevalent chronic respiratory disorder. OSA is significantly more common in men, and has a particularly intimate relationship with obesity, with the prevalence and severity of sleep disordered breathing increasing in parallel with increasing body mass index. The sentinel study of OSA prevalence was the Wisconsin Sleep Cohort study, which assessed sleep breathing in a middle-aged, community-based population in the mid-western United States. When defined by an AHI ≥5 events/hour, the prevalence of OSA within this cohort was 24% in men and 9% in women aged 30–60 years of age. The prevalence of OSA with associated excessive daytime sleepiness (i.e. OSAS) was estimated at 3% to 7% in adult men and 2% to 5% in adult women. However, these data date back to the early 1990s, with an epidemic of obesity engulfing both the developing and developed world in the intervening years. More recent population data suggest a concomitant increase in the occurrence of OSA, with a recent update of the Wisconsin Sleep Cohort study identifying OSAS in 14% of men and 5% of women, while moderate to severe OSA (AHI ≥15) was found in 49% of middle-aged Swiss men. While there is rather marked variance in these data, it is nonetheless clear that there is a large cohort of individuals in the general population with significant, undiagnosed sleep apnoea. OSA is particularly common in a number of patient cohorts, including those with T2DM, resistant hypertension, end-stage renal disease and heart failure. In surgical populations, OSA is common, and may be undiagnosed in up to 60% of cases, with a particularly high prevalence seen in bariatric surgery cohorts.

Clinical Features

Daytime sleepiness is generally considered to be the cardinal symptom of OSA, but its presentation can be significantly more protean than might be expected. Common nocturnal symptoms include sleep disruption, nocturnal choking and dyspnoea, nocturia and night sweats; bed partners will often complain of snoring and may report witnessed apnoeic events. Excessive daytime sleepiness is common in men with more severe OSA, but quite marked sleep disordered breathing may be present even in the absence of this. This is particularly the case in female patients, who may be able to maintain wakefulness without difficulty, and in whom fatigue may be the most prominent daytime symptom. Other daytime symptoms include early morning headaches, irritability and poor concentration. Untreated OSA is associated with reduced quality of life scores, and with a significantly increased risk of road traffic and workplace accidents.

The impact of these symptoms on an individual with OSA may be significant, but of greater concern from a population health perspective is the relationship of OSA with cardiovascular and metabolic disease. Obstructive events occurring during sleep lead to intermittent hypoxaemia (IH) and hypercapnia, increased sympathetic outflow, high swings in intrathoracic pressure and eventually arousal from sleep. Repetitive, chronic IH causes oxidative stress and systemic inflammation, generating a profoundly atherogenic milieu and, combined with sympathetic excitation, can lead to endothelial dysfunction and subsequent clinically overt cardiovascular disease. Nocturnal hypoxaemia and sympathetic excitation also appear to have a detrimental effect on liver and adipose tissue function, leading to insulin resistance, glucose intolerance and dyslipidaemia.

The strongest evidence in this field links OSA and hypertension, with longitudinal data showing a roughly threefold increase in incident hypertension in patients with moderate or severe OSA compared with non-apnoeic subjects. Risks of stroke, coronary artery disease, cardiac arrhythmia and heart failure also appear greater in subjects with untreated significant OSA, independent of confounding demographic, anthropometric and clinical factors. Similarly, OSA severity predicts the presence of T2DM in both cross-sectional and longitudinal analyses, and diabetic patients with severe OSA have higher HbA1c levels and are more likely to have poorly controlled T2DM

than their non-apnoeic counterparts, irrespective of the effects of obesity. OSA may also play a role in carcinogenesis, with the risk of cancer incidence and death markedly higher in subjects with more severe OSA and nocturnal hypoxaemia. Overall, untreated severe OSA is associated with a three- to fivefold increased risk of death, with the bulk of this attributable to increased cardiovascular mortality.

In addition to the increased load on the respiratory muscles caused by upper airway obstruction, the impact of morbid obesity on the lower respiratory tract is significant. Obesity causes an increased load on the respiratory muscle pump that impacts on the work of breathing and requires high levels of neural respiratory drive. Elevated intra-abdominal pressures in obesity impose a pre-load on the diaphragm during inspiration, particularly in the supine posture. These forces contribute to a reduced transpulmonary pressure gradient in the thoracic compartment and affect operational lung volumes. Morbidly obese subjects breathe at low lung volumes, close to the residual volume, their functional residual capacity shifts towards a less favourable part of the pressure–volume curve with a reduced compliance. At low lung volumes, the closing volume of the airway increases airway resistance further and contributes to an intrinsic positive end expiratory pressure.

Treatment

The best-established treatment for OSA is nocturnal continuous positive airway pressure (nCPAP) therapy, which provides a pneumatic splint to maintain upper airway patency during sleep, inflates the chest, and reduces work of breathing and neural respiratory drive. Effective use of nCPAP leads to improvements in daytime sleepiness and quality of life measures, reduces blood pressure measurements and may lead to reductions in cardiovascular mortality. However, patient acceptance of, and adherence to, nCPAP therapy is relatively poor, with up to 50% of patients being non-compliant with treatment after 1 year.

Weight loss can lead to improvements in sleep breathing, but in practice – outside of the context of bariatric surgery – significant degrees of weight loss are difficult to achieve and maintain. Relatively established alternative treatment modalities for OSA include use of mandibular advancement dental devices and, in some cases, upper airway surgery. However, these approaches require careful patient selection, may be limited by poor patient acceptability, and are of uncertain long-term efficacy. Recent evidence suggests that stimulation of the upper airway musculature during sleep may be a viable long-term therapeutic approach, either via an implantable hypoglossal nerve stimulator, or via the transcutaneous delivery of electrical stimulation. However, careful patient selection for these treatments remains critical, and data supporting their long-term efficacy are needed.

Peri-operative Outcomes and OSA

Initial reports of an association between a diagnosis of sleep apnoea and an increased risk of peri-operative complications first emerged over two decades ago, but it was not until more recent years that a significant body of literature exploring this putative relationship emerged. There remains a relative paucity of high-quality studies in this field, but available data appears to suggest that patients with OSA are at increased risk of adverse anaesthetic outcomes.

Airway Management

A limited number of studies have evaluated the impact of a diagnosis of OSA on airway management. An analysis of 50 000 consecutive patients undergoing general anaesthesia (GA) in a large university-affiliated hospital in the United States identified cases of OSA from review of medical records, and found that a diagnosis of sleep apnoea was associated with a hazard ratio (HR) of 2.4 for an inability to provide mask ventilation. However, the absolute risk was small, occurring in only 20 patients from the 3680 identified as having OSA. A similar study from the Multi-Center Peri-Operative Outcomes Group found an OSA diagnosis conferred a significantly increased likelihood of difficult mask ventilation and difficult laryngoscopy (adjusted odds ratio (OR) 1.59) in a population of nearly 500 000 patients undergoing GA. Similarly, in subjects assessed by questionnaire for risk of OSA in an ambulatory surgery setting, those deemed at high risk for sleep apnoea needed more intubation attempts, had worse laryngoscopic views and had greater requirement for fibreoptic intubation.

Respiratory Complications

Studies assessing the impact of OSA on post-operative respiratory complications can be divided into two broad groups – case control and cohort studies, where the diagnosis of OSA was based on a sleep study or the use of a validated questionnaire, and large-scale population level studies drawn from administrative databases, with the diagnosis of OSA based on chart review or International Classification of Diseases (ICD) coding. Among the former there is a general – but not universal – consensus that the presence of OSA is associated with an increased risk of respiratory failure and other pulmonary complications post-operatively. Perhaps the most compelling recent example of this is a study evaluating post-operative complications in approximately 4000 Canadian patients with objectively diagnosed OSA, who were compared with 16 277 controls at low risk of sleep apnoea. OSA conferred an increased risk of respiratory failure and adult respiratory distress syndrome (ARDS), despite adjustment for confounding demographic, anthropometric and clinical factors. An apparent dose-response effect was observed, with subjects with severe OSA at the highest risk for respiratory complications (adjusted OR 2.69).

A substantial proportion of the published literature using administrative data has failed to show a meaningful association between sleep disordered breathing and post-operative respiratory complications. For example, in a large population (n = 91 028) of patients undergoing bariatric surgery in the United States, OSA was not associated with an increased risk of post-operative respiratory failure, and was even seen to confer a lower risk of pneumonia. Conversely, a companion paper to this, published by the same authors, and examining the records of over one million patients undergoing operative management, identified a significant relationship between OSA and respiratory failure following orthopaedic, prostate, abdominal or cardiovascular surgery.

With such apparent divergence in the published literature, one can lean to an extent on two recently published meta-analyses, both of which suggest a greater than twofold risk of post-operative respiratory complications in OSA patients when compared with non-apnoeic subjects. Both of these analyses were confined to studies using some objective confirmation of OSA, but are supported by a recent systematic review, including studies drawn from administrative data, which drew similar conclusions.

A sub-group of patients with sleep disordered breathing at particularly high risk of post-operative respiratory difficulties appears to be that with obesity hypoventilation syndrome (OHS), generally characterised by a combination of significant obesity, OSA, nocturnal hypoventilation and daytime hypercapnia. OHS occurs in up to 30% of severe OSA patients, and in a retrospective, chart-based study from the United States, it was associated with a markedly increased likelihood of acute or chronic respiratory failure (adjusted OR 10.9), need for tracheostomy (adjusted OR 3.8) and ICU transfer (adjusted OR 10.9).

Cardiovascular Complications

An increased risk of adverse cardiovascular outcomes has been identified in studies based on both objective clinical assessment of OSA and those using administrative data. Patients with previously undiagnosed severe OSA – subsequently confirmed by a sleep study – had an adjusted OR of 2.4 of post-operative cardiac arrest or shock when compared to matched controls in a large Canadian cohort study. Similarly, a study of 277 patients undergoing coronary artery bypass grafting, which assessed risk of OSA using a validated questionnaire, identified an adjusted OR of 2.18 for post-CABG (coronary artery bypass graft) atrial fibrillation (AF).

A number of well-conducted studies based on administrative databases also support a relationship between OSA and post-operative AF, an association observed in both cardiac and non-cardiac surgery. These are far from uniform findings, however, and many authors have not observed any increase in risk of post-operative cardiovascular complications. Nonetheless, the available meta-analyses and systematic reviews of these data suggest a significantly increased likelihood of cardiovascular issues arising in the post-operative OSA patient.

Resource Utilisation

Orthopaedic patients with OSA appear to be at significantly increased risk of ICU admission postoperatively, with increased healthcare utilisation costs occurring in parallel with this. While a similar effect has been reported in general surgical cohorts, other studies have suggested that a diagnosis of sleep apnoea may have no measureable impact on postoperative resource utilisation, or may even be associated with reduced healthcare costs. Once again, meta-analysis data suggest a detrimental role for OSA, with an adjusted OR of 2.81 for post-operative ICU transfer in OSA patients.

Post-operative Mortality

Few data support a link between OSA and increased risk of peri-operative death. One report did identify a significant increase in post-operative mortality in orthopaedic patients with OSA, but a majority of studies have failed to confirm this finding. A number of authors have even reported an apparent – and rather surprising – protective effect of sleep disordered breathing on mortality risk. However, many of these data are derived from large administrative databases, without objective confirmation of the presence or absence of sleep apnoea, and remain vulnerable to a large number of potential biases.

Screening for OSA in Peri-operative Populations

As discussed in detail above, the gold standard for the diagnosis of OSA is nocturnal PSG, but its high cost and the high prevalence of undiagnosed sleep disordered breathing in general and surgical populations make it an impractical screening tool. Even the most straightforward method of providing an objective diagnosis of OSA – home oximetry testing – is relatively costly and resource intensive to justify its use in all patients undergoing pre-operative assessment. The recognition that OSA is both common and potentially harmful in surgical populations has led to the development of a number of screening methods and questionnaires to allow better selection of subjects for pre-operative sleep studies.

The most widely used questionnaire in sleep medicine is the Epworth sleepiness scale (ESS) score, which asks the patient to score their likelihood of falling asleep across a range of eight everyday activities, generating a score between 0 and 24, and is available as a pictorial or online questionnaire. A score of ≥10 is generally considered to be consistent with subjective excessive daytime sleepiness (EDS), and may warrant further investigation. Increasing daytime sleepiness is associated with an increase in likelihood of associated sleep apnoea. However, the ESS does not discriminate between the many different potential aetiologies of EDS, has a questionable relationship with objective measures of daytime sleepiness and its utility as a predictive tool in the identification of OSA remains uncertain, particularly in obese subjects. Hence, use of the ESS alone as a screening tool for OSA in surgical cohorts is not generally recommended.

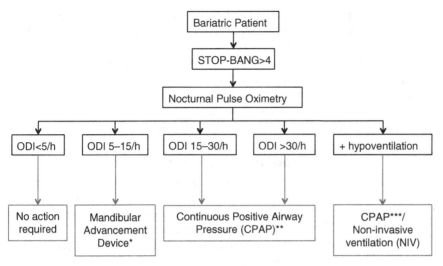

Figure 14.1 Pragmatic approach to screen for sleep-disordered breathing using home oximetry and to treat morbidly obese patients prior to elective general anaesthesia. ODI, oxygen desaturation index. * Mandibular advancement device, if symptomatic, not required for sedation.** Initial CPAP therapy trial,*** if uncontrolled to consider NIV.

Conversely, the STOP-BANG questionnaire has by now been well validated as a method of identifying subjects at high risk of OSA. STOP-BANG consists of questions addressing the presence or absence of snoring, daytime tiredness, observed apnoeic episodes and a history of high blood pressure, along with assessment of demographic and anthropometric variables (body mass index >35 kg/m^2, age >50 years, neck circumference >40 cm and male gender), with one point awarded for each variable. In the initial validation study in an adult surgical population, a cut-off score on the STOP-BANG of ≥3 conferred a sensitivity of 92.9% and 100% for the identification of moderate-severe and severe OSA, respectively. Several subsequent studies have confirmed its utility as a screening tool for undiagnosed OSA in both sleep clinics and in pre-operative assessment clinics, with a recent meta-analysis finding that a sensitivity of 94% and 96% for the detection of moderate-severe or severe OSA, respectively. Moreover, it would also appear that the higher the STOP-BANG score, the greater the likelihood of the subject having clinically significant OSA. While STOP-BANG has an excellent negative predictive value (NPV) for the presence of OSA, this is at the cost of a relatively low degree of specificity, with a pooled specificity in studies of surgical patients of <30%. Notably however, the specificity and positive predictive value of the questionnaire increases markedly with higher STOP-BANG scores, with positive predictive values (PPV) >80% for a score of 8.

Other questionnaires in mainstream clinical practice include the American Society of Anesthesiology (ASA) checklist and the Berlin questionnaire. These appear to have almost identical performance characteristics in surgical patients: the former, comprised largely of similar variables to the STOP-BANG questionnaire, has been shown to have a sensitivity of 87.2% for the identification of severe OSA, with an NPV of 90.9% and a PPV of 27.9%. The Berlin questionnaire, originally validated in a primary care setting, classifies patients as low or high risk for OSA, based on their responses in three clinical categories: snoring history, daytime sleepiness and a history of hypertension or obesity. Its use in pre-operative screening has been shown to have a sensitivity of 87.2%, an NPV of 92.8% and a PPV of 31.5%.

Overall, the available screening questionnaires provide an effective, if imperfect, way of excluding a diagnosis of OSA in patients due to undergo GA, and facilitate the rational use of more resource-intensive diagnostics, such as home oximetry studies (Figure 14.1).

CPAP Therapy and Post-operative Outcomes

If OSA does lead to an increased risk of adverse anaesthetic outcomes, then peri-operative treatment with nCPAP might be expected to have a beneficial modifying effect on these outcomes. This hypothesis is supported by a number of retrospective studies, perhaps the most informative of which was a Canadian matched cohort study, with OSA confirmed by nocturnal PSG. Within this cohort, patients with a prior diagnosis of OSA, who had been prescribed nCPAP therapy, had a significantly reduced risk of cardiovascular complications (adjusted OR 0.34), with this association confined to patients with at least moderately severe OSA. Similar relationships were observed in a study of 26 842 (2646 with OSA) patients undergoing general or vascular surgery in Michigan, where presumptive diagnoses of OSA were made based on review of medical records and/or a STOP-BANG score ≥3. In this population, untreated OSA conferred an increased risk of cardiopulmonary complications, both compared to patients without a diagnosis of OSA and those with OSA who had been prescribed nCPAP (6.4% versus 4.2%; adjusted OR 1.8). The bulk of this effect was made up of an increased risk of post-operative myocardial infarction (1.4% versus 0.6%) and unplanned reintubation (2.7% versus 1.4%).

There is a relative paucity of prospective controlled studies in this field. A randomised controlled trial (RCT) of 177 largely orthopaedic or general surgical patients with previously untreated moderate-severe OSA (AHI ≥15) diagnosed on pre-operative home PSG, showed that autoadjusting CPAP (APAP) therapy led to a marked reduction in post-operative AHI and nocturnal hypoxaemia compared with controls. No major complications occurred in either study arm, and no reduction in minor complications was observed with APAP treatment. Among 86 patients deemed at high risk of OSA, according to a validated questionnaire, undergoing joint arthroplasty in the Mayo Clinic, post-operative APAP therapy made no difference to length of stay, resource utilisation or post-operative complications. Notably, few significant post-operative adverse events were observed in either group. A recent meta-analysis examining outcomes in 904 OSA patients undergoing surgery, including participants in these two RCTs along with four non-randomised studies, found no significant differences between CPAP and no CPAP groups in rates of post-operative complications or length of hospital stay, but unsurprisingly found that post-operative APAP or CPAP therapy did improve indices of sleep disordered breathing.

It is difficult for any treatment to make a meaningful impact if it is not used. Adherence with CPAP therapy is a major difficulty in general sleep populations, and has been a potentially limiting factor in a number of otherwise well-designed clinical trials assessing the effect of CPAP on cardiovascular

and metabolic outcomes in OSA. It would appear that this also holds true in patients commenced on CPAP therapy in the peri-operative period. In the trial discussed above, only 45% of patients were compliant with APAP therapy by the end of the study period, while median nightly use in a population of 104 patients undergoing surgical management in Chicago was only 2.5 hours.

Summary and Recommendations

Patients with untreated OSA are more likely to experience cardiovascular and respiratory complications of surgery than their counterparts on CPAP therapy, but many questions remain unanswered. Critical areas that need to be addressed by future research include determining the severity of OSA that merits peri-operative treatment, the types of surgery that portend the worst prognosis in OSA patients, and the optimal timing and mode of delivery of PAP therapy. The available evidence suggests that patients with moderate-severe OSA should be offered a trial of treatment for their sleep disordered breathing before undergoing GA, but the peri-operative management of OSA remains a markedly underexplored area.

Further Reading

Abdelsattar ZM, Hendren S, Wong SL, Campbell DA, Jr., Ramachandran SK. The impact of untreated obstructive sleep apnea on cardiopulmonary complications in general and vascular surgery: a cohort study. *Sleep*. 2015;**38**(8): 1205–10.

Chia P, Seet E, Macachor JD, Iyer US, Wu D. The association of pre-operative STOP-BANG scores with postoperative critical care admission. *Anaesthesia*. 2013;**68** (9):950–2.

Chung F, Yegneswaran B, Liao P, et al. STOP questionnaire: a tool to screen patients for obstructive sleep apnea. *Anesthesiology*. 2008;**108**(5):812–21.

Garvey JF, Pengo MF, Drakatos P, Kent BD. Epidemiological aspects of obstructive sleep apnea. *J Thorac Dis*. 2015;**7**(5):920–9.

Finkel KJ, Searleman AC, Tymkew H, et al. Prevalence of undiagnosed obstructive sleep apnea among adult surgical patients in an academic medical center. *Sleep Med*. 2009;**10** (7):753–8.

Frey WC, Pilcher J. Obstructive sleep-related breathing disorders in patients evaluated for bariatric surgery. *Obes Surg*. 2003;**13**(5):676–83.

Kaw R, Bhateja P, Paz YMH, et al. Postoperative complications in patients with unrecognized obesity hypoventilation syndrome undergoing elective noncardiac surgery. *Chest.* 2016;**149**(1):84–91.

Kaw R, Chung F, Pasupuleti V, et al. Meta-analysis of the association between obstructive sleep apnoea and postoperative outcome. *Br J Anaesth.* 2012;**109**(6):897–906.

Kent BD, McNicholas WT, Ryan S. Insulin resistance, glucose intolerance and diabetes mellitus in obstructive sleep apnoea. *J Thorac Dis.* 2015;**7**(8):1343–57.

Kent BD, Ryan S, McNicholas WT. Obstructive sleep apnea and inflammation: relationship to cardiovascular co-morbidity. *Respir Physiol Neurobiol.* 2011;**178**(3):475–81.

Kheterpal S, Martin L, Shanks AM, Tremper KK. Prediction and outcomes of impossible mask ventilation: a review of 50,000 anesthetics. *Anesthesiology.* 2009;**110**(4):891–7.

Kheterpal S, Healy D, Aziz MF, et al. Incidence, predictors, and outcome of difficult mask ventilation combined with difficult laryngoscopy: a report from the multicenter perioperative outcomes group. *Anesthesiology.* 2013;**119**(6):1360–9.

Meurgey JH, Brown R, Woroszyl-Chrusciel A, Steier J. Perioperative treatment of sleep-disordered breathing and outcomes in bariatric patients. *J Thorac Dis* 2018;**10**(Suppl 1):S144–52.

Mutter TC, Chateau D, Moffatt M, et al. A matched cohort study of postoperative outcomes in obstructive sleep apnea: could preoperative diagnosis and treatment prevent complications? *Anesthesiology.* 2014;**121**(4):707–18.

Nagappa M, Mokhlesi B, Wong J, et al. The effects of continuous positive airway pressure on postoperative outcomes in obstructive sleep apnea patients undergoing surgery: a systematic review and meta-analysis. *Anesth Analg.* 2015;**120**(5):1013–23.

Opperer M, Cozowicz C, Bugada D, et al. Does obstructive sleep apnea influence perioperative outcome?: a qualitative systematic review for the society of anesthesia and sleep medicine task force on preoperative preparation of patients with sleep-disordered breathing. *Anesth Analg.* 2016;**122**(5):1321–34.

Pengo MF, Steier J. Emerging technology: electrical stimulation in obstructive sleep apnoea. *J Thorac Dis.* 2015;**7**(8):1286–97.

Reed K, Pengo MF, Steier J. Screening for sleep-disordered breathing in abariatic population. *J Thorac Dis* 2016;**8**(2):268–75.

Singh M, Liao P, Kobah S, et al. Proportion of surgical patients with undiagnosed obstructive sleep apnoea. *Br J Anaesth.* 2013;**110**(4):629–36.

Steier J, Martin A, Harris J, et al. Predicted relative prevalence estimates for obstructive sleep apnoea and the associated healthcare provision across the UK. *Thorax.* 2014;**69**(4):390–2.

Steier J, Jolley CJ, Seymour J, et al. Increased load on the respiratory muscles in obstructive sleep apnea. *Respir Physiol Neurobiol.* 2010;**171**(1):54–60.

Steier J, Jolley CJ, Seymour J, et al. Neural respiratory drive in obesity. *Thorax.* 2009;**64**(8):719–25.

Steier J, Lunt A, Hart N, Polkey MI, Moxham J. Observational study of the effect of obesity on lung volumes. *Thorax.* 2014;**69**(8):752–9.

Chapter 15

Risk Assessment and Stratification for Obesity

Andrew Chamberlain and Jonathan Redman

Introduction

The European Surgical Outcome Study (EuSOS) showed that elective surgery is not without significant risk, with the mortality rate in the UK being 3.6%. Up to 30% of patients presenting for surgery are obese, and this group provides an increasing challenge to our healthcare systems.

Obesity is a known risk factor for several medical co-morbidities, including cardiovascular disease and diabetes, as well as being associated with several malignancies. It is therefore important to perform a detailed, accurate risk assessment in this patient group, which requires:

- identification and optimisation of the key co-morbidities and modifiable risk factors;
- risk stratification by the use of a pertinent scoring system;
- undertaking of relevant investigations to quantify the co-morbidities (these are often guided by a history from the patient);
- assessment of functional capacity.

Mortality in the Obese Individual

The 2014 National Bariatric Surgical Database showed the observed in-hospital mortality rate for obese patients after primary surgery was 0.07%. The recorded surgical complication rates for primary operations is 2.9%, which is much lower than that for many other planned operations. This is significantly different from the EuSOS data, but it is essential to remember that many more obese individuals present for non-bariatric surgery, and much of what will be discussed is based upon data not specific to obesity, but based on what we know about the general adult population.

Identifying Risk

In order to perform an accurate risk assessment, it is essential to identify any risk factors that affect

Table 15.1 A summary of important risk factors and their potential implications

Risk Factor	Implications
BMI	Inaccurate assessment of adiposity Waist circumference or waist:hip ratio predictive Moderate obesity can play a protective role (paradox) Outcomes worse with BMI >40 kg/m^2
Age	Increase risk over 65
Cardiovascular	Heart failure most significant predictor of post-op morbidity
Metabolic syndrome	Increase in cardiovascular, respiratory, neurological and renal complications
Diabetes	Poor glycaemic control associated with increased morbidity
OSA	High risk if STOP-BANG ≥5
Surgical	Low-risk <1% to high-risk >5% mortality depending on type of surgery

outcome, such as age and functional capacity, and more specifically those which are potentially modifiable, which if managed correctly may decrease an individual's risk and improve outcome (Table 15.1).

BMI and the Obesity Paradox

BMI is a descriptor of obesity, and it is suited for population-level studies; however, its use can result in inaccurate assessment of adiposity, as weight does not distinguish lean muscle from fat mass. For example, a person with central obesity (excessive visceral fat) and increased surgical risk may have a normal

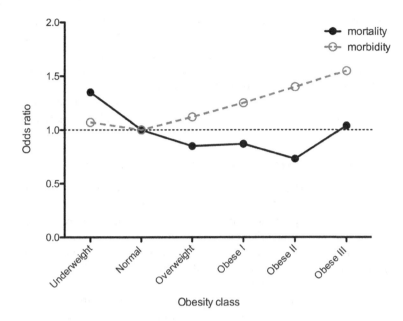

Figure 15.1 Obesity class odds ratio for mortality and morbidity demonstrating the obesity paradox (adapted from Mullen J, Moorman D and Davenport D. The obesity paradox: body mass index and outcomes in patients undergoing nonbariatric general surgery. *Ann Surg.* 2009;250(1):166–72.)

BMI. This raises the question about the utilisation of other indices to measure the central obesity such as waist circumference or waist-to-hip ratio. These measurements more accurately estimate central obesity, known to increase cardiac risk.

It is thought that overweight and obese individuals are at increased risk of complications following surgery, however this may not be true, with evidence suggesting that overweight and moderately obese patients may have better survival rates than those with a normal weight, whilst underweight individuals (BMI <18 kg/m^2) have the worst outcomes. This is known as the obesity paradox (see Figure 15.1). This was illustrated in a large prospective multicenter analysis of over 110 000 patients undergoing non-cardiac surgery, where it was found that overweight (OR, 0.85; 95% CI, 0.75–0.99) and moderately obese (OR, 0.73; 95% CI, 0.57–0.94) patients had a significantly lower risk of death than patients with a normal BMI.

The mechanism for the obesity paradox is unknown, but it is postulated that visceral adipose tissue generates a low-grade inflammatory response preparing the host for the insult of surgery.

Age

Age has consistently been shown to be a significant predictor of outcomes after major surgery. As the population is ageing as a whole and the incidence of obesity increases then a greater proportion of patients presenting for surgery will be higher risk.

A prospective cohort study of over 500 000 general surgical patients undergoing non-cardiac procedures observed a 3% mortality rate for patients aged less than 80 years compared to 8% for those greater than 80 years (p<0.001). In addition, complication rates were also higher in this group (20% versus 12.1%, p<0.001), and the occurrence of post-operative complications in the elderly increased post-operative mortality (26% versus 4%, p<0.001). This same increase in mortality is seen in the elderly undergoing bariatric surgery both in the short and long term.

Cardiovascular Risk Factors

The presence of obesity is associated with numerous cardiac co-morbidities including:

- hypertension;
- ischaemic heart disease;
- arrhythmias – notably atrial fibrillation;
- right and left heart failure.

Ischaemic heart disease is often considered the primary peri-operative risk factor for cardiac complications following surgery; however, in terms of post-operative outcome, the presence of heart failure is a stronger predictor than ischaemic heart disease, heart failure being associated with a doubling of 30-day mortality and re-admission rates, whilst the presence of ischaemic heart disease did not confer such an increase compared to the control group.

Cardiac arrhythmias and conduction defects are a common finding in the pre-operative setting. These are more prevalent with increasing body weight and their presence should prompt further clinical investigation. Atrial fibrillation is the most common tachyarrhythmia, particularly in older patients. Patients with a history of AF who are clinically stable rarely require treatment modification, but may need adjustment to their anti-coagulation based on their stroke risk.

Metabolic Syndrome

Metabolic syndrome is discussed elsewhere, but must be highlighted as a key peri-operative risk factor. Obese patients with metabolic syndrome show a significantly increased mortality rate (see Figure 15.2).

Metabolic syndrome consists of dyslipidaemia, hypertension, central obesity and insulin resistance. Compared with normal weight individuals undergoing non-cardiac surgery, patients with metabolic syndrome have: a threefold increase in risk of cardiac and pulmonary complications, a doubling of coma and stroke risk, and a significant risk of acute kidney injury.

Diabetes

Obesity is associated with increased insulin resistance, and also forms a part of the metabolic syndrome. Poor glycaemic control in the peri-operative period is associated with increased morbidity and hence good glycaemic control is essential. Its presence also confers increased cardiovascular risk, increased risk of stroke, renal impairment, poor wound healing and increased risk of infection. Guidelines published by the Association of Anaesthetists from Great Britain and Northern Ireland suggest that elective patients with HbA1c levels of greater than 69 mmol/mol be postponed to allow optimisation to take place, regardless of BMI.

Obstructive Sleep Apnoea

The identification of OSA pre-operatively is essential to allow successful treatment and reduce peri-operative complications. Simple assessment using the STOP-BANG questionnaire will allow identification of those at high risk of OSA and those with a score of ≥5 should be considered as high risk for OSA and investigated further, with referral to a respiratory physician. Patients with undiagnosed OSA, or those unable to tolerate CPAP are at highest risk of peri-operative respiratory and cardiovascular morbidity, while patients fully compliant with CPAP (usually indicated by symptomatic benefit) are at lower risk of peri-operative events.

Surgical Factors

Surgical magnitude clearly has an effect on the risk associated with surgery to the individual (Table 15.2). The use of laparoscopic surgery has been shown to be beneficial by causing less tissue damage, fluid shifts and post-operative pain than an equivalent open procedure; however, it has not been shown to confer a survival advantage.

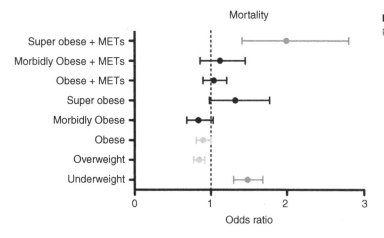

Figure 15.2 Effect of metabolic syndrome on post-operative mortality.

Table 15.2 Risk of MI and cardiac death within 30 days of surgery

Low risk (< 1%)	Intermediate risk (1–5%)	High risk (>5%)
Breast	Abdominal	Aortic and major vascular surgery
Dental	Carotid	Peripheral vascular surgery
Endocrine	Peripheral arterial angioplasty	
Eye	Endovascular aneurysm repair	
Gynaecology	Head and neck surgery	
Reconstructive	Neurological / orthopaedic – major (hip and spine surgery)	
Orthopaedic – minor (knee surgery)	Pulmonary renal/liver transplant	
Urologic – minor	Urologic – major	

Adapted from Boersma E, Kertai MD, Schouten O, et al. Perioperative cardiovascular mortality in noncardiac surgery: validation of the Lee cardiac risk index. *Am J Med*, 2005;118(10):1134–41.

The Use of Scoring Systems

Numerous scoring systems exist to help risk stratify patients pre-operatively, both specifically for those undergoing bariatric surgery, and for the surgical population as a whole, although the latter rarely includes a measurement of BMI (Table 15.3).

Bariatric Scoring Systems

Obesity Surgical Mortality Risk Score (OS-MRS)

OS-MRS is a scoring system for risk assessment and stratification in bariatric surgery. OS-MRS assigns a point to each one of five pre-operative variables, and based on this score, the patient is allocated a risk class (see Table 15.4). This simple tool can be

Table 15.3 Examples of useful risk scoring systems

Bariatric scoring systems	Non-bariatric scoring systems
Obesity surgery mortality risk score (OS-MRS)*	ASA
Edmonton obesity staging system (EOSS)*	Lee's revised cardiac risk index
	P-POSSUM
	American College of Surgeons surgical risk calculator*

*includes obesity-related parameters

easily calculated in the pre-assessment clinic and patients with OS-MRS of 4 or more should be considered high risk.

Edmonton Obesity Staging System (EOSS)

The less well-known EOSS system categorises obese patients into one of five stages incorporating obesity-related co-morbidities and functional status, and is used to guide surgical and non-surgical treatment decision options for the patient. A retrospective study has shown an EOSS ≥2 correlates with a higher mortality; however, further validation is required.

Non-Bariatric Scoring Systems

ASA Grading

The American Society of Anaesthetists physical status classification system is the most commonly used scoring system amongst anaesthetists in the UK. It relies on subjective assessment of a patient's co-morbidity. Simple and easy to use, it makes no risk modification for operative procedure and subject demographics (age and BMI for example). Also, inter-observer reliability of the score has been questioned due to the substantial subjective element. It therefore has a low PPV for individual risk and is best placed for predicting cohort risk.

Lee's Revised Cardiac Risk Index

RCRI is a key part of the American Heart Association guidelines, used to estimate a patient's risk of cardiac complications in non-cardiac surgery. Each of the six risk

Table 15.4 Obesity surgical mortality risk score

Risk factor	Score	
BMI >50 kg/m^2	0–1	**Mortality risk**
Male gender	0–1	**Class A (0–1 points) 0.26%**
Age >45 years	0–1	**Class B (2–3 points) 1.33%**
Hypertension	0–1	**Class C (4–5 points) 4.34%**
Risk factors for pulmonary embolism (PE):	0–1	**As score increases, mortality and post-operative complications increase.**
• Previous venous thromboembolism (VTE)		
• Vena caval filter		
• Hypoventilation (OSA)		
• Pulmonary hypertension		

Adapted from Thomas H, Agrawal S. Systematic review of obesity surgery mortality risk score: preoperative risk stratification in bariatric surgery. *Obes Surg*. 2012;22(7):1135–40.)

Table 15.5 Lee's revised cardiac risk index

Risk Factor	Score	
History of ischaemic heart disease	0–1	**Risk for cardiac death, non-fatal MI, and non-fatal cardiac arrest:**
History of congestive heart failure	0–1	
History of cerebrovascular disease (stroke or transient ischemic attack)	0–1	**0 = 0.4%**
History of diabetes with pre-operative insulin use	0–1	**1 = 0.9%**
Pre-operative creatinine >2 mg/dl or 176.8 μmol/l	0–1	**2 = 6.6%**
Intrathoracic, intraperitoneal, or suprainguinal vascular surgery	0–1	**≥3 = >11%**

Adapted from Lee TH, Marcantonio ER, Mangione CM, et al. Derivation and prospective validation of a simple index for prediction of cardiac risk of major noncardiac surgery. *Circulation*. 1999;100(10): 1043–9.

factors within the RCRI carry equal weighting, and the risk of peri-operative cardiac complications increases with the number of risk factors present (see Table 15.5). It is able to discriminate moderately well between those at low and high risk of peri-operative cardiac events, and in addition can allow decisions to be made regarding pre-operative cardiac interventions. It does not take into account whether the patient is obese.

Physiological and Operative Severity Score for the Enumeration of Mortality and Morbidity (POSSUM)

Of all the current scoring systems used in the peri-operative setting, POSSUM is probably one of the most widely adopted. Its purpose was to allow for risk adjustment between differing surgeons and

units, hence allowing fair comparison of outcomes rather than relying on crude mortality and morbidity rates. POSSUM comprises 12 physiological variables and 6 operative parameters for its calculation. These parameters are weighted and the score gives a percentage prediction of post-operative morbidity and mortality. There is a tendency to overpredict mortality in low-risk patients, which has led to a modification with the Portsmouth POSSUM (P-POSSUM). Once again, this scoring system does not take into account whether the patient is obese.

The American College of Surgeons Surgical Risk Calculator

This contemporary scoring system from the US uses 21 patient-specific variables (including

BMI) to calculate risk of a major adverse cardiac event (MACE), death, and eight other outcomes within 30 days following surgery. This risk calculator may offer the best estimation of surgery-specific risk of a MACE and death, but has only been validated in the National Surgical Quality Improvement Program population in the US to date (www.riskcalculator.facs.org).

Investigations

Most routine pre-operative investigations do not help to predict peri-operative risk and rarely lead to a change in management. Local guidelines and protocols will help avoid unnecessary tests, but there will be situations where more advanced investigations are justified, and novel blood tests may also aid risk stratification.

Biomarkers

One of the most promising biomarkers is B-type natriuretic peptide (BNP) and its precursor N-terminal pro-B-type natriuretic peptide (NT-proBNP). These are peptides secreted by cardiac ventricular myocytes in response to ventricular wall stress and ischaemia. Elevated levels of BNP are seen in patients with heart failure, and correlate with prognosis both in cardiac failure and after acute myocardial infarction. In the general surgical population, there is growing evidence of their predictive ability for short- and long-term adverse cardiac events and mortality. They have also been shown to have a high NPV, but care must be taken with obese patients, as there can be a paradoxical reduction in BNP levels.

Echocardiography

The use of echocardiography in the peri-operative setting to predict cardiac risk is controversial. It is useful to detect anatomical abnormalities, assess valve function and determine if there is any regional wall abnormality. In obese patients, there is often important pathology identified attributable to systemic hypertension (left ventricular hypertrophy and diastolic dysfunction) pulmonary hypertension and right-sided heart failure. There is an assumption that with increased body habitus, a transthoracic approach will not yield good-quality images, however in the majority of patients this is not the case and image quality is usually more than sufficient.

Routine echocardiography is performed at rest and therefore does not reflect the dynamic cardiac response that occurs during surgery. A stress echocardiogram can be performed to observe any stress-inducible myocardial ischaemia; this yields a greater PPV for cardiac risk assessment when compared to static tests.

Functional Capacity

Measuring functional capacity is a key part of predicting risk. The rationale is that surgery is associated with a stress response and a resultant increase in oxygen consumption, which continues days after surgery. To meet these demands, there is an increase in oxygen delivery from an increased cardiac output to prevent oxygen debt. Individuals who are unable to meet these demands have been shown to have a worse post-operative outcome. Measuring functional capacity can be either subjective, by using patient-centred questionnaires, or objective, where specific markers of oxygen uptake can be measured.

Subjective Approach

Various tools are available to correlate levels of activity with oxygen consumption. The Duke activity status index is a simple questionnaire, asking what the patient's maximal level of exertion is for 12 differing activities. From this, their oxygen consumption in terms of metabolic equivalents (METs) is estimated. One MET equates to 3.5 ml/kg/min of oxygen consumption, and represents basal oxygen consumption. Varying degrees of exercise are assigned a number of METs, and achieving >4 METs (stair climbing, swimming) marks good aerobic fitness and lower risk for major surgery. Unfortunately, there is a tendency for patients to overestimate their ability and hence their peri-operative risk.

Objective Approach

Cardiopulmonary Exercise Testing

CPET is seen as the gold standard for measuring functional capacity, and there is growing evidence demonstrating its ability to predict peri-operative outcome. It is a non-invasive incremental exercise test in which breath-by-breath gas analysis allows calculation of oxygen consumption, carbon dioxide production and minute ventilation. There are numerous variables that can be calculated, but in terms of

Table 15.6 Typical threshold values obtained at CPET indicating low risk values

Parameter	Value
Anaerobic threshold	>11 ml.kg^{-1}
Peak VO$_2$	>15.8 ml.kg^{-1}
VE/VECO$_2$	<34

Adapted from McCullough PA, Gallagher MJ, deJong AT, et al. Cardiorespiratory fitness and short-term complications after bariatric surgery. *Chest.* 2006;130(2):517–25.

risk assessment, there are three that have been found to be most predictive (Table 15.6):

- *Anaerobic threshold (AT)* is the oxygen consumption at which, with increased exercise, aerobic metabolism is unable to sustain adequate ATP synthesis. After AT is reached, aerobic metabolism does not cease, rather anaerobic supplementation begins, consequently increasing blood lactate levels. AT is effort independent, and can be improved with training.
- *Peak oxygen consumption (VO$_2$ peak)* is the maximal oxygen consumption that an individual obtains during CPET.
- *Ventilatory equivalents for carbon dioxide (VE/VCO$_2$)* are described by the ratio of minute ventilation (VE) to the amount of CO$_2$ produced. They are unitless numbers that describe the efficiency of the cardiorespiratory system to exchange gas.

There is growing evidence supporting the use of CPET as a risk stratification tool, but most of the studies to date have been observational and unblinded. In the bariatric population, there have been two publications demonstrating increased post-operative complications and length of hospital stay in those individuals with poor functional capacity. With increasing body weight, interpreting the data can be difficult as the majority of the variables are indexed and based on total body weight.

CPET is, however, labour intensive, requiring significant resources. Alternatives are available, but do not provide the same level of detail. The 6MWT, ISWT and stair climbing test can all be used in situations where CPET is not available. The stair climbing test measures the vertical height an individual can ascend. Values <12 m achieved have correlated with poor surgical outcome.

The 6MWT measures how far the individual can walk on the flat at a normal pace in 6 minutes, with median values of 500 m seen in healthy subjects. The ISWT uses an audio signal to direct the walking pace back and forth between two cones 10 m apart. The walking speed is increased every minute and the test ends when the patient cannot reach the turning point. This test has a greater correlation with peak oxygen uptake than the 6MWT, but is more dependent on patient motivation. The 6MWT and ISWT have been validated and are reproducible in the obese population.

Patients with poor functional capacity should be counselled on alternative treatments where possible. Appropriate organisation should be in place for those who are deemed high risk to have critical care admission post-operatively.

Conclusions

With the increase in obesity prevalence, risk scoring amongst the bariatric population remains underinvestigated. Although scoring systems are available, there are few that are bariatric-specific, and of those which are available, only OS-MRS has been validated. Regardless of which scoring system is used, risk stratification through appropriate pre-operative assessment, identification/optimisation of key co-morbidities such as OSA, metabolic syndrome and cardiac disease are essential to reduce patient risk.

Further Reading

Boersma E, Kertai MD, Schouten O, et al. Perioperative cardiovascular mortality in noncardiac surgery: validation of the Lee cardiac risk index. *Am J Med.* 2005;118(10) 1134–41.

Flum DR, Salem L, Broeckel Elrod., et al. Early mortality among medicare beneficiaries undergoing bariatric surgical procedures. *JAMA.* 2005;294(15): 1903–8.

Glance LG, Wissler R, Mukamel DB, et al. Perioperative outcomes among patients with the modified metabolic syndrome who are undergoing noncardiac surgery. *Anesthesiology.* 2010;113(4):859–72.

Gurunathan U, Myles PS. Limitations of body mass index as an obesity measure of perioperative risk. *Br J Anaesth.* 2016;116(3):319–21.

Hennis PJ, Meale PM, Hurst RA, et al. Cardiopulmonary exercise testing predicts postoperative outcome in patients undergoing gastric bypass surgery. *Br J Anaesth.* 2012;109 (4):566–71.

Lerakis S, Kalogeropoulos AP, El-Chami MF, et al. Transthoracic dobutamine stress echocardiography in patients undergoing bariatric surgery. *Obes Surg.* 2007;17 (11):1475–81.

McCullough PA, Gallagher MJ, deJong AT, et al. Cardiorespiratory fitness and short-term complications after bariatric surgery. *Chest.* 2006;130(2):517–25.

Mullen J, Moorman D, Davenport D. The obesity paradox: body mass index and outcomes in patients undergoing nonbariatric general surgery. *Ann Surg.* 2009;250 (1):166–72.

Thomas H, Agrawal S. Systematic review of obesity surgery mortality risk score: preoperative risk stratification in bariatric surgery. *Obes Surg.* 2012;22(7):1135–40.

Peri-operative Anaesthetic Implications in the Obese Child

Helen Smith and Liam Brennan

Introduction

Childhood obesity is a global public health problem. Between 1980 and 2013, the worldwide incidence of childhood obesity had increased by 47% with developed countries demonstrating the greatest upsurge. In England, the incidence of obesity is more than 20% amongst 5-year-olds, rising to 30% by age 11 years, with 82% of these becoming obese adults. Combating obesity, particularly its prevention, is central to healthcare strategy for England. It is an epidemic that is a major societal challenge as it places considerable strain on existing services. The cost to the UK economy of obesity was estimated at £15.8 billion per year in 2007, including £4.2 billion in costs to the NHS.

Extensive published literature exists about the anaesthetic implications for the obese adult, but until 15 years ago there was very little on anaesthetic management of the obese child. This has been redressed in recent years with an explosion of articles focusing on childhood obesity in the peri-operative period. This demonstrates that not only is the problem growing, but that those involved in anaesthetising obese children are struggling with the challenges they frequently encounter.

Besides the clinical issues, childhood obesity raises questions about potential safeguarding (child protection) concerns that are an issue for all healthcare professionals involved in caring for children, including anaesthetists.

Definition

Defining childhood obesity has been a challenge. The adult criteria of a body mass index greater than 30 kg/m^2 is not relevant to growing children. However, epidemiological work led by Cole et al., drawing on data from close to 200 000 children worldwide has produced centile curves taking into account age and gender. Childhood obesity is defined as position on or above the body mass index curve that passes through the 30 kg/m^2 point at 18 years of age.

Aetiology

Undoubtedly the commonest cause of childhood obesity worldwide is calorie intake in excess of output compounded by an increasingly sedentary lifestyle with less outdoor play. Children with simple obesity are more than often >50th centile for height whereas a child who is <5th centile is more like to be syndromic. Only a small percentage of cases are due to endocrine and genetic diseases such as hypothyroidism, Cushing's, Bardet–Biedl or Prader–Willi syndromes. An alteration of leptin production or interference with the leptin receptor has been demonstrated in a number of genetic disorders associated with obesity. The polypeptide hormone, leptin, is produced within adipocytes and interacts with receptors in the central nervous system, most importantly in the hypothalamus. When the body is in a positive energy state, there is a rise in the leptin level, which increases satiety.

Co-morbidities

Co-morbidities related to childhood obesity may well be significant, but are all too frequently underdiagnosed. Hypertension, type 2 diabetes, asthma, obstructive sleep apnoea (OSA), gastro-oesophageal reflux disease (GORD) and non-alcoholic steatohepatitis (NASH) may be found regularly in children with a raised BMI (Table 16.1).

All respiratory variables are decreased in the obese child, particularly forced vital capacity (FVC) and functional residual capacity (FRC) with the resultant high closing volume potentially leading to atelectasis, air trapping and intra-pulmonary right to left shunting, leading to hypoxaemia. Reduced static lung volumes and impaired diffusion capacity correlate with the level of obesity. OSA is a major problem associated with obesity and one particular study has demonstrated a rate in the obese child as high as 17%. In addition, obesity-related hypoventilation with CO_2 retention and chronic hypoxaemia has been described

Table 16.1 Co-morbidities associated with childhood obesity

RESPIRATORY	ASTHMA AND BRONCHIAL HYPERREACTIVITY ↑UPPER RESPIRATORY TRACT INFECTIONS OBSTRUCTIVE SLEEP APNOEA
Cardiovascular	Hypertension Left ventricular wall thickening
Endocrine	Type 2 diabetes Metabolic syndrome Dyslipidaemia
Gastrointestinal	Gastro-oesophageal reflux Non-alcoholic steatohepatitis
Neurological/ psychological	Pseudotumour cerebri Low self-esteem

in some children. Asthma and associated bronchial reactivity have a greater incidence in the obese child, with around 30% of obese children aged 8–18 years suffering, matched by increasing severity according to the degree of obesity. This is compounded by an increased susceptibility to upper respiratory tract infections.

There is a close link with hypertension, elevated triglycerides, low HDL-cholesterol and glucose intolerance, which cumulatively is known as the paediatric metabolic syndrome associated with obesity. In the USA, this syndrome is present in 30–50% of overweight adolescents. In the United Kingdom, there is a large increase in the number of children developing type 2 diabetes, a disease that traditionally only affected adults, with children as young as 7 years old now developing the disease.

A further problem for the obese child with type 2 diabetes is the potential to develop significant liver disease. NASH in obese children is reasonably common, but frequently underdiagnosed; 6% of overweight and 10% of obese children within the USA have been shown to have elevated liver enzymes. Hyperinsulinaemia with its inhibitory effect on free fatty acid oxidation leads to fat accumulation in the liver. Of those children who have NASH diagnosed following a liver biopsy, 95% also meet the criteria for insulin resistance. Over time this may lead to more significant liver-related problems, with implications for altered drug handling and life-threatening issues such as portal hypertension and end-stage liver disease.

GOR is more common in the overweight child, with 20% suffering symptoms as compared to 2% of

normal weight. However, a study of 1000 day-case patients aged 2–12 years showed no increase in gastric fluid volume or gastric acidity in the child with raised BMI and no cases of pulmonary aspiration, leading to a recommendation that the standard starvation guidelines should apply to the obese child.

Childhood obesity leads to cardiovascular changes with an increased heart rate, greater resting and reactive hyperaemic blood flow, larger brachial artery diameter, suggesting an adaptive hyperaemic state. There is also an increased left ventricular wall thickening, which is an independent risk factor for morbidity and mortality. This strength of association between obesity and wall thickening increases with age. Childhood obesity appears to confer a lifetime risk of cardiovascular disease with an important effect on cardiac structure, which persists into adult life. A reduction in cholesterol and blood pressure does help to reduce the morbidity and mortality risks, even if weight is not reduced. Although this highlights the importance of preventative and treatment measures for obesity, it also highlights the potentially serious peri-operative implications for children who have been severely obese for a prolonged period of time.

Psychological Aspects

The obese child may be of substantial weight and height, but psychologically can be much younger than they look. In addition, the psychological abuse they may well suffer from peers can lead to a more immature response to stressful situations. A recent study redefines obesity in adolescence as a multilayered brain disorder with compromised motivation and control, an imbalance between reward, emotional memories and cognitive control. The low esteem that is felt by these children may not only lead to further obesity, but can be explained by disrupted functional connectivity within the brain. It is important for the anaesthetist to be fully aware of the potential psychological issues when building a relationship with the obese paediatric patient and their parents/carers, particularly adolescents who may well have the added insecurity of body image associated with puberty.

Pre-assessment

In terms of pre-assessment there are disorders related to childhood obesity dependent upon the extent and longevity of the problem.

As mentioned above, asthma, hypertension, metabolic syndrome, type 2 diabetes, fatty liver and OSA may be present. The associated conditions need to be optimised whenever possible, the peri-operative plan and risks discussed with the patient and parents, as well as the intra-operative team and any special arrangements for post-operative care organised well in advance, particularly if high dependency unit (HDU) or ICU care is a requirement.

Diagnosis of the surgical condition may be problematic and can lead to a late diagnosis, making the need for emergency surgery an even greater challenge for the anaesthetist.

Pharmacology

Obesity affects the pharmacokinetics of most anaesthetic agents, however child-specific data is lacking. A study by Burke in 2014 showed that due to lack of data and recommendations for dosage in the obese child there have been significant gaps in understanding. As a direct result, obese children are more likely to receive medication outside the recommended range than those of normal weight. The most important consideration in drug dosing of the obese child are lean, total and ideal body weights (Table 16.2).

For calculation of ideal body weight (IBW) and lean body weight (LBW):

IBW = BMI @ 50th percentile × (height in metres)^2

LBW = IBW × 0.3 (TBW – IBW)

The prediction of which category of body weight to use for an individual drug in a specific child is problematic. The volume of distribution for some highly lipophilic drugs is increased in obesity, but for others is decreased. Generally, hydrophilic drugs should be administered according to the IBW. However, the most studied drug in the obese child is succinylcholine, which should be dosed according to the TBW as there is an increase in the level of pseudocholinesterase. Special consideration needs to be taken of those children with NASH and obesity-associated glomerulonephritis, where elimination of drugs may be highly complex. There are, in addition, certain important drugs where the data is insufficient, for example, midazolam. Clearly, overdosing risks prolong recovery from anaesthesia and cardiorespiratory depression whilst underdosing may be associated with accidental awareness during anaesthesia.

Induction

Securing vascular access may be a major problem in some obese children. The use of local anaesthetic creams to facilitate awake cannulation may lead to even greater difficulty, particularly if it leads to vasoconstriction (e.g. EMLA). This may lead to the greater use of inhalational induction for the most obese patients. The potential airway concerns, such as difficult bag-mask ventilation in the obese child may lead to a challenging induction without intravenous access. The need for two appropriately trained anaesthetists at induction may be required, particularly when difficult ventilation is anticipated alongside difficult intravenous cannulation. If the child is distressed, then added airway secretions might add to the complexity of the clinical scenario. The potential risk of gastro-oesophageal reflux and aspiration has not been demonstrated in the obese paediatric population. There is, however, a concern about a more

Table 16.2 Intravenous drug dosage in the obese child

Drug	Profile	Induction according to	Maintenance according to
Thiopental	Lipophilic	LBW	
Propofol	Lipophilic	LBW	TBW
Succinylcholine	Hydrophilic	TBW	
Non-depolarising neuromuscular blocking agents	Hydrophilic	IBW	IBW
Fentanyl, alfentanil, sufentanil	Lipophilic	TBW	LBW
Morphine	Lipophilic	IBW	IBW
Remifentanil	Lipophilic	LBW	LBW

Total body weight (TBW), ideal body weight (IBW), lean body weight (LBW).

reactive airway, with the risk of bronchospasm and laryngeal spasm cited as recurring problems. The ability to manage these episodes is compounded by the increased weight on the chest and abdomen requiring increased inspiratory pressure to achieve adequate ventilation.

Airway Maintenance

Maintenance of the airway depends upon the type of surgery as well as the condition of the patient. Due to increased airway reactivity in the obese child, some authors advocate the use of a laryngeal mask airway. Others are concerned about the theoretical risks of reflux, aspiration and atelectasis, and only perform tracheal intubation. There has been concern about potential difficult intubation with some authors reporting multiple attempts at laryngoscopy in the more obese child, while others not finding any difficulty compared to matched non-obese peers. The greater weight on the chest and abdomen from adipose tissue may lead to severe atelectasis and difficulty in maintaining good oxygenation and CO_2 clearance without intermittent positive pressure ventilation (IPPV) and the use of positive end expired pressure (PEEP). This is particularly important in those children managed in the lithotomy, Trendelenberg or prone positions, where diaphragmatic splinting may occur.

Difficult mask ventilation, airway obstruction and oxygen desaturation with an overall increase in critical respiratory events are encountered during anaesthesia for the obese child. Particular associated risk factors are: procedures that include the airway, children under the age of 10 years and presence of OSA. High BMI and sleep disordered breathing are independent predictors of laryngospasm during the peri-operative period. What is evident is that obese children who have sleep disordered breathing are at greater risk of airway problems. However, severe obesity alone in the paediatric population is a significant risk factor for peri-operative adverse events. The increased incidence of asthma and airway reactivity makes this group of children particularly challenging. This can lead to airway problems in recovery and a longer post-operative stay. In addition, some studies have shown a higher requirement for unexpected overnight stay in hospital following anaesthesia, even for minor surgical procedures.

Monitoring

As in adults, obesity may compromise the ability to adequately monitor the patient in the peri-operative period. Of particular importance is the need for an appropriately sized non-invasive blood pressure (NIBP) cuff; undersized cuffs produce inaccurate data showing falsely high recordings. For the more severely obese child the conical shape of the limbs may render the NIBP cuff unusable and arterial monitoring may need to be instituted, particularly for more major surgery. An added advantage of this is blood gas analysis can be undertaken and assist with the management of ventilation. In the obese child, there is a greater discrepancy between the end tidal and the arterial CO_2 levels. Pulse oximetry may be affected by the increase in body mass, ear probes or wrap-around finger probes may assist with this problem. The bispectral index (BIS) monitor is increasingly being used, of particular importance in the obese child, especially when undertaking total intravenous anaesthesia (TIVA) due to the altered pharmacology and to mitigate against the risk of accidental awareness during general anaesthesia. Higher tissue resistance associated with excess adiposity can produce falsely low voltage ECG readings.

Pain Management

The indiscriminate use of peri-operative opioids may lead to prolonged stay in post-operative recovery, overnight hospital stays or even require paediatric intensive care unit (PICU) admission, especially in those overweight children with sleep disordered breathing. The advantage of regional anaesthesia is a reduction in the potential respiratory depression, as well as better pain relief, with post-operative pulmonary function returning to normal levels faster than with the use of opioids. The use of regional analgesia is advocated where possible, but technical difficulties may make this problematic. The challenges are obscured anatomical landmarks, increased depth to neurovascular bundle and positioning. The increasing use of ultrasound in performing regional blockade may mean that a good analgesic result is far more likely in the obese child than before sonographic equipment and skills were widely available. Poor patient compliance means that the majority of blocks will be performed in the anaesthetised child. The most important factor is optimal positioning of the patient for the intervention, in addition to availability of the correct equipment (e.g. longer needles).

Positioning

Positioning obese children may be problematic and older paediatric patients with high BMI will require the same range of adjuvants to enable safe movement without harming patient or staff. The inability to move the obese child easily as compared to the non-obese child with added facilities such as airbed transfers needs careful preparation, particularly in facilities that do not routinely manage morbidly obese patients. The equipment required includes operating tables of sufficient width and weight limits alongside relevant straps and padding for positioning. These are not part of everyday practice for dedicated paediatric teams and need specific consideration. Appropriate patient supports may be difficult to source and require time and planning to enable surgery to take place.

The increased duration of surgery due to surgical access problems make positioning of the patient and placement on the operating table very important, with good padding of all susceptible areas and clear attention to detail. Nerve damage is more likely in the obese child. The adipose tissue is less well-perfused and therefore prolonged surgery can lead to tissue ischaemia unless the utmost care is undertaken to pad affected areas and good perfusion maintained by attention to fluid therapy and maintenance of mean arterial pressure.

Fluid Management

The blood vessels within fat tissue are multiple and bleed easily, making excessive blood loss an increased risk in the obese child. This, alongside the difficulties of managing fluid therapy according to lean body weight rather than total body weight, presents a particular challenge for the anaesthetist.

Post-operative Care

As highlighted above, children with a raised BMI can be challenging in the peri-operative period. They may have a prolonged stay within the post-operative recovery area, with an increased requirement for unexpected overnight stay in hospital, particularly related to airway issues such as upper airway obstruction. Indeed, for those undergoing surgery involving the airway, overnight hospitalisation is recommended, particularly those with sleep disordered breathing.

Consideration of the HDU or PICU for those with potentially life-threatening complications, those who have high opioid requirements and ongoing monitoring needs such as those with obstructive sleep apnoea undergoing emergency laparotomy is necessary. The increased need for HDU/PICU has implications for planning for the procedure (as well as cost) particularly in a district general hospital where these facilities may not be present.

Bariatric Surgery

Prevention appears to be the most important factor in the management of childhood obesity. Lifestyle changes for the whole family, eating healthily and exercise with less sedentary activity are the mainstay of treatment. However long-term weight loss is difficult to attain.

Bariatric surgery has demonstrated a reversal of metabolic complications and cardiac structural and functional changes of the more severely obese adolescent. Until recently bariatric surgery was not considered in children, but there are currently two centres in the UK that offer weight reduction therapy as a surgical option. Guidelines for clinicians when considering weight-loss surgery in children have been produced by the UK National Institute for Health and Clinical Excellence (NICE) in 2006 (Table 16.3). Childhood obesity confers an increased lifetime risk of cardiovascular disease. The onset of type 2 diabetes with associated complications is significant. Both type 2 diabetes and hypertension are reversible with weight loss. The seriousness of the effects of childhood obesity on future health is why this had been offered for certain categories of paediatric patients. In the UK, only those fulfilling the NICE criteria are considered for surgery, and almost exclusively adolescents over 16 years old.

The procedures available are no different to those undertaken in adults. Surgery is associated with complications, including gastro-intestinal perforation, wound infection, gastric band slippage and obstruction. Nausea and vomiting alongside gastro-oesophageal reflux are longer-term side effects that can emerge with certain procedures.

The implication for anaesthesia is twofold; firstly, peri-operative management of such cases and secondly anaesthetising children who have undergone such procedures in the past. The centres that offer bariatric surgery are equipped with specialist teams with equipment and expertise, including

Table 16.3 NICE guidelines for bariatric surgery in children

- Bariatric surgery may only be considered for young people in exceptional circumstances
- Need to have achieved/nearly achieved physiological maturity
- The young person commits to the need for long-term follow-up
- Should be undertaken only by a multidisciplinary team that can provide paediatric expertise in:
  - Pre-operative assessment
  - Dietetic advice
  - Management of co-morbidities
  - Intra-operative management (paediatric surgeon and anaesthetist)
  - Post-operative care (including PICU)
  - Psychological support (child psychologist)
  - Plastic surgery

multidisciplinary team evaluation (which includes a psychologist) with screening for associated co-morbidities.

Child Safeguarding

The increased incidence of childhood obesity and the recognised complications of this problem have led to concerns regarding the possibility of child neglect and therefore the potential for child safeguarding (child protection) concerns. Currently, although childhood obesity in isolation is not a child safeguarding issue, persistent failure to engage in weight loss programmes despite repeated emphasis to the parents of the risk to the child's health indicates possible child neglect. What is becoming clear both in the UK and the USA is that obesity may be part of wider concerns about neglect and emotional abuse, particularly in the younger child. When agencies explore such concerns, assessment needs to include family and environmental factors.

As anaesthetists, we have an important role in child protection. Any concerns that emerge from our involvement with the family need discussion with senior paediatric colleagues, usually the designated clinician with child protection responsibilities. In such cases it is important not to tackle the parents or child directly, but to work through the appropriate designated child protection structure in place for the facility in which the child is being managed.

Further Reading

Burke CN, Voepel-Lewis T, Wagner D, et al. A retrospective description of anesthetic medication dosing in overweight and obese children. *Paediatr Anaesth.* 2014;24:857–62.

El-Metainy S, Ghoneim T, Aridae E, et al. Incidence of perioperative adverse events in obese children undergoing elective general surgery. *Br J Anaesth.* 2011;106:359–63.

Lin C. Impact of obesity in pediatric anesthesia. *Adv Anesth.* 2007;25:79–101.

Marcus CL, Curtis S, Koerner CB, et al. Evaluation of pulmonary function and polysomnography in obese children and adolescents. *Pediatr Pulmonol.* 1996;21:176–83.

Mortensen A, Lenz K, Abildstrom H, et al. Anesthetizing the obese child. *Pediatr Anesth.* 2011;21:623–9.

Nafiu OO, Reynolds PI, Bamgbade OA, et al. Childhood body mass index and perioperative complications. *Paediatr Anaesth.* 2007;17:426–30.

National Institute for Health and Clinical Excellence (NICE). *Obesity: Clinical Guideline 43.* London: National Institute for Health and Clinical Excellence; 2006.

Owen J, John R. Childhood obesity and the anaesthetist. *Contin Edu Anaesth, Crit Care Pain.* 2012;12:169–75.

Ross PA, Scott GM. Childhood obesity: a growing problem for the pediatric anesthesiologist. *Semin Anesth, Periop Med Pain.* 2006;25:142–8.

Setzer N, Saade E. Childhood obesity and anesthetic morbidity. *Paediatr Anaesth.* 2007;17:321–6.

Shield JPH, Crowne E, Morgan J. Is there a place for bariatric surgery in treating childhood obesity? *Arch Dis Child.* 2008;93:369–72.

Smith HL, Meldrum DJ, Brennan LJ. Childhood obesity a challenge for the anaesthetist? *Pediatr Anesth.* 2002;12: 750–61.

Tait AR, Voepel-Lewis T, Burke C, et al. Incidence and risk factors for perioperative adverse respiratory events in children who are obese. *Anesthesiology.* 2008;108:375–80.

Ward and Operating Room Equipment for the Obese

Paul Ayrton and Andrew Lewitt

Introduction

Manual handling of any load is recognised as potentially hazardous; in UK law the Manual Handling Operations Regulations 1992 help to define within a hospital trust how it should operate and what systems should be in place to ensure the safety of anyone who may have some involvement in moving loads.

This is achieved primarily through a robust risk assessment process to reduce the risks involved in handling activities to the lowest level achievable. Risk assessments are critical in determining the actions that need to be taken to ensure that any handling activity is performed as safely as possible.

Peri-operative handling of the morbidly obese patient is a dynamic process: an episode that runs from admission to discharge, where planning for the latter needs to be instigated on admission in order to avoid later delays. There are measures available that can facilitate this process, whilst simultaneously promoting patient and staff safety, and building the patient's confidence in the organisation's ability to deliver safe, effective and suitable care in all circumstances.

There are numerous publications that address anaesthetic and surgical components of obesity care. However little or no reference is made to the movement and positioning of the patient. There is limited published material specific to the manual handling of the obese patient. Much of what follows is based on practical experience and problem-solving by the University Hospitals of Leicester Manual Handling Service.

Much depends on assessment of the patient, e.g. in pre-assessment clinic, where information can be gathered about their anthropometrics and mobility. This, combined with information on the procedure they are to undergo and likely effect on post-operative recovery, should inform the receiving ward and/or operating department as to whether specialist equipment or techniques may be required and to what degree.

The patient's individual manual handling assessment should be a dynamic process, with changes documented and communicated to all parties involved in the patient's management throughout the episode. *Remember*: the weight of the patient is not the only determining factor in how to approach care.

Consideration should also be given to the increased amount of space required for the safer provision of care. This factor has been identified over a variety of tasks, including lateral transfer and urgent interventions such as resuscitation.

Selecting the Most Appropriate Bed

A patient entering hospital via a pre-assessment clinic should already have equipment needs identified for the whole of their hospital episode. It is likely their capabilities will change, if only for a short period. Specialised equipment may therefore be necessary for a period post-operatively that was not required pre-operatively.

For a standard ward, the minimum equipment requirements include:

- A bedside chair of suitable weight capacity, seat width and seat height (ideally also height-adjustable) and with a seat cushion offering low to moderate pressure relief.
- A four-section electric profiling bed of appropriate weight capacity. This may be the standard ward bed or a more specialist bed that can be increased/decreased in width independently at each section and in two stages, to better fit the patient's body shape and with the greatest range of height to facilitate safer care and promote patient independence throughout their stay.
- The bed should have a matching, suitable sleep surface that expands with the bedframe.
  The mattress itself may have an impact upon a patient's post-operative mobility; our experience suggests that although an alternating/low air loss mattress may be indicated from a tissue viability

perspective, their very nature may impact upon the patient's ability to move. A foam mattress is likely to have a firmer surface to assist with patient movement within the bed.

- A commode/shower chair (the toilet/wet-room facility must have suitable width of access to allow easy entrance and exit with the occupied commode chair).
- A means of recovering a fallen patient who is unable to get up from the floor independently, e.g. a heavy duty mobile hoist system such as the Liko Viking XL (safe working load (SWL) 300 kg), a mobile lifting platform such as the 'MD350 lifter' (SWL 349 kg) or air-powered lifting device such as 'Hover-jack' (SWL 450 kg). Only those who are both trained and competent in its safe and appropriate use must use these items of equipment.

There is a variety of bariatric beds available that can be used. The appropriate type may be determined by the capabilities and characteristics of the patient. Many patients may well be within the given SWL of a standard bed (often 180 kg), but their shape may mean that the bed is too narrow to accommodate them post-operatively, should they need to be moved and repositioned by nursing/medical staff. It is likely therefore that a wider bed is necessary. Equally, a shorter patient may struggle with access to and from a wider bed if the bed does not go low enough. This may impact on post-operative mobilisation.

Our experience suggests that although there are various types of bariatric beds available, the most flexible type is a four section, with each section extendable and a very low minimum height. This type of bed allows the greatest number of options within the ward environment, and can, if necessary, be used as the operating table to accommodate the patient's size.

Transporting a Patient to Theatre

The options available for getting an obese patient to the operating department are:

- patient walks to the department;
- patient is moved in a wheelchair;
- patient is moved on a bed/trolley.

Despite their size and weight, most obese patients are capable of walking to theatre. This should be the default option. However, they may become breathless if the distance they have to walk is considerable. This may have a clinical impact and therefore may not be appropriate.

There may also be dignity issues. Larger (5XL) gowns should be available for use, which provide suitable cover for the patient. The patient may feel self-conscious walking along the hospital corridor in only a theatre gown and (perhaps) dressing gown.

Transfer to the theatre department via hospital wheelchair would reduce the likelihood of breathlessness becoming a factor. The caveat here is that the wheelchair is of the appropriate size and SWL for the patient, in good serviceable condition and that the appropriate numbers of staff are present to move the chair safely.

Another factor to consider is the patient's ability to get onto the theatre table/trolley. Some surfaces can be quite high, and the patient's own height and/or shape may make it difficult for them to climb onto the table/trolley independently. The use of a step – this needs to be of sufficient depth and width for the patient – or other means of raising the floor surface is an option, but this can raise its own problems; some people, especially if their mobility is limited, may find the height too much and struggle to climb onto the step. This may make the use of a wheelchair for transport inappropriate and they will have to be moved via bed or trolley.

Using a trolley to transfer may incur additional manual handling tasks, i.e. getting the patient onto the trolley in the ward environment. Another problem may be caused by the width of the patient, for example there are trolleys that have a SWL of 318 kg, but a mattress width of 67 cm. These would be too narrow for a patient with a hip width of greater than this and will impact on the patient's comfort during transfer. Subsequent transfer to the theatre table may be difficult, as there is limited space in which to tilt the patient onto their side in order to position a transfer board adequately.

It is our experience that most theatre patients who do not walk to theatre will be transported on their bed. The potential problem with this is the total load weight and how easy it is to move the bed with the patient in situ. Whilst having a very low minimum height can be advantageous when mobilising a patient from the bed post-operatively, some bariatric low beds may be quite difficult to move with a patient weighing in excess of 200 kg because of the small castor size necessary to achieve the minimum height

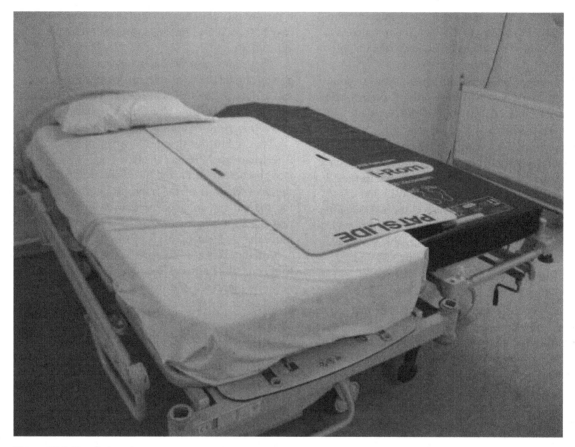

Figure 17.1 Transfer board.

of the bed. It is necessary therefore to ensure sufficient personnel are available to assist with the transport. This becomes a greater problem if an extreme emergency situation develops and there are other items, such as intravenous fluid stands and gas cylinders to be moved as well.

Transferring from Bed/Trolley to the Operating Table

Techniques employed in transferring a bariatric patient from a bed/trolley to the operating table will depend upon the equipment required. A fully mobile patient may be able to transfer from one surface to another, whereas a dependent patient is likely to require significant assistance. Several options can be considered in the latter case, depending upon the patient's clinical condition, shape and weight. A patient may be transferred efficiently using a basic bridging board and slide sheets (Figures 17.1 and 17.2) and the number of staff required, depending on the patient's level of consciousness; the weight rating of the board must be considered, along with the size of any gap between the two surfaces. If the patient has already been sedated and requires airway management support then four staff plus the airway person may be sufficient. More staff should be used if deemed appropriate. The movement should be quick and controlled, occurring in two or more stages.

With a much heavier patient (e.g. 200+ kg), using a transfer board may be effective, but may well involve a significant increase in number of staff and physical effort required. It may be necessary to use the bed sheet to assist the move, with some staff pushing the patient across whilst one or more staff on the receiving side holds the bed sheet and uses a step back

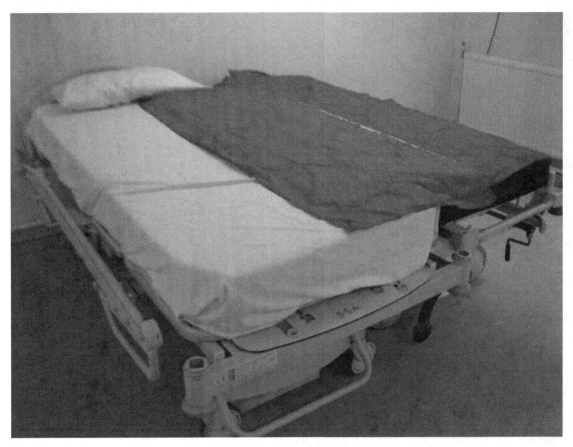

Figure 17.2 Slide sheets and board.

action to pull the patient over. An alternative may be an air-assisted transfer device (Figure 17.3), using an inflating mattress and air pump to create a thin cushion of air underneath the patient. This allows the transfer to take place at any speed, and therefore with a much greater level of control. The number of staff needed for the move may be the same or less than with a basic transfer board, even though the patient may be of a significant weight. With the patient already anaesthetised, an extra person is required to manage the airway. The use of this type of air system would allow reasonably easy adjustments of the patient on the table by inflating the transfer device and moving as little or as far as necessary.

Transferring the post-operative patient back to a bed does potentially pose other problems. If the patient is very tall, incorrect positioning on the bed may mean that the patient's ability to breathe may be compromised.

It should always be considered that although the operating table may have the capacity to take a patient (many tables will take up to 450 kg), the patient's shape might make it unsafe to use the table. A patient's width may be such that part of their body overhangs the edge(s) of the table. This may make the patient unstable on that surface. It will be necessary to ensure that tables capable of taking the patient's weight also have the capacity to extend the width of the operating surface to accommodate patient size/shape. Several manufacturers produce tables that can accommodate weight up to 450 kg and have side extensions to give support along the patient's torso and hips.

There also needs to be consideration of using the table to its best advantage for the surgeon. For example, has the table the capability to split the leg section, allowing the surgeon greater/alternative access?

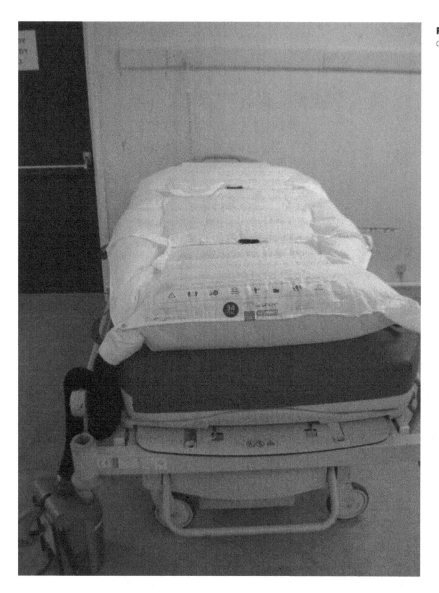

Figure 17.3 Air transfer mattress deployed.

Alternatively, it may be considered more appropriate/practical that the surgery should take place on the bed itself rather than on an operating table. This would reduce the need to transfer the patient at all. However, it may compromise the safety of the surgeon and/or anaesthetist and of the patient if either is not able to safely undertake their clinical roles.

Airway Management

Airway management of an obese patient may present problems. Thorough pre-operative assessment should highlight this. Most obese patients will prove straightforward, but there will be those whose weight at the upper torso will impact upon their ability to breathe effectively, and the size and shape of the patient's neck and shoulders may make it difficult to undertake airway procedures. This could be more difficult the larger the patient is, and the ability of the patient to lie flat will also have an implication for procedures.

If the patient is able to lie flat, but airway control proves inadequate it may be necessary to tilt the head backwards to assist; this may be difficult. Options include some support to raise the shoulders from the patient surface, which could

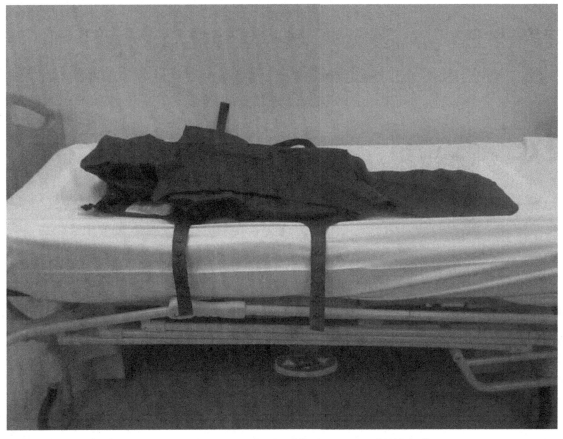

Figure 17.4 Wedge deflated. (Image – Trust's own, reproduced with kind permission of CJ Medical.)

be an ad-hoc system of a pillow underneath the shoulders. From a safe handling perspective this means placement should take place whilst the patient is conscious, otherwise it requires undesirable manual lifting of the head, neck and shoulders once the patient is anaesthetised. Neither option is particularly good and from a handling perspective, the latter is poor practice as it involves the physical lifting of a heavy load (i.e. the upper body). This could be as much as 62% of the entire body weight. The use of a foam wedge-type device would require the same actions in order to insert the wedge correctly. This type of action involves pulling, pushing, lifting and potentially working away from the handler's centre-of-gravity, all of these being factors for increasing the risk of a musculo-skeletal injury to staff.

An existing alternative is available in the form of an air wedge system that is positioned underneath the patient and inflated and deflated to allow the chest, head and neck to be altered to the required angles and facilitate the 'ramped' position.

The air wedge (Figures 17.4 and 17.5) can be used on a bed, as the patient's weight will help to hold it in place; it is designed with securing straps for use on an operating table and is relatively narrow. It is essential the patient be positioned centrally on the device prior to inflation. With a wider patient this may prove difficult, causing them to tilt to one side as it is inflated, therefore this must be considered before using the device. The wedge should be removed prior to transfer from one surface to another as they are not designed for this action, and doing so may compromise the safety of the patient.

There should also be several options considered pre-operatively, so that in the event of an unexpected situation arising there are alternatives already available. These will have to be based upon the patient's

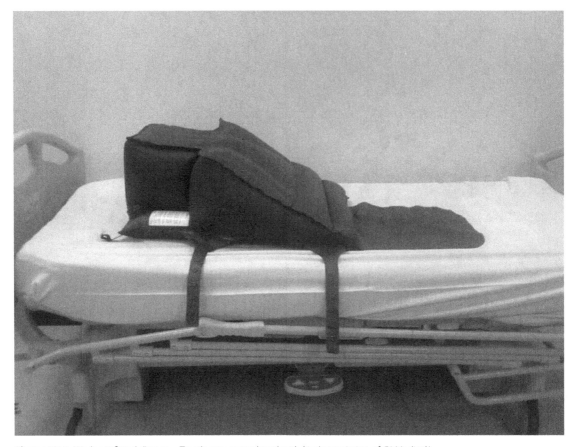

Figure 17.5 Wedge inflated. (Image – Trust's own, reproduced with kind permission of CJ Medical.)

clinical condition and the likely needs/requirements during intubation.

In emergency circumstances there may be no option but to physically lift the patient. This should always be a last resort.

Prone Position

The prone position is a high-risk challenge in the obese patient. Of primary concern is the control of the manoeuvre, whilst taking care that the patient's limbs are correctly positioned to avoid entrapment, and intravenous cannulae and tracheal tube are not dislodged. The patient must be safely received onto the destination surface. Historically, the technique evolved into what was popularly termed 'flip-and-catch', with the anaesthetised patient being rolled over towards the operating table and onto the outstretched arms of receiving staff, who then completed the transfer into the final position on the table. Ad hoc solutions have been devised using slidesheets and additional transfer

aids. Bespoke, commercially available systems are also available that offer considerable control of the manoeuvre during the turn to prone and subsequent repositioning on the operating surface, whilst at the same time reducing operator effort and physical risk. These of course carry financial considerations, but given that not every patient would require this level of intervention they are cost and time-efficient.

The Deceased Obese Patient

When an obese patient dies during their hospital stay, a judgement has to be made on their suitability for the standard hospital concealment trolley. Should the size of the patient dictate that this is unsuitable, careful consideration should be given to other methods of transport that maintain patient dignity, staff safety and consideration of members of the public. It has long been recognized that transporting the deceased obese patient on a bed and concealing the death is totally unsuitable. Covering

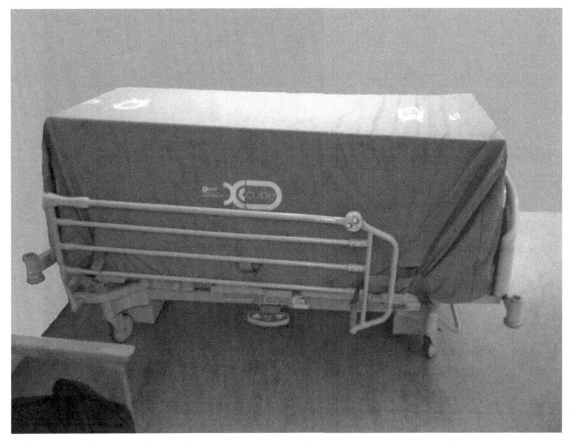

Figure 17.6 XcCube deployed.

the patient with a sheet to their shoulders and applying an Oxygen mask to the face in an attempt to affect a 'live' patient being treated is not acceptable. This challenges the right of the patient to be treated with dignity after death, and is traumatic for the staff involved in the process.

There are limited choices of suitable concealment trolleys, and whilst bespoke solutions are possible we have experienced some success when investing in a versatile alternative – the 'XcCube'™ (Figures 17.6 and 17.7). This is a system comprising a fibreglass tubular frame that extends in length, width and height sufficient to match the size of the bed and conceal the deceased, and a dedicated cover that goes over both the frame and the bed, secured in place with elasticated corners and integral straps. The cover is impermeable to light and the apparatus is placed inside the head and foot ends of the bed, allowing the head and foot-boards to be used to guide and control the bed during transport to and from the department.

Patient Discharge from Hospital

At some point post-operatively the patient will be discharged home. If planning is left until the patient is fit for discharge, there may be a significant delay to this process, sometimes as much as 1–2 weeks. If ambulance transport is required, a bariatric vehicle may be needed, as these are equipped to cope with the larger patient (greater internal space, reinforced ramp, winch to assist with transferring the trolley into the vehicle, wider heavy duty trolley).

There will be a requirement prior to discharge for the ambulance service to visit the patient in hospital and to assess their home environment. Such issues as external access to the house, internal access to rooms, step(s) etc. will have to be reviewed to ensure that the transfer home goes smoothly.

Where significant problems are identified (unsuitable home environment, wider beds, mattresses,

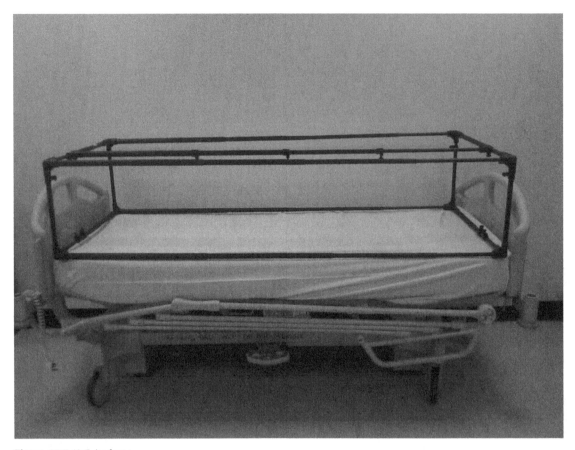

Figure 17.7 XcCube frame.

chairs, etc.) then multiagency meetings may need to take place to ensure the ultimate discharge can occur. This process can be time-consuming and slow down planning, so it is important to commence arrangements as soon as possible.

Conclusion

Obese patient handling can be challenging, but it doesn't have to be difficult. Preparation and planning, in combination with a risk assessment process, is the key to safe and successful handling of these patients.

Communication and cooperation between different teams and specialists is vital to achieving the best outcome from patient and staff safety perspectives. All arrangements for the patient's pathway from admission to discharge should commence at the earliest stage possible.

Use of appropriate equipment and sourcing manual handling expertise, training and advice will significantly reduce the risks and problems involved with obese patient handling.

Further Reading

Al-Benna S. Perioperative management of morbid obesity. *Br J Periop Nurs.* 2011;**21** (7):225–33.

Hignett S, Chipchase S, Tetley A, et al. *Risk assessment and process planning for bariatric patient handling pathways.* Health & Safety Executive, Research Report RR573; 2007.

HMSO. *Manual Handling Operations Regulations 1992 – Guidance on Regulations.* L23; 1992, 1998, 2004.

Rush A., Cookson K. People handling for bariatrics: a systems approach. In *The Guide to the Handling of People, 6th edn,* (ed. Smith J). Sunbury-on-Thames: Backcare; 2011:217.

Sharpe NH, Briody K, Love S. *Safer Moving and Handling in the Perioperative Environment.* Towcester, UK: National Back Exchange; 2014:10, 28, **38–41**.

Tözeren A. *Human Body Dynamics: Classical Mechanics and Human Movement.* London: Springer Science & Business Media; 1999.

Patient and Operating Room Preparation for the Obese

Rhodri Birtchnell and Nick Kennedy

Patient Preparation

Pragmatically, although nearly all anaesthetists regularly manage obese patients, it is important to have a pre-operative screening process in place to identify early potentially high-risk patients, e.g. those with very high BMI (>40), and those with significant obesity related co-morbidities. This allows early review by senior clinicians, organisation of appropriate investigations, an opportunity to discuss risk, gain consent, build a rapport and educate patients about the procedure, and formulate an individualised management plan. Many morbidly obese patients are aware they are higher risk for anaesthesia and are consequently often quite anxious. Information about the particular importance of early mobilisation, stopping smoking, CPAP compliance, pre-operative weight loss goals, potentially limited use of opiates (managing pain expectations) and possible critical care admission can also be provided.

Guidance from the Royal College of Anaesthetists (2016) regarding provision of anaesthesia services in the morbidly obese population is summarised in Table 18.1.

Respiratory System Considerations

Sleep disordered breathing (SDB) is more prevalent in the obese population and encompasses two conditions; obstructive sleep apnoea (OSA) and obesity hypoventilation syndrome (OHS). For every unit increase in BMI, the adjusted odds ratio for developing OSA is 1.14 (95% CI 1.1–1.19).

The American Society of Anesthesiologists gives prominence to the need for pre-operative diagnosis and management of SDB. Unplanned re-intubation, emergent ICU admission and myocardial infarction are significantly greater in OSA patients not treated with positive airway pressure therapy pre-operatively. Early diagnosis and treatment of OSA also has long-term health benefits for patients (improvement in daytime somnolence and the incidence of cardiovascular complications after 8 weeks of therapy). Increasing the number of hours use each night results in better neurocognitive, cardiovascular and mortality outcomes, although self-reported utilisation can correlate poorly with actual CPAP use (poor compliance in up to 50%).

Although the gold standard diagnostic tool for OSA is overnight polysomnography (PSG), it is time-consuming and costly, which can significantly delay surgery. A convenient and inexpensive alternative is nocturnal oximetry to determine undiagnosed SDB using the oxygen desaturation index (ODI).

Several screening test questionnaires are available in order to predict patients at high risk for OSA. This

Table 18.1 Summary of guidance on anaesthesia of the morbidly obese

Patient dignity must be maintained by ensuring appropriate equipment and clothing is available and by staff attitudes to obesity.
Nominated anaesthetic lead for obese patients undergoing surgery in every hospital.
Operating lists should include the patients' weight and body mass index (BMI).
The WHO Surgical Safety Checklist should include obesity-related issues such as correct equipment and manual handling (operating table, intubation, hoists, beds, positioning aids and transfer equipment).
Emergency surgery should be conducted with experienced surgeons and anaesthetists (typically at a consultant level), in order to minimise operative time.
Bariatric patients should be considered for level 2 or 3 nursing care post-operatively.

Table 18.2 STOP-BANG scoring questionnaire

STOP-BANG criteria:
- Snoring
- Tiredness
- Observed apnoea
- Pressure (hypertension)
- BMI >35
- Age >50
- Neck circumference >40 cm
- Gender (Male)

facilitates more selective referral of patients with a high disease probability for further testing. The Berlin questionnaire has the greatest diagnostic accuracy for OSA, and the Epworth sleepiness scale the poorest. The STOP-BANG questionnaire (Table 18.2) is considered an excellent bedside method for predicting severe OSA, has a simple eight-point linear scale and does not require additional investigations. Referral triggers vary between centres, but generally >5 warrants referral for sleep studies.

The incidence of bronchial asthma is increased in the obese population, approximately double that of lean, although the exact mechanism is not known. It may reflect the generalised pro-inflammatory state associated with excessive weight, termed 'obesity-induced airway hyper-reactivity' and thus differentiating it from other asthma aetiologies. This patient group demonstrates poorer control (particularly in obese women), greater morbidity and is relatively resistant to steroid therapy.

Smoking increases the risk of venous thromboembolism and mortality in patients undergoing major surgery, and increases the risk of anastamotic breakdown and wound infection.

Cardiovascular System Considerations

Obese patients exhibit an elevated circulating blood volume proportional to body surface area, resulting in increased pre-load and cardiac output. Initial compensatory mechanisms are increased; left heart diastolic filling and left ventricular hypertrophy. Stroke volume remains essentially fixed, hence obese individuals are only able to raise cardiac output during exercise by increasing heart rate. Ultimately systolic dysfunction ensues when the heart can no longer respond to increased demand, a process known as obesity-induced cardiomyopathy. Pulmonary hyper-

tension as a consequence of SDB can lead to right ventricular enlargement and eventual cor pulmonale.

Hypertension is more prevalent and may result in concentric left ventricular hypertrophy. Such remodelling may also impair diastolic function, increasing the risk of peri-operative congestive heart failure.

Arrhythmias, particularly atrial fibrillation (AF) may be encountered, and each unit increase in BMI correlates with a 3–8% higher risk of new AF onset. Obesity is also an independent risk factor for stroke, coronary artery disease, myocardial infarction and sudden death.

Evaluation of cardiovascular performance may be problematic, as morbidly obese patients have limited ability to perform physical activity, fitness levels being similar to lean patients with advanced heart failure. The sedentary nature of some individuals may mask underlying angina or exertional dyspnoea. Some patients may preferentially have become accustomed to sleeping in a chair and hence not describe classical symptoms of orthopnoea and paroxysmal nocturnal dyspnoea. Limb adiposity may impede movement from skin friction when exercising, although cardiopulmonary exercise testing (CPET) can be achieved prior to bariatric surgery. There is a significant association between CPET performance and post-operative outcome following gastric bypass surgery. Pre-operative anaerobic threshold (AT) below 11 ml/kg/min predicts both post-operative morbidity and prolonged hospital length of stay. Radioisotope perfusion scanning or transoesophageal dobutamine echocardiography are alternatives to evaluate the presence of ischaemic heart disease in those unable to perform simple exercise stress testing.

Increased chest wall fat can result in low volume heart sound auscultation and sub-optimal transthoracic echo imaging. Sub-epicardial adipose can be difficult to delineate from pericardial effusion with ultrasound (pseudopericardial effusion).

Electrocardiographic changes of obesity include low QRS voltage (from adiposity-increased distance to the recording electrodes) and a leftward axis (from horizontal displacement of the heart by the elevated diaphragm). LVH by voltage criteria is often underdiagnosed in obese patients. There is a low frequency of diagnostic ECG findings in patients demonstrated to have LVH by echocardiography. Some advocate the use of the R wave in aVL and S wave in V3 to diagnose LVH by voltage in this patient group. Combined amplitudes of

>35 mm in men and >25 mm in women showed an overall accuracy of 76%.

Metabolic and Endocrine Considerations

The metabolic syndrome (MetS) is a combination of central obesity, hypertension, atherogenic dyslipidaemia and high fasting glucose concentration. Table 18.3 shows the five diagnostic criteria, three of which are required for diagnosis.

MetS increases the risk of type 2 diabetes and cardiovascular disease. It is an independent predictor of post-operative complications following non-cardiac surgery, including adverse cardiac events (two- to threefold risk increase), pulmonary complications (1.5–2.5-fold risk increase), acute kidney injury (three- to sevenfold risk increase), stroke and sepsis. Interestingly, MetS does not increase perioperative complication risk in bariatric surgery.

BMI strongly predicts the development of type 2 diabetes, with a fivefold risk increase for BMI >25, 28-fold for BMI >30 and 93-fold for BMI >35. These patients are more prone to surgical wound infection, warranting stringent control of hyperglycaemia and an HbA1c level below 69 mmol/mol (8.5%) prior to elective surgery. Bariatric surgery has been shown to eliminate the need for diabetic medications post-operatively, with remission rates of type 2 diabetes of 55 to 95%.

Sub-clinical hypothyroidism is correlated with increasing BMI, and hence more prevalent in obese patients, and pre-operative thyroid function tests may be indicated.

Gastrointestinal Considerations

The prevalence of gastro-oesphageal reflux disease (GORD) and hiatus hernia is greater in the obese population, but this does not translate into a greater risk of aspiration. Routine use of antacid pre-medication is not now required. Patients with a gastric band, however, are at greater risk of aspiration, due to oesophageal dysmotility and dilatation above the band. They require antacid prophylaxis and the use of rapid sequence induction for endotracheal tube placement.

Risk Management

The obesity surgery mortality risk score (OS-MRS; Table 18.4) is a validated mortality scoring system in bariatric surgery used to stratify patients into three risk groups.

OS-MRS allows for rational elective use of higher-level care facilities. The majority of patients can be managed at ward level post-operatively, but class C patients will require a high-dependency bed to be booked in advance.

Prediction of unplanned ICU requirement after bariatric surgery has also been estimated (Table 18.5). Revision surgery is the most significant risk factor for emergent ICU admission, with open surgery, diabetes mellitus, chronic respiratory disease and obstructive sleep apnoea also showing strong associations. This calculation may also aid the planning of higher-level care requirements for obese patients requiring emergency surgery, particularly if the probability estimation is large.

Table 18.3 Diagnostic criteria for metabolic syndrome

Increased waist circumference	>102 cm men, >88 cm women
Elevated triglycerides (or on drug Rx)	>150 mg/dl (1.7 mmol/l)
Reduced high-density lipoprotein-cholesterol (or Rx)	<40 mg/dl (1.0 mmol/l) men <50 mg/dl (1.3 mmol/l) women
Hypertension (or on drug Rx)	>130 mmHg SBP >85 mmHg DBP
Elevated fasting glucose (or on Rx)	>100 mg/dL (5.6 mmol/l)

Table 18.4 The obesity surgery mortality risk score (1 point for each risk factor)

- BMI >50
- Hypertension
- Age >45
- Risk factors for PE: previous VTE, pre-operative vena cava filter, obesity hypoventilation syndrome, right heart failure/pulmonary hypertension
- Male

Class A	Score 0–1	Low risk
Class B	Score 2–3	Intermediate risk
Class C	Score 4–5	High risk

Table 18.5 Prediction of unplanned ICU admission

Field	Points
Revisional surgery	100
COPD	75
OSA	60
Open surgery	55
Diabetes mellitus (DM)	35
Totals	Risk of unplanned admission (%)
110 (e.g. DM + COPD)	10
135 (e.g. OSA + COPD)	20
>160 (e.g. Revision + COPD or OSA)	>30

Examination

Radiological imaging provides the most accurate determination of central (visceral) fat deposition, although waist circumference offers a close approximation. Measurement taken at the superior point of the iliac crest (greater than 88 cm in women and 102 cm in men), or a waist:hip ratio >1 in men (>0.85 in women) reflects central adipose deposition.

BMI is a weak predictor for difficult and failed tracheal intubation, but remains a high risk factor for difficult mask ventilation (DMV), reportedly up to 13% of cases. Other predictors of DMV include limited mandibular protrusion, Mallampati (MP) score >3, neck circumference >46 cm and male gender.

Airway examination of neck circumference (NC) should be measured level with the thyroid cartilage. An MP score >3 plus NC >40 cm may predict a difficult direct laryngoscopy. NC >50 cm carries a 20% risk of difficult intubation. Thyromental distance (TMD) is measured from the thyroid notch to the mentum. An NC to TMD ratio >5 has the highest predictive accuracy of difficult intubation.

Operating Room Preparation

A safety briefing is an obligatory part at the start of an operating list. In addition to the compulsory generic checklist it is recommended the following additional specific considerations relating to morbidly obese patients are included:

- Operating table and adjuncts are weight tolerant
- Electric bed is available

- Hover mattress is in theatre
- Appropriate airway kit
- Staffing numbers (peri- and post-op) to safely manage patient
- Specific issues of positioning large patient
- Drugs and dosing regimens
- Post-operative care location and availability
- Diabetes mellitus management
- Length of surgery
- Potential break in surgery to reposition patient to avoid crush injury.

Recovery room staff need to be briefed about OSA/CPAP therapy, analgesic plan and post-operative care level and location. Sufficient staff must be immediately available for the duration of the operation should the patient need to be moved in an emergency

Patient Transportation

Patients should be encouraged to mobilise wherever possible, walking to theatre and positioning themselves on the operating table, to avoid unnecessary manual handling by staff. Those unable to walk to theatre should be highlighted in advance. Specific bariatric wheelchairs or increased weight-tolerant hospital beds may be required. Special hoists are utilised in some centres when the patient is unable to self-transfer onto the operating table.

A hover mattress, placed deflated underneath the patient prior to surgery, is highly recommended to transfer the patient back onto their bed post surgery. All obese patients should be nursed on an electric bed post-operatively.

Operating Table

Specially designed electric tables with a high weight tolerance are required, with the ability to add extensions (Figure 18.1). Side extensions offer a greater surface area for the patient and individual leg extensions allow for surgical access peri-operatively. Padded arm supports keep the upper limbs away from the body and provide anaesthetic access. Footplates are required to prevent patient slippage whilst positioning in steep reverse Trendelenburg for intubation and ventilation. Lower limbs are also often bound to the table for added security. The table must be checked to ensure these movements are functioning correctly before the start of the list.

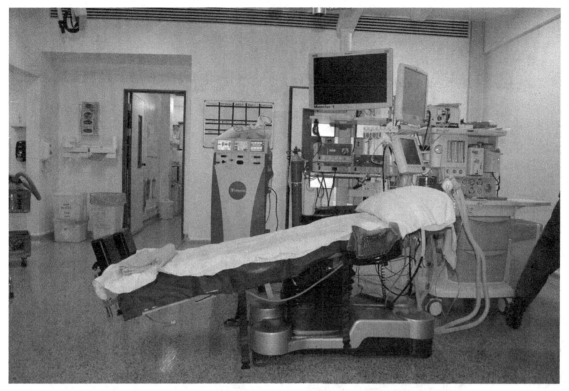

Figure 18.1 Bariatric operating table with footplates and padded arm supports. The hinged lower limb section facilitates surgical access between the legs peri-operatively.

Patient Positioning

The best laryngoscopic view is obtained with a ramped upper torso and the external auditory meatus horizontally aligned with the sternal notch (Figure 18.2). This position also aids with mask ventilation under general anaesthesia as it better maintains patency of the pharynx allowing unobstructed airflow. Bespoke devices specifically designed to aid ramping are available; however, correct positioning can be achieved by appropriate adjustment of the theatre table and use of additional pillows.

Cushioning of pressure areas is vital. Increased body weight significantly increases the risk of compressive nerve, soft tissue and muscle injury. Brachial plexus stretch injury and ulnar neuropathy are the most frequent injuries. Lithotomy position and excessively raised abdominal insufflation pressure increase the potential for compression damage to the lateral femoral cutaneous nerve. Rhabdomyolysis is a rare compression complication involving muscle groups in contact with the operating table (gluteal, lumbar and shoulder). Patients with BMI >50, prolonged surgery (>3–4 h), and particular surgical positions (lithotomy and lateral decubitus) are risk factors.

Venous Access

Peripheral access can be achieved in the vast majority of patients, ultrasound may be helpful in difficult cases. Siting of two cannulae is recommended, particularly if TIVA is being used. Central venous catheters are seldom required and insertion is potentially risky in the morbidly obese. Obese subjects poorly tolerate the supine or head-down position required to site central venous cannulae.

Pharmacology and Weight Calculation

Total body weight (TBW) is the weight as physically measured by scales. However, with increasing obesity, fat mass becomes a disproportionately larger component of TBW than lean tissue.

The concept of ideal body weight (IBW) originated from life insurance studies, which derived the weight for a given height and gender associated with the lowest rate of mortality. IBW calculation in

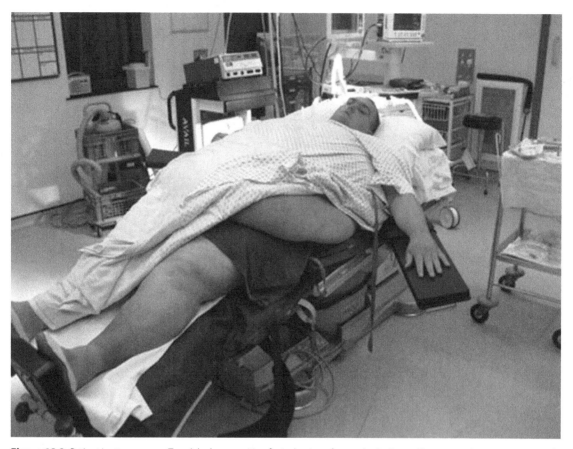

Figure 18.2 Patient in steep reverse Trendelenburg position for induction of anaesthesia. Extra pillows ramp the upper torso to align the external auditory meatus horizontally with the sternal notch.

morbidly obese patients can lead to underdosing of pharmacological agents, as this underestimates the lean tissue component.

Lean body weight (LBW) is the difference between TBW and fat mass and is calculated using specific formulae, e.g. as derived by Janmahasatian et al. It is the ideal weight scalar for drug dosing in morbidly obese patients, as drug clearance increases proportionally with LBW.

Male LBW (kg) = 9270 × TBW (kg) / (6680 + (216 × BMI (kg/m^2))

Female LBW (kg) = 9270 × TBW (kg) / 8780 + (244 × BMI(kg/m^2))

In general, lipophilic drugs have an increased volume of distribution in obese patients, whereas hydrophilic drug pharmacokinetics remain relatively unchanged. Dosing scalars for the majority of anaesthetic medications are based on LBW, with the exception of suxamethonium and neostigmine that are dosed on TBW.

Pharmacokinetic (PK) models used in target-controlled infusion (TCI) pumps were not derived from an obese patient cohort, therefore caution must be exercised when programming the pump. The Marsh model is linearly related to TBW and can lead to excessively large initial loading doses in the morbidly obese, with potential haemodynamic compromise. The Schnider model may also lead to underdosing of propofol administration if TBW rather than adjusted body weight (ABW) is entered. Owing to the inverted parabolic shape of the 'James' equation used to calculate LBW, once a BMI of 37 (females) and 42 (males) is exceeded then LBW becomes underestimated, with potential even for negative values in the super-obese. Use of an ABW improves the performance of both Marsh and Schnider PK models.

ABW = IBW (kg) + 0.4 (TBW (kg) − IBW (kg))

(NB: in this instance   IBW = 22 × height^2)

Monitoring

Full monitoring in line with AAGBI recommendations is mandatory for all obese patients. Depth of anaesthesia (DOA) monitoring is mandatory when using TCI of propofol. This is especially important as there is an increased risk of awareness under anaesthesia in the obese population, especially when using TCI techniques using corrected (hybrid) weights in the standard pharmacokinetic models (Marsh, Schnider) that were not originally derived from an obese population.

A standard sized non-invasive blood pressure cuff is likely to overestimate the arterial pressure in an obese patient. Often no upper arm cuffs will fit obese patients. Forearm cuffs are a useful alternative, which are an accurate and validated means of assessing blood pressure. Arterial line placement is not routinely required for the obese surgical patient.

Peripheral nerve stimulation to assess neuromuscular blockade can be problematic in obese patients. Excess wrist adiposity may result in supramaximal current requirements (>70 mA) to elicit a motor response, which some devices are unable to deliver. In this instance the face would be the recommended monitoring location.

Summary

The following are useful principles:

- Actual body weight is important in relation to manual handling, theatre equipment (particularly operating table) and bed.
- BMI is important for drug dosing, and as a generally understood measure of obesity.
- The concept of 'apple' and 'pear' shapes, together with airway appearance, are useful for surgical/anaesthetic risk assessment

Further Reading

Chung F, Subramanyam R, Liao P, et al. High STOP-BANG score indicates a high probability of obstructive sleep apnoea. *Br J Anaesth*. 2012;**108**(5): 768–75.

Hodgson L, Murphy P, Hart N. Respiratory management of the obese patient undergoing surgery. *J Thorac Dis*. 2015;**7** (5):943–52.

Ingrande, J, Lemmens HJM. Dose adjustment of anaesthetics in the morbidly obese. *Br J Anaesth*. 2010;**105**: i16–23.

Nightingale CE, Margarson MP, Shearer E, et al.; Members of the Working Party. Peri-operative management of the obese surgical patient 2015. *Anaesthesia*. 2015;**70**:859–76.

Morgan DJR, Ho KM, Armstrong J, Baker S. Incidence and risk factors for intensive care unit admission after bariatric surgery: a multicentre population-based cohort study. *Br J Anaesth*. 2015;**115**(6):873–82.

Poirier P, Giles TD, Bray GA, et al. Obesity and cardiovascular disease: pathophysiology, evaluation, and effect of weight loss. *Circulation*. 2006;**113**: 898–918.

Tzimas P, Petrou A, Laou E, et al. Impact of metabolic syndrome in surgical patients: should we bother? *Br J Anaesth*. 2015;**115**(2):194–202.

Chapter 19

Induction of General Anesthesia and Positioning in Obesity

Tiffany S. Moon

Pre-Induction and Positioning

Prior to induction of general anaesthesia in the obese patient (Table 19.1), special accommodations must be considered in order to account for the altered anatomy and physiology. An example of such altered physiology includes the reduction in functional residual capacity (FRC) that is further reduced when adopting the supine position. Obese patients are at risk of rapid oxygen desaturation owing to the reduced FRC and the cephalad movement of the diaphragm in the supine position. In order to reduce this risk and to facilitate improved laryngoscopic views, several different methods have been proposed.

The ideal head and neck placement is achieved when an imaginary horizontal line extending from the external auditory meatus to the sternum is obtained. To achieve this in obese patients, the

Table 19.1 Body mass index categories

BMI (kg/m^2)	Description	Obesity Class
18.5–24.9	Normal	
25.0–29.9	Overweight	
30.0–34.9	Obesity	I
35.0–39.9	Obesity	II
>40	Extreme obesity	III

'ramped' position, in which the shoulders and the upper torso are supported and elevated, has been proposed and validated by comparative studies. (Figure 19.1). In addition, improved laryngeal exposure can be achieved in the ramped position as compared to the sniffing position, which can help decrease

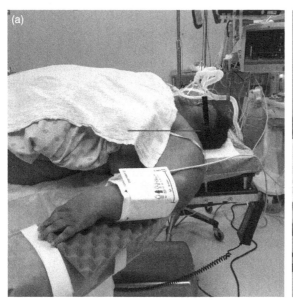 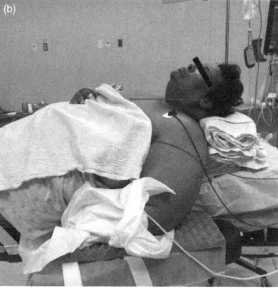

Figure 19.1 (a) Obese patient in the supine position on the operating table. The solid line is used to indicate that the external auditory meatus is not on the same horizontal plane as the sternum. (b) Obese patient in the ramped position using a foam wedge and stacked blankets. The solid line is used to show the ideal alignment of the external auditory meatus to the sternum on the same horizontal plane.

the incidence of difficult intubation. Establishing the horizontal plane from the external auditory meatus to the sternum can be achieved with either table elevation or by ramping patients with stacks of blankets; these two techniques are comparable in facilitating tracheal intubation. In some circumstances, adjusting the table rather than moving the patient may be safer for the patient and less cumbersome for operating room staff. Other alternatives to blankets include use of commercial inflatable supports such as the Troop Elevation Pillow®, which can help to raise the upper torso.

Pre-oxygenation is a critical practice that prepares patients for the subsequent period of apnoea during laryngoscopy and intubation. The combination of 100% O_2 administration and head-up position (reducing the abdominal contents pressing on the diaphragm) delays the apnoea to desaturation time. Studies have demonstrated the importance of proper patient positioning of the obese individual during the pre-induction period. A seated position rather than the supine position protects against rapid desaturation, extending the safe apnoeic period by approximately one minute. In the reverse Trendelenburg position, the head is elevated relative to the legs, to facilitate the displacement of the abdomen away from the chest, which further increases the apnoea to desaturation time.

Administration of continuous positive airway pressure (CPAP) can protect against prolonged periods of apnoea in potentially difficult laryngoscopies. Positive end expiratory pressure (PEEP) combined with recruitment manoeuvers help to reduce atelectasis. For example, applying PEEP prior to tracheal intubation has been demonstrated to lengthen the time until oxygen desaturation (i.e. increased safe apnoeic period) compared to those not receiving any PEEP. Limited data currently supports nasal or buccal insufflation of oxygen to prolong the safe apnoeic period. Specifically, the administration of 5 l/min O_2 through nasal prongs extends the time that SpO_2 remains at or above 95%. The lowest SpO_2 reached by those who had oxygen insufflated was also higher than that reached by those who did not have oxygen insufflated. Similarly, the buccal approach prevents rapid desaturation among obese patients and is proposed to be an alternative to nasal insufflation when this method is contraindicated. In addition, maintenance of PEEP at 10 cmH$_2$O after induction improves oxygenation by decreasing the A–a gradient similar to the improvements observed with the reverse Trendelenburg position.

The use of a rapid sequence induction (RSI) technique can be used to decrease gastric aspiration. There is much debate regarding the necessity of routinely undertaking RSI for morbidly obese patients. One major point of contention is the use of cricoid pressure. Whilst cricoid pressure is intended to reduce the risk of aspiration, it can distort the laryngoscopic view obtained. The evidence supporting its benefits are inconsistent. Recent reviews suggest only using RSI for obese patients who have specific co-morbidities that place them at greater risk for aspiration, such as symptomatic gastro-esophageal reflux and emergency surgery.

Induction Drugs and Dosing Modifications

Induction of anaesthesia is most commonly performed with intravenous anaesthetic agents. Obesity increases cardiac output, which causes prolonged induction time when performing an inhalational induction. Combined with the potential for airway difficulties, results in this being a poor choice of induction. Commonly used intravenous drugs (propofol, etomidate, benzodiazepines, opioids and neuromuscular blockers) have altered pharmacokinetics and pharmacodynamics in the obese population, necessitating special care to ensure safe and effective dosing.

Many drugs used by anaesthetists are dosed by total body weight (TBW) in normal weight patients. However, in obese patients, more suitable dosing scalars include ideal body weight (IBW) and lean body weight (LBW). Ideal body weight can be calculated using height, gender and body frame. Devine's formula is commonly used to determine IBW. However, IBW does not directly relate to body composition changes that occur among obese individuals. This relationship is achieved using LBW calculations, which associates gender, TBW and body fat mass. Lean body mass in obese patients does not increase linearly as TBW increases (Figure 19.2). Adipose tissue makes up approximately 60–80% of the extra weight gained by obese patients. Obese patients also have a higher cardiac output than lean patients. However, since cardiac output is more closely correlated with LBW than TBW, dosing drugs by TBW in obese patients can result in a relative overdose. Thus, it is necessary to understand each drug's pharmacological properties to determine correct dosing.

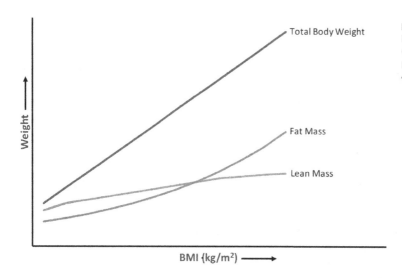

Figure 19.2 Schematic of total body weight, lean mass and fat mass as BMI increases. (Adapted from Lemmens HJ. Perioperative pharmacology in morbid obesity. *Curr Opin Anaesthesiol.* 2010;23:485–91.)

Propofol

A fast onset and short duration of action make propofol a very common induction agent for patients of all sizes. It is a highly lipophilic drug and has a large volume of distribution. The clinical effects of propofol include vasodilation and myocardial suppression. In non-obese patients, the dosing of propofol is based on TBW, but studies have shown that this should not be the case in obese patients.

The plasma concentration of propofol is strongly correlated with the patient's cardiac output. Obese patients have a higher cardiac output than lean patients, which leads to an increased clearance of propofol. This suggests that higher doses of propofol are required to achieve the same level of anaesthesia in obese patients as in lean patients, but because increases in fat outpace the increase in lean mass, administering bolus doses of propofol by TBW in obese patients can result in hypotension or cardiovascular collapse. Studies show that administering propofol to obese patients based on LBW results in a time to loss of consciousness that is roughly equal to control groups of lean patients who were dosed by TBW. Some authors have expressed concern regarding the potential for inadequate anaesthesia when dosing propofol by LBW and suggest that an intermediate dosing scalar is needed. One proposed model is the lean-scaled weight, which is calculated as a percentage of BMI and falls as BMI increases.

Etomidate

Etomidate is suggested for patients who are haemodynamically unstable because of its minimal effects on cardiovascular function. There have been no specific studies that aim to determine the correct dosing scalar to use for etomidate in obese patients. The drug's pharmacokinetics are similar to propofol, so it is currently recommended that bolus doses of etomidate should also be dosed according to LBW. Of note, etomidate has been shown to cause transient adrenal suppression through its inhibition of 11-beta-hydroxylase, which may lead to decreased circulatory stability, delayed wound healing and muscle weakness. These effects may be more pronounced in obese patients and care should be taken if administration is considered in the critically unwell.

Benzodiazepines

Given their sedative, anxiolytic and amnesic properties, benzodiazepines are commonly administered as premedication. Benzodiazepines are lipophilic drugs with a volume of distribution that is markedly increased in obese patients. Midazolam is the drug of choice in this category, as it is short-acting and has minimal respiratory and cardiovascular effects. Dosing recommendations for benzodiazepines in obese patients vary. Some authors recommend dosing by TBW, while others suggest that initial dosing should be based on LBW followed by titration to the desired effect.

Opioids

Opioids provide potent pain relief, but appropriate dosing is vital to minimise potentially fatal side effects. Opioids are associated with both central and obstructive apnoea, which can lead to decreased oxygen saturation. Since obesity compromises respiratory and cardiovascular function, the effects of opioids are more pronounced. Patients with obstructive sleep apnoea, a common co-morbidity associated with obesity, may have an exaggerated response to the effects of opioids. Nearly half of the documented adverse respiratory events attributed to opioids occur in obese patients.

Fentanyl

The plasma concentration of fentanyl is affected by cardiac output, which is correlated with LBW. Studies involving pharmacokinetic models that dose fentanyl according to TBW show that higher than necessary doses were administered. Clearance of fentanyl has been shown to have a strong correlation with a derived pharmacokinetic mass that rises linearly until 100 kg and plateaus around 140 kg. This pharmacokinetic mass is closely correlated with LBW. Thus, it is recommended that dosing of fentanyl be determined by LBW.

Remifentanil

Remifentanil is a high-potency opioid with unique pharmacokinetics. Its metabolism is organ-independent, which leads to a large reduction in drug concentration 5–10 minutes after an infusion is discontinued. These properties make remifentanil a good choice for obese patients, especially those with associated co-morbidities that impair hepatic and renal function. Furthermore, its rapid elimination is advantageous in obese patients with obstructive sleep apnoea, who have an increased sensitivity to the effects of residual systemic opioids. Using LBW or IBW to dose remifentanil produces similar results in both obese and lean patients.

Neuromuscular Blocking Agents

Neuromuscular blockade facilitates intubation and optimises surgical access. Commonly used drugs in this category include suxamethonium, rocuronium and vecuronium.

Suxamethonium

Suxamethonium is a depolarising neuromuscular blocking agent that has a short onset and duration of action. It is frequently used to facilitate a rapid sequence induction and intubation. Its short duration of action is advantageous in the event of a difficult airway and failed intubation attempts, where return to

spontaneous ventilation may be necessary to prevent severe hypoxaemia. The duration of action of succinylcholine is dependent on pseudocholinesterase activity and extracellular fluid space, both of which are increased in obese patients. Higher doses are needed to overcome these factors. This is consistent with comparisons of different weight scalars for suxamethonium demonstrating optimal intubating conditions when dosed according to TBW. Suxamethonium is unique in that it is the only neuromuscular blocking drug advised to be dosed according to TBW.

Rocuronium and Vecuronium

Rocuronium and vecuronium are non-depolarising neuromuscular blocking agents. Both drugs have similar pharmacokinetic and pharmacodynamic profiles in obese and lean patients. However, dosing based on TBW in obese patients can prolong their duration of action, potentially making emergence and recovery from anesthesia more difficult. Conversely, dosing based on IBW can potentially result in less than optimal intubating conditions. Authors have recommended that it is acceptable to dose these drugs according to IBW or LBW and titrating to effect.

Dexmedetomidine

Dexmedetomidine is an alpha-2 agonist with both sedative and analgesic effects. It can cause cardiovascular depression, but one of the main advantages is that it has minimal respiratory effects. Dexmedetomidine is commonly given as an adjunct to general anaesthesia, but it also has value as an alternative to propofol in monitored anaesthesia care cases. Some providers use dexmedetomidine because it can reduce the need for opioids, reducing the risk of post-operative respiratory complications. It has been shown that dosing by TBW in obese patients results in higher serum concentrations than in lean patients. Thus, it is suggested that dexmedetomidine should be dosed by LBW instead of TBW.

Conclusion

With the increasing prevalence of obesity, it is important for anaesthetists to recognise the associated physiological, pharmacodynamic and pharmacokinetic changes. Pre-induction positioning and oxygenation are critical to prevent rapid desaturation and to offset

Table 19.2 Drug dosing in obese patients

Drug	Dosing Scalar	Notes
Propofol	LBW	Differs from maintenance infusion dosing (TBW) Some authors suggest using lean-scaled weight instead
Etomidate	LBW	Minimal effects on haemodynamics, but potential to cause adrenal suppression
Midazolam	LBW	Titrate to effect
Fentanyl	LBW	Patients with OSA may have sensitivity to opioids
Remifentanil	IBW	Rapid organ-independent metabolism reduces risk of post-operative respiratory depression
Succinylcholine	TBW	Dosing based on TBW results in optimized intubating conditions
Rocuronium Vecuronium	IBW or LBW	Titrate to effect for optimal intubation conditions
Dexmedetomidine	LBW	Can cause cardiovascular suppression, titrate to effect

reductions in FRC. Additionally, the unequal increases in fat tissue and lean mass, increased cardiac output and impaired clearance of some drugs necessitate careful consideration of drug dosing (Table 19.2). Proper preparation and induction techniques are paramount to the safe anaesthetic care of this patient population.

Further Reading

Aceto P, Perilli V, Modesti C, et al. Airway management in obese patients. *Surg Obes Relat Dis.* 2013;9:809–15.

Altermatt F R, Munoz HR, Delfino AE, Cortinez LI. Pre-oxygenation in the obese patient: effects of position on tolerance to apnoea. *Br J Anaesth.* 2005;95:706–9.

Collins JS, Lemmens HJ, Brodsky JB, Brock-Utne JG, Levitan RM. Laryngoscopy and morbid obesity: a comparison of the 'sniff' and 'ramped' positions. *Obes Surg.* 2004;14:1171–5.

Dong D, Peng X, Liu J, et al. Morbid obesity alters both pharmacokinetics and pharmacodynamics of propofol: dosing recommendation for anesthesia induction. *Drug Metab Dispos.* 2016;44:1579–83.

Friesen JH. Estimating the induction dose of propofol in morbid obesity: striking a happy medium. *Br J Anaesth.* 2016;116:730–1.

Gander S, Frascarolo P, Suter M, Spahn DR, Magnusson L. Positive end-expiratory pressure during induction of general anesthesia increases duration of nonhypoxic apnea in morbidly obese patients. *Anesth Analg.* 2005;100:580–4.

Harbut P, Gozdzik W, Stjernfalt E, Marsk R, Hesselvik JF. Continuous positive airway pressure/pressure support pre-oxygenation of morbidly obese patients. *Acta Anaesthesiol Scand.* 2014;58:675–80.

Heard A, Toner AJ, Evans JR, Palacios AM, Lauer S. Apneic oxygenation during prolonged laryngoscopy in obese patients: a randomized, controlled trial of buccal RAE tube oxygen administration. *Anesth Analg.* 2016;124 (4):1162–7.

Ingrande J, Brodsky JB, Lemmens HJ. Lean body weight scalar for the anesthetic induction dose of propofol in morbidly obese subjects. *Anesth Analg.* 2011;113:57–62.

Ingrande J, Lemmens HJ. Dose adjustment of anaesthetics in the morbidly obese. *Br J Anaesth.* 2010;105(Suppl 1): i16–23.

Lam KK, Kunder S, Wong J, et al. Obstructive sleep apnea, pain, and opioids: is the riddle solved? *Curr Opin Anaesthesiol.* 2016;29:134–40.

Lemmens HJ. Perioperative pharmacology in morbid obesity. *Curr Opin Anaesthesiol.* 2010;23:485–91.

Lemmens HJ, Brodsky JB. The dose of succinylcholine in morbid obesity. *Anesth Analg.* 2006;102:438–42.

Leykin Y, Miotto L, Pellis T. Pharmacokinetic considerations in the obese. *Best Pract Res Clin Anaesthesiol* 2011;25:27–36.

Rao SL, Kunselman AR, Schuler HG, Desharnais S. Laryngoscopy and tracheal intubation in the head-elevated position in obese patients: a randomized, controlled, equivalence trial. *Anesth Analg.* 2008;107:1912–8.

Chapter 20

The Rapid Sequence Induction: Myth and Obesity

Jay B. Brodsky

Introduction

'Rapid sequence induction' (RSI) is a general term used to describe a variety of techniques, each of which is intended to produce the rapid onset of general anaesthesia, along with neuromuscular blockade in order to provide optimal tracheal intubating conditions as quickly as possible. Since it involves both anaesthetic induction and tracheal intubation, it is sometimes referred to as RSII. The goal of RSI is to minimise the time interval between the onset of apnoea and loss of protective airway reflexes until the successful placement of a cuffed endotracheal tube to protect the airway from aspiration. Thus, an RSI is routinely performed on patients with full stomachs, either in emergency situations or when preoperative fasting guidelines have not been followed. Surgical patients with significant gastro-oesophageal reflux disease, ileus, acute abdomen, term pregnancy, diabetes mellitus with associated autonomic neuropathy, impaired levels of consciousness and neurologic conditions with loss of gag reflexes undergo RSI. Obesity, by itself, is often cited as an indication for RSI.

The components of 'traditional' RSI consist of preoxygenation, followed by intravenous administration in very quick succession of both a rapid onset anaesthetic induction agent and a muscle relaxant. Traditional RSI is always combined with the application of cricoid pressure, the so-called Sellick manoeuvre. Positive-pressure bag-mask ventilation is avoided until successful tracheal intubation is accomplished. For elective procedures, prophylactic administration of agents to reduce and neutralise gastric fluid and to increase gastric emptying time are often used.

Although anaesthetists have employed some form of RSI for nearly 50 years, its clinical indications remain controversial, and accepted protocols on the correct way to perform RSI do not exist. There are as many strong advocates for the continued practice of traditional RSI with cricoid pressure, as there are others who believe that RSI is associated with significant risks to the patient, without evidence that it effectively reduces aspiration.

Lack of Standardisation

There is no agreement on how to perform RSI. What is the best patient position to pre-oxygenate and induce anaesthesia? Is a head-up position (better to protect against aspiration from gastric reflux) preferable to a head-down position (better to protect against aspiration from vomiting)? Which anaesthetic induction agent (thiopental, propofol, etomidate, ketamine) should be used? Should a predetermined bolus dose of these drugs be administered, or is titration to loss of consciousness a better method to induce anaesthesia? When to administer, and what dose of different neuromuscular blocking agents should be given? If suxamethonium is used should the patient be allowed to fasciculate or should a de-fasciculation dose of a non-depolarizing neuromuscular blocker be administered first? If rocuronium is used, is a priming dose indicated? Will bag-mask ventilation result in gastric insufflation? Is complete avoidance of bag-mask ventilation really necessary, or can the patient be given positive-pressure breaths at low peak pressures (<20 cmH$_2$O) during an RSI to avoid hypoxaemia? Finally, and probably most controversial of all, is cricoid pressure actually effective in preventing aspiration? A complete discussion of the many different RSI methods is beyond the scope of this chapter and the reader is referred to the further reading.

Efficacy in Preventing Aspiration

The simplest definition of pulmonary aspiration is inhalation of material into the airway below the vocal cords. Peri-operative aspiration can be further defined as the presence of bilious secretions or particulate matter in the tracheobronchial tree, and/ or the presence on post-operative chest roentgenogram of an infiltrate that was not present pre-operatively. The actual incidence of aspiration during anaesthesia is unknown. A rate of 0.03% has been reported for all patients undergoing general anaesthesia. Aspiration events occur considerably more frequently at the time of induction during emergency surgery, even though many of these patients undergo RSI. The true incidence may be higher than reported, since an unknown number of anaesthetised patients have silent, unrecognised aspiration without clinical sequelae. There is no data to support (or refute) the use of RSI to lower the risk of aspiration. Despite the lack of consistency on how to perform RSI, or even in the absence of definitive evidence that RSI is effective, traditional RSI with cricoid pressure is considered the 'standard of care' for the induction of anaesthesia and tracheal intubation in patients believed to be at risk for pulmonary aspiration.

RSI and Obesity

Historically, traditional RSI has been a routine part of the anaesthetic management of morbidly obese patients, based on the belief that all obese patients are at increased risk for gastric aspiration. How and when did this association between obesity and aspiration risk originate? It can be traced to a study, published over 40 years ago, which reported that fasting obese patients had a larger volume (>25 ml) of more acidotic (pH <2.5) gastric fluid than similar lean patients. Since the severity of the pneumonitis following aspiration depends on the volume and acidity of the material aspirated, Vaughan's study identified obese patients as being at increased risk for aspiration and pulmonary injury. This report influenced the anaesthetic management of morbidly obese patients for many years.

Several subsequent studies have failed to repeat these findings. The gastric contents of non-pre-medicated, non-diabetic fasting obese patients (BMI >30 kg/m^2) without significant gastro-oesophageal pathology are not different from lean surgical patients. Similarly, the volume of gastric fluid and pH measurements were identical in obese and normal weight subjects. Therefore, obesity per se should not be an indication for RSI.

Obese patients, like everyone else, can and do have associated co-morbidities that may predispose them to pulmonary aspiration. These include symptomatic gastro-oesophageal reflux disease and hiatal hernia, diabetes mellitus with autonomic neuropathy (gastroparesis), term pregnancy and emergency surgery. Many morbidly obese patients do complain of heartburn and acid reflux. Diabetes mellitus, either type 1 or type 2 (which is very common in obesity), can be associated with autonomic neuropathy with delayed gastric emptying of both fluids and solids. But what is the evidence that even with these co-morbidities, obese patients benefit from RSI?

There are concerns that bariatric procedures predispose patients to developing de novo gastro-oesophageal reflux or exacerbate pre-existing reflux symptoms.

A single study of obese patients, all of whom had previously undergone a gastric banding procedure and were now having plastic surgery, reported a higher incidence of intra-operative aspiration compared to control, normal-weight patients undergoing similar procedures. There are also isolated case reports of patients who had gastric banding surgery, and after prolonged pre-operative fasting, aspirated on induction of general anaesthesia for subsequent surgery even when RSI had been performed.

Sleeve gastrectomy has now become the primary surgical procedure for weight loss. Some studies have reported that it is frequently associated with development of new symptoms of gastro-oesophageal reflux, while others claim resolution of pre-existing reflux symptoms after the same operation. Intractable gastric reflux can occur after sleeve gastrectomy, and is an indication for conversion to gastric bypass. Roux-en-Y gastric bypass consistently results in long-lasting improvement in gastro-oesophageal reflux, and presumably a decrease in the risk of aspiration during subsequent anaesthetics. Unlike gastric banding, to date there have been no reports of aspiration during induction of anaesthesia in patients who have previously undergone sleeve gastrectomy or Roux-en-Y gastric bypass. Despite this, many anaesthetists continue to practice RSI on any patient who has previously undergone a bariatric surgical procedure, while others recommend RSI only for patients who have had a restrictive procedure.

The 4th National Audit Project (NAP4) review of airway management complications in the UK did report that aspiration, the most frequent cause of anaesthesia-related airway mortality, occurred in a 'disproportionate' number of obese patients. Mortality from all causes was extremely rare, approximately 1 death per 180 000 general anaesthetics. The study did not identify obesity per se as an aspiration risk, rather unfamiliarity with the appropriate airway management of obese patients, poor clinical judgement and failure to prepare for potential difficulty with tracheal intubation all contributed to these events.

With the possible exception of the sub-set of morbidly obese patients who have had gastric banding procedures, there is no evidence that obese patients are at aspiration risk during anaesthetic induction, although RSI continues to be recommended for routine induction and airway management of all morbidly obese surgical patients. There is increasing recognition that RSI is unnecessary in the majority of fasted obese patients, especially those with no other risk factors.

Potential Risks of RSI

Since aspiration during general anaesthesia is extremely rare, concerns have been raised as to whether the potential risks of RSI are greater than its presumed benefits.

The 5th National Audit Project (NAP5) found that awareness during surgery occurred most often during the induction of anaesthesia. Approximately half the reported instances of awareness happened during urgent or emergency procedures, many involving RSI. A 'fundamental reassessment' of RSI, both the indications for its use and a standard definition on how to perform it, was recommended. Titration of the anaesthetic induction agent until loss of consciousness is achieved, not a component of traditional RSI where bolus doses of induction and paralysing drugs are given in quick succession, would probably markedly reduce the incidence of awareness events.

The effectiveness of whether cricoid pressure actually achieves its aim has been questioned. Applying too low a force can lead to incomplete occlusion of the oesophagus, while too excessive a force can compress the trachea and limit laryngeal visualisation. By deforming airway anatomy, cricoid pressure can make tracheal intubation more difficult, something to be avoided in morbidly obese patients. The incidence of failed intubations with direct laryngoscopy is increased when cricoid pressure is applied. Cricoid pressure is difficult to perform correctly, potentially dangerous and is probably unnecessary.

Previously, the routine prophylactic administration of agents to reduce and neutralise gastric fluid and to increase gastric emptying time was recommended for all obese patients. An oral non-particulate antacid was also given before anaesthetic induction. The volume of gastric fluid can be reduced and the pH neutralised with H2 receptor antagonists (cimetidine, ranitidine, famotidine). Premedication with H2 blockers is more effective than proton pump inhibitors (PPIs) in reducing gastric volume and increasing gastric fluid pH. Prokinetic drugs (metoclopramide) also can decrease gastric volume. The European Society of Anaesthesiology and the American Society of Anesthesiologists have published guidelines on reducing the risk of peri-operative aspiration. Both societies do not recommend the routine use of antacids, metoclopramide or H2 antagonists before elective surgery. These agents can be given to patients (lean or obese) with high risk for acid reflux, but their actual effectiveness is unknown.

Since obesity by itself is not a risk factor for pulmonary aspiration, obese patients without co-morbid conditions (diabetes mellitus with gastroparesis, symptomatic gastro-oesophageal reflux) can follow the same fasting guidelines as non-obese patients and be allowed to drink clear liquids up until 2 hours before elective operations.

Anesthetic Induction in Obesity

The indication for performing RSI is to reduce the risk of aspiration. As the name implies, during a 'rapid sequence' induction, all medications are administered in rapid sequence. As noted, traditional RSI is not indicated in most obese patients since they are not at any greater risk of aspiration than their normal-weight counterparts. However, for obese patients it is important to establish an airway quickly, not to prevent aspiration, but to avoid hypoxaemia.

The usual supine position for induction of anaesthesia must be avoided. An obese patient lying flat experiences a marked decrease in functional residual capacity (FRC), total respiratory system and pulmonary compliance, and consequently experiences larger ventilation/perfusion (V/Q) mismatch than a normal-weight patient. The decreased lung volume results in reduced oxygen reserves. The 'safe apnoea period' (SAP), that is, the length of time following paralysis and apnoea until the onset of hypoxaemia is much shorter in obese compared to lean patients. It is best to secure the airway quickly, since an apnoeic obese patient's haemoglobin will desaturate very rapidly once muscle relaxants are given.

Induction of general anaesthesia in every obese patient should be performed in the 'ramped' or 'head-elevated laryngoscopy position' (HELP). In this position the patient's head, shoulders and upper body are elevated so an imaginary horizontal line can be drawn from the sternum to the ear. This position improves the view during direct laryngoscopy, potentially resulting in more rapid and successful tracheal intubation. In addition, the operating table should be tilted in a reverse Trendelenburg position, which will further prolong SAP, thus allowing the anaesthetist more time, if needed, to intubate the trachea.

Obese patients should be pre-oxygenated until their oxygen saturation (SpO_2) is 100% and their end-tidal O_2 is >90% for several minutes. Traditional RSI bag-mask ventilation is avoided because of concerns that it will cause insufflation of the stomach and increase the risk of aspiration. Even with the application of cricoid pressure, clinically significant gastric insufflation does not occur during normal bag-mask ventilation. The incidence of oxygen desaturation (SpO_2 <95%) is as high as 35% in patients of all sizes undergoing traditional RSI. For obese patients, with a markedly shortened SAP, the risk of hypoxemia may be even greater, especially if initial attempts at tracheal intubation fail. Unlike traditional RSI, anaesthetic induction of obese patients should include positive-pressure ventilation with the application of PEEP prior to tracheal intubation. Pre-intubation bag-mask ventilation will decrease atelectasis and increase SAP by as much as 50%.

Many practitioners of traditional RSI avoid giving opioids prior to induction of anaesthesia. Current evidence suggests that addition of an opioid before RSI actually improves conditions. Short-acting opioids (fentanyl, remifentanil, alfentanil) should be given to supplement induction agents and decrease the incidence of awareness.

In contrast to traditional RSI, assessment of adequate depth of anaesthesia following administration of induction agents should be performed before administering neuromuscular blocking agents. Giving fixed doses of induction agents and muscle relaxants can lead to underdosing and awareness, or overdosing with potentially severe haemodynamic changes. Following pre-oxygenation, the anaesthetic induction agent should be titrated to loss of consciousness. The patient's clinical condition determines choice of induction agent. For the obese patient, as in normal-weight individuals, adjustment of drug doses is based on lean body weight and not total body weight.

An oral airway is placed. The patient, in the ramped position with the operating table tilted in reverse Trendelenburg, is ventilated by mask. An inhalation agent can be added at that time.

Muscle relaxants are administered after demonstration that bag-mask ventilation is possible. Either suxamethonium or rocuronium are currently used. Suxamethonium provides superior intubation conditions compared to rocuronium. However, 'clinically acceptable intubation conditions' are not different between suxamethonium and rocuronium when propofol is used as the induction agent.

Unlike traditional RSI, there should be no need to rush, since mask ventilation continues during the induction sequence until the patient is completely paralysed and optimal conditions for tracheal intubation are achieved. If a difficult tracheal intubation is anticipated, traditional RSI should not be attempted. As there are no accepted definitions of what actually constitutes a 'difficult intubation', the decision on how to establish an airway is based on the experience of the anaesthetist, the availability of 'difficult airway' resources, and the presence of additional help if needed. Weight or BMI alone do not predict poor laryngoscopic view. For most obese patients, conventional direct laryngoscopy is usually successful. The increasing use of video-laryngoscopy for routine tracheal intubation has presumably led to an even greater success rate in morbidly obese patients. Application of cricoid pressure can actually increase the degree of difficulty and time required for intubation when using a video-laryngoscope, which in turn may cause hypoxemia in obese patients with reduced oxygen reserves and short SAP. Few obese patients require awake fibre- or video-bronchoscopy for tracheal intubation. However, a second-generation supraglottic airway should always be readily available to serve as a bridge if initial tracheal intubation or bag-mask ventilation efforts fail.

Conclusion

For many decades a traditional RSI technique consisting of cricoid pressure and the administration of fast-acting anaesthetic induction and neuromuscular paralysing agents, given in rapid succession, was routinely performed on obese surgical patients. RSI was believed to be necessary because of the misperception that all obese patients were at increased risk for aspiration and pulmonary injury during anaesthetic induction. There is no evidence that this actually is the case. Traditional RSI is not without risks (awareness, under-and overdosing of drugs, impaired visualisation during laryngoscopy, SpO_2 desaturation), and these risks are potentially greater than the low risk of aspiration. Unless the obese patient has clinically significant co-morbidities (symptomatic gastric reflux, emergency surgery, term pregnancy, diabetes with gastroparesis, previous gastric banding surgery), there is no reason to perform an RSI. In the majority of obese patients induction of anaesthesia and tracheal intubation should include placing the patient in a head-up position, adequate pre-oxygenation, administration of fast-acting opioids to supplement the anaesthetic induction agent, titration of the induction agent until loss of consciousness is achieved, avoidance of cricoid pressure and continued bag-mask positive pressure ventilation following the administration of a neuromuscular blocking agent until the patient is fully paralysed and ready for tracheal intubation. Although often called 'modified' RSI, these steps differ from what is historically considered true RSI. Rather than mislead by suggesting that a 'rapid sequence' is involved, the sequence for the anaesthetic induction and tracheal intubation of a morbidly obese patient would be better described as 'controlled intravenous induction and intubation'.

Further Reading

Algie CM, Mahar RK, Tan HB, et al. Effectiveness and risks of cricoid pressure during rapid sequence induction for endotracheal intubation. *Cochr Database Syst Rev.* 2015;**11**: CD011656.

Altermatt FR, Muñoz HR, Delfino AE, et al. Pre-oxygenation in the obese patient: effects of position on tolerance to apnoea. *Br J Anaesth.* 2005;95:706–9.

American Society of Anesthesiologists Committee. Practice guidelines for preoperative fasting and the use of pharmacologic agents to reduce the risk of pulmonary aspiration: application to healthy patients undergoing elective procedures: an updated report by the American Society of Anesthesiologists Committee on Standards and Practice Parameters. *Anesthesiology.* 2011;114:495–511.

Boyce JR, Ness T, Castroman P, et al. preliminary study of the optimal anesthesia positioning for the morbidly obese patient. *Obes Surg.* 2003;13:4–9.

Brodsky JB, Lemmens HJ, Brock-Utne JG, et al. Morbid obesity and tracheal intubation. *Anesth Analg.* 2002;94: 732–6.

Brown JPR, Werret GC. Bag-mask ventilation in rapid sequence induction: a survey of current practice among members of the UK Difficult Airway Society. *Eur J Anaesthesiol.* 2015;32:446–8.

Collins JS, Lemmens HJ, Brodsky JB, et al. Laryngoscopy and morbid obesity: a comparison of the 'sniff' and 'ramped' positions. *Obes Surg.* 2004;14:1171–5.

De Almeida MC, Pederneiras SG, Chiaroni S, et al. Evaluation of tracheal intubation conditions in morbidly obese patients: a comparison of succinylcholine and rocuronium. *Rev Esp Anestesiol Reanim.* 2009;56:2–8.

El-Orbany M, Connolly LA. Rapid sequence induction and intubation: current controversy. *Anesth Analg.* 2010;110: 1318–25.

Freid EB. The rapid sequence induction revisited: obesity and sleep apnea syndrome. *Anesthesiol Clin North Am.* 2005;23:551–64.

Gaszynski TM, Szewczyk T. Rocuronium for rapid sequence induction in morbidly obese patients: a prospective study for evaluation of intubation conditions after administration 1.2 mg kg^{-1} ideal body weight of rocuronium. *Eur J Anaesthesiol.* 2011;28:609–10.

Harter RL, Kelly WB, Kramer MG, et al. A comparison of the volume and pH of gastric contents of obese and lean surgical patients. *Anesth Analg.* 1998;86:147–52.

Kristensen MA. Airway management and morbid obesity. *Eur J Anaesthesiol.* 2010;27:923–7.

Lam AM, Grace DM, Manninen PH, et al. The effects of cimetidine and ranitidine with and without metoclopramide on gastric volume and pH in morbidly obese patients. *Can Anaesth Soc J.* 1986;33:773–9.

Maltby JR, Pytka S, Watson NC, et al. Drinking 300 mL of clear fluid two hours before surgery has no effect on gastric fluid volume and pH in fasting and non-fasting obese patients. *Can J Anaesth.* 2004;51:111–15.

Neilipovitz DT, Crosby ET. No evidence for decreased incidence of aspiration after rapid sequence induction. *Can J Anaesth.* 2007;54:748–64.

Ovassapian A, Salem MR. Sellick's maneuver: to do or not do. *Anesth Analg.* 2009;109:1360–2.

Smith I, Kranke P, Murat I, et al. Perioperative fasting in adults and children: guidelines from the European Society of Anaesthesiology. *Eur J Anesthesiol.* 2011;28:556–69.

Airway Management in Obesity

Benjamin Millette, Vassilis Athanassoglou and Anil Patel

Background and Epidemiology

According to Health Survey England in 2011, 24% of men and 26% of women in the UK are obese. The prevalence of obesity is increasing and obese patients are more likely to present to hospital because they are more prone to several associated disease processes. Airway management in the obese is therefore a problem that will be encountered by virtually all anaesthetists.

Difficult airways are common in the obese patient population. A BMI >35 is associated with a 34% greater chance of difficult or failed tracheal intubation. A BMI >30 is also an independent predictor of difficult bag-mask ventilation, but does not appear to be an independent predictor of impossible bag-mask ventilation.

There are several aspects of the pathophysiology of obesity that contribute to difficulties in managing the airway. These include:

- difficulties in patient positioning;
- increased neck fat deposition may lead to upper airway obstruction on induction;
- respiratory changes, including reduced functional residual capacity, increased closing capacity and increased oxygen consumption all lead to decreased apnoea to desaturation time compared with lean individuals;
- difficulties in drug dosing that may lead to sub-optimal intubating conditions.
- raised intra-abdominal pressure which may increase the risk of gastric aspiration.

Proper provision of equipment, thorough assessment and expert management of the obese patient based on sound theory and evidence can mitigate these problems.

Associated Pre-morbid Conditions

Obesity is associated with increased insulin resistance and diabetes. Diabetic patients, particularly those with the 'stiff joint syndrome' may be at increased risk of difficult airway management if the jaw and/or cervical vertebrae are affected. This is thought to be due to decreased joint mobility secondary to the glycosylation of collagen.

The prevalence of obstructive sleep apnoea (OSA) in the obese is almost double that of normal weight adults. OSA is an independent predictor of impossible bag-mask ventilation (defined as inability to exchange air during bag-mask ventilation attempts, despite multiple providers, adjuvants and neuromuscular blockade). If untreated, OSA may progress to obesity hypoventilation syndrome. This is associated with chronic hypoxaemia and hypercapnia, which increase the probability of peri-operative respiratory complications. Both are associated with a higher incidence of post-operative desaturation and respiratory compromise. Pre- and post-operative treatment with CPAP can be very effective.

Airway Assessment

History

A full anaesthetic history should be taken and the patient should be specifically questioned regarding the pre-morbid conditions above. Records of previous anaesthetics, especially any involving airway difficulties, can be invaluable in planning the airway management for future surgery and form part of the overall airway assessment. A history of previous difficult airway is a good predictor of future problems. Attention should also be paid to risk factors and history of gastro-oesophageal reflux. The use of the STOP-BANG score to screen for OSA is useful, as presence of OSA is a predictor of impossible bag-mask ventilation with a hazard ratio of 2.4. Surgical procedures involving a shared airway or potentially affecting the airway should prompt a more thorough airway assessment.

Examination

Established examination methods of assessing the likelihood of difficult tracheal intubation such as Mallampati score, mouth opening, thyromental distance and assessment of head, neck and jaw mobility should be performed. Neck circumference should be measured, as a larger neck circumference is associated with increased probability of difficult intubation, as well as difficult mask ventilation. Neck circumference >42 cm is an independent predictor of difficult intubation.

Investigation

In some circumstances pre-operative polysomnography may be appropriate to diagnose OSA. Depending on the surgical pathology, cross-sectional imaging of the head and neck or fibreoptic nasendoscopy may form part of the airway assessment. Point of care ultrasound has been used with increasing frequency to assess the likelihood of difficult airway. Literature demonstrates that sonographically assessed distance from skin to epiglottis of >27.5 mm is a good predictor of Cormack–Lehane grade 3/4 laryngoscopy, especially when used in conjunction with a modified Mallampati score. Ultrasound can also be used to assess depth to cricothyroid membrane if planning an elective cricothyroid puncture (Figure 21.1).

There is as yet no prospectively validated scoring system to assess the probability of difficult airway specifically in the obese patient population.

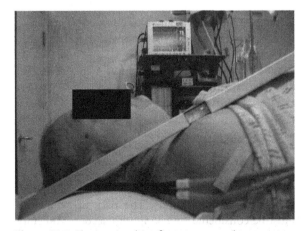

Figure 21.1 Obese patient lying flat – sternum and tragus not level. (Courtesy of Dr V Athanassoglou.)

Pre-oxygenation

Good pre-oxygenation is essential in the obese given their propensity to faster arterial oxygen desaturation. It is traditionally performed via tight-fitting facemask using 100% oxygen. Pre-oxygenation in the 25° head up or sitting position has been shown to be superior to pre-oxygenating in the supine position due to improved lung mechanics. A technique of four vital capacity breaths within 30 seconds is as effective as using 3–5 minutes of tidal volume ventilation.

Both continuous positive airway pressure (CPAP) and non-invasive positive pressure ventilation (NIPPV) have been described as effective pre-oxygenation methods in the obese, but they are not in widespread use.

Use of warmed humidified high-flow nasal oxygen (HFNO) is becoming more widespread in the management of the obese airway. Apnoeic oxygenation can reduce the incidence of desaturation during intubation. This can be facilitated using oxygen via nasal prongs or, more effectively, by HFNO. Apnoeic oxygenation with HFNO has been used to facilitate unhurried airway instrumentation in obese patients.

Use of Supraglottic Airways

Supraglottic airways do not offer as much protection against aspiration of gastric contents as cuffed endotracheal tubes. As such, their elective use is relatively contraindicated in the obese. Second-generation supraglottic airways provide better protection than the first generation. The 4th National Audit Project of the Royal College of Anaesthetists found that obesity was over-represented in adverse anaesthetic events following insertion of a supraglottic airway. The Society for Obesity and Bariatric Anaesthesia (SOBA)/Association of Anaesthetists of Great Britain and Ireland (AAGBI) guidelines suggest that use of supraglottic airways should be reserved for 'highly selected patients, undergoing short procedures and where the patient can be kept head up during surgery'.

Supraglottic airways can be used as an effective rescue technique in the difficult intubation/mask ventilation scenario. Furthermore, they can also be used as a conduit for more advanced airway techniques using a fibreoptic scope with or without an airway exchange catheter.

However, elective insertion of supraglottic devices should, wherever possible, be avoided in the obese patient, except as part of airway rescue techniques.

Tracheal Intubation

Proper patient positioning is crucial to successful tracheal intubation in the obese. Adjusting the head height to place the patient in a ramped position so that the tragus and sternum are at the same level helps to improve laryngoscopy view and maximise safe apnoea time (Figures 21.1 and 21.2). This can be achieved very simply by elevating the head end of the operating table and use of pillows. Purpose-built devices such as the Oxford Head Elevating Laryngoscopy pillow/Troop Elevation Pillow can also be used.

An appropriate dose of muscle relaxant should be administered to optimise intubating conditions. Suxamethonium should be dosed based on total body weight, whereas non-depolarising muscle relaxants should be dosed based on lean body weight. Suxamethonium fasciculations may increase oxygen consumption and decrease safe apnoea time; therefore in the setting of a rapid sequence induction, rocuronium may be more appropriate. Rocuronium also has the added advantage of being immediately reversible with the use of sugammadex should problems arise.

Videolaryngoscopy is associated with high success rates in the obese. It is associated with better laryngoscopic views and faster time to intubation compared to direct laryngoscopy. However, ease of laryngoscopy will to a degree be operator dependent and related to experience.

Depending on the initial airway assessment, fibreoptic intubation may be the airway management of choice. This can be more technically and ergonomically challenging in the obese given difficulties in patient positioning, anatomical changes in airway, airway obstruction and faster time to desaturation.

FONA (Front of Neck Access)

Emergency cricothyroidotomy can be much more difficult in the obese owing to difficulty identifying anatomy and positioning the patient. Current Difficult Airway Society (DAS) guidelines recommend cricothyroidotomy using a scalpel, gum elastic bougie and cuffed size 6 mm endotracheal tube. If the cricothyroid membrane is palpable then a transverse incision through the membrane is recommended. If it is impalpable then a vertical 8–10 cm incision is

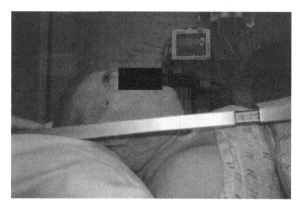

Figure 21.2 Obese patient ramped – sternum and tragus level. (Courtesy of Dr V Athanassoglou.)

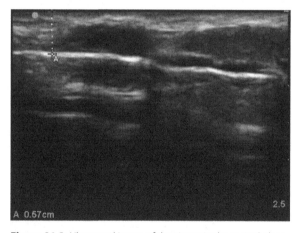

Figure 21.3 Ultrasound image of the airway in the sagittal plane showing the distance to the trachea. (Courtesy of Dr V. Athanassoglou.)

recommended followed by blunt dissection of tissues with the fingers in order to identify laryngeal anatomy to perform the procedure.

Ultrasound is also emerging as a useful tool to identify cricothyroid anatomy and airway depth (Figure 21.3). While this may be of limited use in the emergency situation, it has the potential to greatly assist elective cricothyroid puncture.

Extubation

Obese patients are at higher risk of tracheal extubation-related complications. The risks of extubation must be considered by taking into account difficulty of airway, presence of airway trauma, aspiration risk and surgical factors.

Perform Awake Extubation
Pre-oxygenate with 100% oxygen
Suction as appropriate
Insert a bite block (e.g. rolled gauze)
Position the patient appropriately
Antagonise neuromuscular blockade
Establish regular breathing
Ensure adequate spontaneous ventilation
Minimise head and neck movements
Wait until awake (eye opening/obeying commands)
Apply positive pressure, deflate the cuff & remove tube
Provide 100% oxygen
Check airway patency and adequacy of breathing
Continue oxygen supplementation

Figure 21.4 DAS awake extubation guideline. (Courtesy of Dr Anil Patel and the Difficult Airway Society.)

Awake extubation is recommended and should be managed according to DAS guidelines (Figure 21.4). CPAP or NIPPV can be useful to maintain oxygenation following tracheal extubation, particularly in those patients who have OSA or have undergone long procedures.

Recovery Room Management

Appropriate monitoring should be maintained in the recovery room. The patient should be managed in the sitting position or with head up tilt to minimise the risk of respiratory compromise. Supplemental oxygen should be administered until the patient is fully awake, mobile and at baseline oxygen saturations. CPAP/NIPPV or HFNO can also be used in order to maintain oxygenation if appropriate. The patient should be closely monitored for hypoventilation, especially if opiates have been administered. High dependency care is appropriate for those requiring ongoing monitoring or those requiring respiratory support that cannot be provided on a general ward.

Further Reading

Kheterpal S, Han R, Tremper K, et al. Incidence and predictors of difficult and impossible mask ventilation *Anesthesiology.* 2006;**105**(11):885–91.

Kheterpal S, Martin L, Shanks AM, Tremper KK. Predictions and outcomes of impossible mask ventilation: a review of 50,000 anesthetics. *Anesthesiology.* 2009;**110**:891–7.

Kristensen M. Airway management and morbid obesity. *Eur J Anaesthesiol.* 2010;**27**(11):923–7.

Lundstrøm LH, Møller AM, Rosenstock C, Astrup G, Wetterslev J. High body mass index is a weak predictor for difficult and failed tracheal intubation: a cohort study of 91,332 consecutive patients scheduled for direct laryngoscopy registered in the Danish Anesthesia Database. *Anesthesiology.* 2009;**110**(2669):1.

Nightingale CE, Margarson MP, Shearer E, et al. Perioperative management of the obese surgical patient 2015. *Anaesthesia.*2015;**70**:859–76.

Patel A, Nouraei SAR. Transnasal Humidified Rapid-Insufflation Ventilatory Exchange (THRIVE): a physiological method of increasing apnoea time in patients with difficult airways. *Anaesthesia.* 2015;**70**(3):323–9.

Pinto J, Cordeiro L, Periera C, et al. Predicting difficult laryngoscopy using ultrasound measurement of distance from skin to epiglottis. *J Crit Care.* 2016;**33**:26–31.

Riad W, Vaez MN, Raveendran R, et al. Neck circumference as a predictor of difficult intubation and difficult mask ventilation in morbidly obese patients: a prospective observational study. *Eur J Anaesthesiol.* 2016;**33**(4):244–97.

Romero-Corral A, Caples S, Lopez Jimenez F, Somers V. Interactions between obesity and obstructive sleep apnoea. *Chest.* 2010;**137**(3):711–19.

Teoh WH, Kristensen M. Utility of ultrasound in airway management *Trends Anaesth Crit Care.* 2014;**4**(4):84–90.

Yumul R, Elvir-Lazo OL, White PF, et al. Comparison of three video laryngoscopy devices to direct laryngoscopy for intubating obese patients: a randomised controlled trial. *J Clin Anesth.* 2016;**31**:71–7. www.das.uk.com/guidelines/das_intubation_guidelines (accessed February 2017).

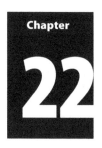

22

Maintenance of General Anaesthesia in Obesity

Bjorn Heyse and Luc De Baerdemaeker

Total Intravenous Anaesthesia (TIVA) versus Inhalational Anaesthesia

Outcome and patient's perception of quality of recovery are important determinants for anaesthetists to select a type of anaesthesia that fits their patient.

Studies on the differences in anaesthetic outcome between these two techniques in lean and obese patients have great difficulty in demonstrating superiority of one technique over the other.

The overall incidence of post-operative nausea and vomiting (PONV) after bariatric surgery is still high and depends on the risk factors and the type of bariatric procedure. Even when TIVA was used with dual anti-emetic prophylaxis, 24 h cumulative incidence of PONV was 45% (34–60%). Studies on inhalational anaesthesia and laparoscopic gastric banding reported a cumulative 24 h incidence of 23.3% when triple anti-emetic prophylaxis was used. The avoidance of opioids and higher dosage of dexamethasone (0.1 mg/kg IBW) and ondansetron (8 mg) have an additional reducing effect.

In a meta-analysis on post-operative recovery in the morbidly obese, the authors reported the fastest return of consciousness with desflurane, followed by sevoflurane, isoflurane and propofol. Despite reports of improved post-operative pain with TIVA, no significant difference was reported in visual analogue scores or in length of stay in the recovery room.

A few studies in non-obese patients demonstrated less impact on post-operative pulmonary functions when inhalational anaesthesia was used.

Even though TIVA does carry some advantages over inhalational anaesthesia, its use is still low (Table 22.1). Data on its use in morbidly obese patients are sparse, as is research on optimisation of TIVA for challenging patients such as the obese. Improved knowledge in the field of pharmacology, interactions, pharmacodynamic monitoring, target-controlled infusions (TCI) systems and closed-loop technology did give it a boost. However,

this did not facilitate it becoming the preferred anaesthesia technique for any type of procedure or patient.

TCI systems use pharmacokinetic/pharmacodynamics models to deliver (in a computerised way) a variable infusion rate of a drug in order to achieve and maintain an appropriate drug concentration in the plasma compartment or in the effect-site compartment. Over decades of use, this technology has matured and proven itself as safe as other conventional TIVA techniques.

The problem with the use of TCI systems in the obese is that obese patients were excluded in the original study population that generated the data to develop these models. Unfortunately, in the models that do use lean body mass (LBM) as a covariate, the James equation was used. The problem with this equation is that starting from a certain total body weight (TBW), the calculated LBM starts to decline, allowing for underdosing. The manufacturers have solved this problem by limiting the input of total body weight to the value where LBM reaches its maximum.

Commercially available TCI systems are being used for the administration of the hypnotics propofol and midazolam, and opioids such as fentanyl, remifentanil, sufentanil and alfentanil.

As a general safety rule, whenever there is uncertainty over the pharmacokinetics of a drug in a particular patient population, pharmacodynamic monitoring can be very useful to help titrate this drug during the maintenance phase.

Hypnotics: Propofol and Midazolam

For the first 10 minutes of pharmacokinetics of propofol the initial volume of distribution V1 is not significantly influenced by obesity and is closely related to LBM. This helps to explain why the induction dose of propofol should be calculated on LBM and the continuous infusion on TBW.

The manual BET (bolus, elimination, transfer) scheme published by Roberts et al. for the delivery of

Table 22.1 Pro and cons of TIVA and inhalational anaesthesia

Inhalational agents	Total intravenous agents
Favourable pharmacokinetics	No risk of malignant hyperthermia
Rapid induction of anaesthesia when initial IV access failed	Less occupational and environmental hazard
Easy adjustment of depth of anaesthesia	Antidotes available for some agents
Predictable and safe recovery	No real time pharmacokinetic monitoring
Inter-individual dose variation small compared to IV agents	High inter-individual dose requirements
Less awareness using end tidal anaesthetic concentration guided (ETAG) anaesthesia	Cardiovascular stability of some IV agents is superior
High degree of controllability	Recovery without shivering or agitation, clear headed
Monitoring of end tidal concentrations to reflect brain concentration during steady state	Less post-operative nausea and vomiting (PONV)
Elimination by exhalation	Awareness (infusion of neuromuscular blocking agent (NMBA))
No true allergies to the molecule	Post-operative respiratory depression
Volatile induction of anaesthesia in adults with non-pungent agents	Patient acceptance
	Quality of recovery better?
Only needs a vaporiser/injector, which is integrated in the ventilator	Cumbersome: pumps, syringes, extension lines, one-way valves
	Provision of anaesthetics is separated from the ventilator

propofol was designed to achieve and maintain a plasma propofol concentration of 3 μg/ml. Although practical, these manual regimens could not assure adequate anaesthesia in all patients in all circumstances, as reported in the NAP5 on accidental awareness during general anaesthesia. When using the BET scheme with adjusted body weight (ABW) = IBW + 0.4 (TBW – IBW), the mean duration of periods with BIS >60 was 13.74 ± 21.74% of total anaesthesia time.

The Marsh model for propofol adjusts all the volumes of the three-compartment model according to the total weight input of the patient and the rate constants are fixed. In severely obese patients, this results in a large induction dose of propofol, creating haemodynamic instability. In an attempt to overcome haemodynamic and accumulation issues, clinicians have used ABW as the weight input. Some studies showed improved accuracy when ABW was applied, whereas others failed to do so. When using ABW as an input for the Marsh model, it is advisable to monitor depth of anaesthesia.

In the Schnider model, V1 and V3 are fixed. V2, k_{12} and k_{21} are age dependent and most importantly,

the elimination rate constant k_{10} is the only parameter dependent on LBM. When TBW is used as input, the device will stop at the value where maximum value of LBM is reached (from the James equation). Without this pragmatic solution, the infusion rate to compensate for the estimated metabolised propofol would otherwise increase exponentially, with a risk of overdosing. Performance of the Schnider model in the obese improves when ABW is utilised as input weight.

Another approach is to develop models specifically for the obese or to develop a general-purpose model that performs well over a wide range of patient groups and clinical conditions such as the experimental Eleveld model. Provided that this pharmacokinetic model is expanded with a pharmacodynamic model derived from the same population and after validation, it has the potential to become the definitive 'universal' model for TCI administration of propofol.

For midazolam, the peripheral volume of distribution increases with TBW according to a power function and clearance does not change with weight. For this reason, the initial bolus dose can be calculated on TBW, but the continuous infusion should be adjusted

125

to IBW. Alternatively, a fixed bolus dose of 2 mg and a fixed maintenance dose of 3.5 mg/h, adapted to clinical needs, can be used. No studies on the performance of midazolam TCI using Greenblatt's model in obese patients exist.

Opioids: Remifentanil, Fentanyl, Sufentanil, Alfentanil

Remifentanil, with its rapid onset and a constant context-sensitive half-life, has become the opioid of choice for TIVA for both obese and non-obese patients.

When using manual infusions, Egan and co-workers have shown that remifentanil should be calculated on LBM. For TCI administration, the Minto model performs well, but is hampered by the use of the James equation to calculate LBM. The input of the fictitious height from the formula published by La Colla improves the predictive performance of the model. With fictitious height as an input, the James equation will calculate a value for LBM that equals LBM according to the Janmahasatian equation for LBM.

The Shafer and Scott–Stanski pharmacokinetic models used for fentanyl TCI were derived from a non-obese study population. Shafer and colleagues advised to only use their model in the range of 1 SD of the mean weight (69 kg ± 17 kg). Both models overestimate the measured plasma concentration of fentanyl when TBW is used in the obese. Shibutani et al. studied the accuracy of both models in obese patients and used a non-linear regression analysis on the non-linear relationship between performance error and TBW to calculate correction factors for both models.

The pharmacokinetic mass = $52/[1 + (196.4 \times e^{-0.025TBW} - 53.66)/100]$ is a correction factor that will convert TBW into a fentanyl dosing weight that will correct the error between Shafer's predicted and measured fentanyl plasma concentrations and should be used as input when using fentanyl TCI with the Shafer model. Fentanyl dosing normalised to pharmacokinetic mass is a very practical dosing weight for manual infusions of fentanyl for clinicians not using computerised infusion pumps. From 52–100 kg pharmacokinetic mass increases linearly and for every 10 kg increase of TBW, 6.5 kg needs to be added to the reference weight of 52 kg. Beyond 100 kg TBW,

the graph starts to curve and flattens out between 140 to 200 kg, where the pharmacokinetic mass only varies from 100–108 kg, respectively.

For sufentanil, Schwartz et al. advised using TBW for calculating the loading dose in the obese and to 'prudently reduce' the maintenance dose without further specification. The Gepts model used for sufentanil TCI was studied in morbidly obese patients and performed well up to a BMI of 40. Above this, the predicted plasma concentrations were higher than the measured plasma concentrations because clearance of sufentanil increased with BMI. Clinicians should take this into account when using sufentanil TCI.

For manual alfentanil infusion schemes, IBW or LBM can be used because alfentanil has a lower clearance and far less redistribution compared to an opioid such as sufentanil. Pérus et al. studied the performance of the alfentanil TCI models published by Maître, and Scott and Stanski in obese patients and concluded that the Scott and Stanski model performed poorly in obese patients. The Maître model underestimates the measured plasma concentration, but is still within acceptable limits, although users have to be cautious when using higher target concentrations.

Volatile Anaesthetics for Maintenance

Obesity only moderately affects the uptake and wash out of isoflurane, sevoflurane and desflurane. The minimum alveolar concentration (MAC) value of all agents is unchanged for the lean and the obese patient. The molecule with the lowest blood gas partition coefficient will yield the quickest pharmacokinetics, even in the obese. Fat solubility of an agent is often regarded as an important factor influencing the choice of volatile agents. The wash in and wash out times of a tissue is determined by its time constant τ and is calculated as:

$$\tau_{tissue} = (volume_{tissue}. \lambda_{tissue/blood})/flow_{tissue}$$

It is the time needed to reach 63% of equilibrium.

For the fat group, the time constants for bulk fat are 36.6 hours and 20.4 hours for sevoflurane and desflurane, respectively. This means that the partial pressure in the bulk fat after anaesthetics lasting 2–6 hours will be substantially lower than the arterial blood partial pressure, and thus bulk fat will continue to absorb agent rather than releasing it during emergence. Fat will act as a sink, absorbing anaesthetic and potentially prolonging emergence. The fat surrounding well-perfused organs can take up important amounts of anaesthetic by inter-tissue diffusion and has the potential to delay recovery because this fat has a shorter time constant and the same capacity to hold anaesthetic. Partial pressure attaining MAC_{awake} can be reached after 6 hours of anaesthesia in this inter-tissue diffusion group.

Whatever agent is chosen, the anaesthetist should be aware of re-hypnotisation due to hypoventilation at the moment of emergence because alveolar minute ventilation is an important factor both in uptake and elimination of volatile anaesthetics.

To reduce awareness, using end tidal anaesthetic concentration guided (ETAG) anaesthesia in the range of 0.7–1.3 MAC is advised when no brain monitoring is available.

Other Drugs Used During Maintenance of Anaesthesia

After a bolus administration at induction, the maintenance dose of neuromuscular blocking agent depends on the level of muscle relaxation one wishes to achieve and is ideally titrated using neuromuscular transmission monitoring. For deep neuromuscular blockade during laparoscopic procedures, a rocuronium infusion of 0.6 mg/kg/h using LBM is probably the most logical choice, with a sugammadex reversal dose of 4 mg/kg TBW at the end of surgery.

Dexmedetomidine is frequently used in the obese patient in order to reduce or even abolish the intra-operative use of opioids. When using a manual infusion scheme, 0.2 μg/kg/h TBW is recommended. Hanivoort and co-workers managed to develop an optimised three-compartment model using allometric scaling for the continuous infusion of dexmedetomidine with weight as an important co-variate. The model performed well over a wide range of age and weights. Following validation, this model has the potential to be used in future TCI dexmedetomidine administration.

Intra-operative infusions of lignocaine using a bolus dose of 1.5 mg/kg and a continuous infusion of 2 mg/kg/h until end of surgery calculated on ABW can reduce post-operative opioid consumption and improve quality of recovery in morbidly obese patients scheduled for laparoscopic bariatric surgery.

Magnesium can be administered over the course of surgery at a total dose of 80 mg/kg IBW or extrapolated from studies in non-obese with a loading dose of 50 mg/kg IBW and a maintenance dose of 8–15mg/kg/h.

For ketamine, Feld et al. used IBW to administer 0.17 mg/kg/h during maintenance with a maximum total dose of 1 mg/kg. Alternatively, a loading dose of 0.25–0.5 mg/kg IBW can be followed by a continuous infusion of 2–2.5 μg/kg/min IBW.

Combinations and Interactions of Anaesthetic Drugs in the Obese

Combinations of hypnotics and opioids are used to achieve the endpoints of hypnosis, immobility and suppression of autonomic response to noxious stimuli. For each endpoint, different plasma concentrations of hypnotics and opioids are possible to achieve the desired end point. Hypnotics and opioids interact and the interactions between these different combinations have been described and modelled. In non-obese patients, Vuyk et al. have determined the optimal combinations of propofol and different opioids that allow clinicians to set TCI concentrations or manual infusion rates that will obtain 50% and 95% probability of no response to surgical stimuli and the fastest awakening times. No studies have explored the efficiency of these recommendations in the obese.

With the introduction of pharmacodynamic monitoring, anaesthetists can select combinations of plasma concentrations or end tidal concentration of both hypnotics and opioids that will guarantee with a degree of certainty that the pharmacodynamic effect will stay within a pre-set desired target. Software such as Navigator and Smartpilot are even able to make predictions on when and how the desired endpoints will be reached. This can be done with the anaesthetist as the controller in an open loop or in an automated mode using feedback closed-loop controllers.

Table 22.2 lists the induction dose and maintenance dose of propofol and remifentanil derived from studies aiming to keep depth of anaesthesia monitors within a chosen target.

Nitrous Oxide versus Air

Nitrous oxide is often co-administered with potent anaesthetics, both in TIVA and inhalational anaesthesia. Table 22.3 lists some of the disadvantages and advantages of nitrous oxide that could affect safe anaesthesia in the morbidly obese.

Although nitrous oxide has some interesting characteristics, justifying administration in morbidly

Table 22.2 Propofol, inhaled anaesthetics and opiate combinations in morbidly obese patients

Propofol		Remifentanil		Brain monitor type/target
Induction	Maintenance	Induction	Maintenance	
1.2(1.1–1.6)	5.2(4.1–6)	1.0	0.12(0.07–0.16)	BIS 40–60
2.5	4.8(1.5)	–	–	BIS 40–60
–	6.1(1.8)		0.15(0.07)	BIS 40–50
1.5–2 ABW	3.8(1.0)	0.5	0.34(0.15)	BIS 40–60
	6.53(1.11)		0.36(0.09)	BIS 40–60

Sevoflurane	Desflurane	Remifentanil		
Maintenance	Maintenance	TCI	Maintenance	
0.71(0.22) MAC	0.56(0.15) MAC	4 ng/ml		BIS 45–55
	3.3(1.1) vol% ET	4 ng/ml	0.125 µg/kg/min	BIS 45–55

Induction and maintenance dose are expressed in TBW unless otherwise mentioned. Opioids can be converted using the ratio of equipotency (fentanyl to alfentanil to sufentanil to remifentanil 1:1/70:630:1/2.3).
Data are expressed as mean (SD) or median (range)

obese patients, its use is often discouraged in review articles based on reasons mentioned in Table 22.1.

The advice not to use nitrous oxide in the obese for reasons of hypoxia is mainly based on the higher oxygen consumption of the morbidly obese patient. This could imply that a higher FiO_2 might be needed during anaesthesia and thus limit the use of nitrous oxide at efficient concentrations of 50–70%. The second gas and concentrating effect of nitrous oxide during both the maintenance and emergence phase is underestimated and applies to oxygen as well. Arterial oxygenation during maintenance is actually higher when using oxygen/nitrous oxide compared to oxygen/air mixtures. Hypoxic events during the emergence period are hardly influenced by 'diffusion anoxia' caused by nitrous oxide, but should rather be attributed to pulmonary atelectasis and other co-morbidities. In ASA I patients receiving sedation with only O_2/N_2O, Jeske et al. were not able to detect differences in pulse oximetry compared to patients receiving oxygen or room air during the immediate recovery period.

Theoretically, nitrous oxide might promote atelectasis in poorly ventilated lung regions by gas absorption. A meta-analysis by Sun linked the use of nitrous-oxide-based anaesthesia to pulmonary atelectasis (OR 1.57(1.18–2.10)), yet none of the included studies involved morbidly obese patients or the standard use of recruitment manoeuvers followed by PEEP as preventive measures against atelectasis.

After 2 hours of prolonged laparoscopy with O_2/N_2O anaesthesia at an FiO_2 of 33%, the CO_2 pneumoperitoneum is contaminated by diffusion with 29% of nitrous oxide, a fraction that becomes hazardous with regard to gas embolisation and explosion risk, e.g. intestinal H_2 and CH_4 from an inadvertent bowel perforation during laparoscopy might ignite in this mixture. After 8–10 hours, the intra-peritoneal N_2O equals the end tidal N_2O. One solution is to avoid N_2O during laparoscopy lasting more than 2 hours or to use insufflators with calibrated pneumoperitoneal venting. In one animal study, it has been demonstrated that in case of an inadvertent CO_2/N_2O embolism, no negative impact of nitrous oxide on the haemodynamic consequences of this type of embolism could be detected.

Bowel distension is not an issue during laparoscopic bariatric procedures lasting 90 minutes using O_2/N_2O anaesthesia at a FiO_2 of 50%.

The ENIGMA II trial supports the safety record of nitrous oxide in non-cardiac surgery: no increased risk of death, cardiovascular complications or surgical site infections. The emetic effect depends on duration of administration and can be counteracted by

Table 22.3 List of potential disadvantages and advantages of nitrous oxide (N_2O) in morbidly obese patients

Disadvantages of N_2O	Advantages of N_2O
PONV	Analgesic properties
Expansion of air spaces	Dose reduction of other drugs
Myocardial ischaemia Elevated homocysteine levels	Long-standing safety record
Increased risk of hypoxia	Possible lower risk of awareness
Increased ICP	Second gas and concentrating effect
29 vol% CO_2/N_2O supports combustion	Prevention of acute and chronic pain
Pulmonary atelectasis	Short-acting/low blood/gas solubility
Increases pulmonary artery pressure	Increases sympathetic activity

standard PONV prophylaxis. The trial showed that the use of volatile agents was reduced and nitrous oxide can accelerate both its uptake and clearance.

Adding nitrous oxide to propofol–opioid-based techniques using pharmacodynamics monitoring does not seem to reduce the dose of hypnotics and has no effect on the dosage of opioids. In volatile–opioid-based techniques, however, its addition does lower BIS values and allows a dose reduction of the volatile agents.

Remarkably, many milestone papers on TIVA and inhalational anaesthesia in morbidly obese patients did use the co-administration of nitrous oxide. Whether consensus statements on the safety of nitrous oxide can be expanded to morbidly obese patients requires further studies.

Further Reading

Absalom AR, Mani V, De Smet T, Struys MMRF. Pharmacokinetic models for propofol: defining and illuminating the devil in the detail. *Br J Anaesth.* 2009;103:26–37.

Brodsky JB, Lemmens HJM, Collins JS et al. Nitrous oxide and laparoscopic bariatric surgery. *Obes Surg.* 2005;15:494–6.

Casati A, Marchetti C, Spreafico E, Mamo D. Effects of obesity on wash-in and wash-out kinetics of sevoflurane. *Eur J Anaesthesiol.* 2004;21:243–5.

Cortínez LI, De La Fuente N, Eleveld DJ, et al. Performance of propofol target-controlled infusion models in the obese: Pharmacokinetic and pharmacodynamic analysis. *Anesth Analg.* 2014;119:302–10.

De Baerdemaeker LEC, Jacobs S, Pattyn P, Mortier EP, Struys MMRF. Influence of intraoperative opioid on postoperative pain and pulmonary function after laparoscopic gastric banding: remifentanil TCI vs sufentanil TCI in morbid obesity. *Br J Anaesth.* 2007;99:404–11.

De Oliveira GS, Duncan K, Fitzgerald P, et al. Systemic lidocaine to improve quality of recovery after laparoscopic bariatric surgery: a randomized double-blinded placebo-controlled trial. *Obes Surg.* 2014;24:212–8.

Eleveld DJ, Proost JH, Cortínez LI, Absalom AR, Struys MMRF. A general purpose pharmacokinetic model for propofol. *Anesth Analg.* 2014;118:1221–37.

European Society of Anaesthesiology Task Force on Use of Nitrous Oxide in Clinical Anaesthetic Practice. The current place of nitrous oxide in clinical practice: an expert opinion-based task force consensus statement of the European Society of Anaesthesiology. *Eur J Anaesthesiol.* 2015;32:517–20.

Greenblatt DJ, Ehrenberg BL, Gunderman J, et al. Remifentanil pharmacokinetics in obese versus lean patients. *Anesthesiology.* 1998;89:562–73.

Hawthorne C, Sutcliffe N. Total intravenous anaesthesia. *Anaesth Intensive Care Med.* 2016;17:166–8.

Ingrande J, Brodsky JB, Lemmens HJ. Lean body weight scalar for the anesthetic induction dose of propofol in morbidly obese subjects. *Anesth Analg.* 2011;113(1):57–62

Jabbour HJ, Naccache NM, Jawish RJ, et al. Ketamine and magnesium association reduces morphine consumption after scoliosis surgery: prospective randomised double-blind study. *Acta Anaesthesiol Scand.* 2014;58:572–9.

Alvarez A, Singh PM, Sinha AC. Postoperative analgesia in morbid obesity. *Obes Surg.* 2014;24:652–9.

Juvin P, Vadam C, Malek L, et al. Postoperative recovery after desflurane, propofol, or isoflurane anesthesia among morbidly obese patients: a prospective, randomized study. *Anesth Analg.* 2000;91:714–9.

La Colla L, Albertin A, La Colla G, et al. No adjustment vs. adjustment formula as input weight for propofol target-controlled infusion in morbidly obese patients. *Eur J Anaesthesiol.* 2009;26:362–9.

Liu F-L, Cherng Y-G, Chen S-Y, et al. Postoperative recovery after anesthesia in morbidly obese patients: a systematic review and meta-analysis of randomized controlled trials. *Can J Anaesth.* 2015;62:907–17.

Miller TE, Gan TJ. Total intravenous anesthesia and anesthetic outcomes. *J Cardiothorac Vasc Anesth.* 2015;29 (Suppl 1): S11–15.

Myles PS, Leslie K, Chan MT V, et al. The safety of addition of nitrous oxide to general anaesthesia in at-risk patients having major non-cardiac surgery (ENIGMA-II): a randomised, single-blind trial. *Lancet* 2014;384:1446–54.

Myles PS, Leslie K, Silbert B, Paech MJ, Peyton P. A review of the risks and benefits of nitrous oxide in current anaesthetic practice. *Anaesth Intensive Care.* 2004;32:165–72.

Schnider TW, Minto CF, Struys MMRF, Absalom AR. The safety of target-controlled infusions. *Anesth Analg.* 2016;**122**:79–85.

Sun R, Jia WQ, Zhang P, et al. Nitrous oxide-based techniques versus nitrous oxide-free techniques for general anaesthesia. *Cochr Database Syst Rev.* 2015: CD008984.

Chapter 23

Techniques of Ventilation and the Pneumoperitoneum

Rupert Mason and Mike Margarson

Ventilation

The Fundamental Problem

Work of breathing is increased in the morbidly obese, and this is most marked in the supine position. Most obese patients sleep on their side and a significant proportion sleep in chairs.

Once anaesthetised, and particularly if in the supine position, few patients will breathe adequately unsupported. The development of a degree of atelectasis is common; subsequent hypercapnia and hypoxaemia under anaesthesia in the spontaneously breathing patient are almost inevitable.

The obese patient also has a higher baseline oxygen consumption than an equivalent non-obese patient, in the larger patients some 400 ml/min, compared with the oft-quoted 250 ml/min of the resting normal weight adult. Part of this reflects an increased basal metabolic rate and increased cardiac output, but a significant proportion of this excess relates to the increased work of breathing incurred by the additional fat mass on the chest and abdominal wall, and within the abdomen. This baseline oxygen requirement is in turn posture dependent – most relevant in the immediate post-extubation phase, when anaesthetic agents, opioids and potentially some residual muscle weakness may be present – hence the mantra 'position, position, position', i.e. sit the obese patient up as much as possible.

Fat and Respiratory Mechanics

The quantification of the additional fat mass has been demonstrated in an elegant MRI study, where male patients with an average BMI of 38 had a smaller intra-thoracic volume, and some 10 kg more fat over the anterior chest and abdominal wall than a control group with a median BMI of 25. Many of our patients have BMI values much greater than in this study, and consequently much larger fat masses. Clearly the distribution of fat is very important in determining this work of breathing and potential impairment – 'apples' with their central fat distribution will have a considerably higher work of breathing than 'pears'.

This weight upon the chest coupled with the tendency for the diaphragm to be pushed up, especially in the supine position, tends to compress the lungs; thus leading to areas of complete atelectatic collapse, with adjacent areas of poor ventilation and V/Q mismatching. The extent of this collapse will be reflected in baseline oxygen saturations, and in some patients this can be marked. Clinical top tip: low baseline oxygen saturation of 94% or less should be a global red-flag warning to the anaesthetist of potential trouble.

As part of the reduction in total lung volumes, there will be the reduction in the functional residual capacity, in particular the expiratory reserve volume. The impact of this is primarily recognised in the anaesthetised patient in terms of reduced oxygen stores and the effect upon the safe apnoea time.

However, there is a secondary effect, much less widely recognised. A large reduction in lung volumes means the total amount of volatile agent in the lungs available for absorption will also be markedly reduced. This will result in a concomitant increase in the time taken to achieve effective plasma and hence brain concentrations. This has an obvious, but rarely considered potential impact on risks of accidental awareness.

So the awake obese patient has an increased work of breathing, with a 50–100% increase in oxygen demand and a tendency to atelectasis. Diminish the power of the muscle groups and central drive by administering general anaesthesia and the resulting hypoventilation, hypercapnia and desaturation from a combined shunt and V/Q mismatch is almost inevitable. Only in rare cases will it be safe to allow respiration without endotracheal intubation and positive pressure ventilation. Thus intubation and ventilation should be the default position in anyone with a BMI in excess of 40, and probably is indicated in the majority with even lower levels of obesity, in the BMI 30–40 range.

Exacerbating Factors

In laparoscopic surgery, the tendency to atelectatic collapse secondary to the chest and abdominal wall fat mass is further exaggerated by the influence of the pneumoperitoneum. The surgeon seeking to create an adequate workspace will typically insufflate 4–5 litres of volume into the abdomen, and the cephalad movement of the diaphragm will further reduce lung volumes. It is important to note that it is not just the diaphragm that moves, the entire lung changes shape and moves, and the carina will often move cephalad too. The importance of this being that if an endotracheal tube is close to the carina, with the insufflation of the abdomen one may suddenly find that the carina is pushed up to contact the tip of the tube, triggering bronchospasm and coughing – potentially even endobronchial intubation.

The combination of reduced lung volumes, weight on the chest wall and splinting of the diaphragm mean that in the morbidly obese patient, calculated compliance of the lung is markedly reduced, and even more so in the presence of the pneumoperitoneum. Again, the patient's pattern of fat distribution, the total weight of the patient and posture will all play a role in determining the extent of this change, but it would appear to range from near normal compliance (in those who have a peripheral fat distribution and are managed head up) to lung compliances that may be two- to threefold lower than normal. The clinical relevance here is that a supine obese patient with near normal compliance can manage short periods of spontaneous ventilation, but the vast majority will require ventilatory support with a secured airway for anything but the briefest of procedures.

From the critical care literature, it is clear that collapse and atelectasis with repetitive re-expansion, especially of the dependent parts of the lung, is associated with the release of pro-inflammatory mediators, leading to both pulmonary and extra-pulmonary injury. The prevention of this cyclical change, by the use of adequate levels of PEEP, should reduce this injury by attenuating the inflammatory response. Furthermore, from the critical care world it is accepted that lower tidal volume ventilation clearly improves outcome, and it is probable that tidal volumes greater than 8 ml/kg of lean body weight (often approximated as ideal body weight) should be avoided.

Ventilatory Modes in Morbid Obesity

This is an area with many theoretical advantages of particular modes postulated, but little evidence to support these ideas. With the variation in compliance associated with changes in positioning, pneumoperitoneal pressures and the altering levels of neuromuscular blockade, maintaining minute volume with some variety of volume-controlled mode has many potential benefits. Extrapolating again from the critical care literature, pressure control modes and others with decelerating flow rates may have theoretical advantages in terms of reducing shear stress, but the need for multiple adjustments to compensate for changing compliance make this a challenging mode.

However, despite multiple smaller studies proposing the benefit of one over the other, the evidence that any one mode is superior to others is lacking and in the only sizeable meta-analysis into modes of ventilation in this scenario, there is no apparent benefit to pressure control over the others.

Need for PEEP in Obesity

Various studies have been undertaken into levels of pressure required when ventilating the morbidly obese patient. Some show the inspiratory plateau pressures required to fully recruit atelectatic lung and some show the levels of PEEP required to prevent the re-development of any clinically significant atelectasis. In one of the most elegant of these studies, in a cohort of patients undergoing bariatric surgery, Tusman et al. used a step-wise change in ventilatory pressures to show that the plateau pressures required to re-recruit collapsed lung in his cohort, were between 38 and 48 cmH_2O. Within the same study it was demonstrated that the level of PEEP required to prevent subsequent de-recruitment was as much as 18 cmH_2O in some patients, and that desaturation was occurring in every patient when PEEP fell to 12 cmH_2O.

The protective effect of PEEP during intra-operative ventilation was initially thought likely to be of great importance, but studies designed to show a clinical benefit have been disappointing. One of the largest, the PROVHILO study, in some 900 patients randomised to receive either 2 or 12 cmH_2O of PEEP throughout the period of surgery, showed absolutely no difference in the incidence of post-operative pulmonary complications. However, this study excluded obese patients.

As the beneficial effects of PEEP might be most likely seen in the morbidly obese, a specific study focusing on this area is underway. Currently we are awaiting the results of the PROBESE study, which specifically investigated the incidence of post-operative pulmonary complications (and cardiovascular instability) in a cohort of obese patients undergoing a high PEEP strategy with recruitment manoeuvres versus a low PEEP strategy in higher-risk obese patients.

Balance of PEEP versus Pressure Effects: Concept of Permissive Atelectasis

There are obvious potential risks with high levels of PEEP and the use of recruitment manoeuvres. The most obvious of these is to cause cardiovascular compromise, which is particularly accentuated in the head-up position used in laparoscopic upper abdominal surgery. The benefits of the *routine* use of high PEEP have not been conclusively shown, although the PROBESE study may yet demonstrate a value in the truly obese. It is likely that we need to be selective in deciding which patients should receive recruitment manoeuvres and a higher level of PEEP, balancing risk against benefit.

A pragmatic approach of 'intra-operative permissive atelectasis' has been described, whereby lower levels of PEEP are used to prevent alveolar over-distension and to avoid cardiovascular effects, but the inspired oxygen fraction is increased to compensate for degrees of mismatch and shunt resulting from atelectatic changes. But it is also becoming increasingly clear that high concentrations of oxygen for even modest periods of time may be detrimental.

We do not yet know the best balance of PEEP versus oxygen concentrations, and we probably never will achieve a 'one size fits all' strategy.

So we must in each patient consider and tailor our ventilatory strategies, taking into account the patients ability to maintain cardiac output and haemodynamic stability, whilst tolerating modest degrees of atelectasis and hypoxaemia, and aiming for low tidal volumes and inspired oxygen concentrations of 30–40% whenever possible.

Ventilation Summary

Ventilation of the morbidly obese patient requires support at significantly higher inspiratory and end-expiratory pressures than normal, to ventilate, but also to avoid atelectatic collapse of the lung bases. High levels of PEEP will minimise collapse, but the cardiovascular effects can be significant. Unsurprisingly, given the many factors that can impact on post-operative pulmonary complications, there is no good evidence to support unselected use of recruitment manoeuvres and high levels of PEEP.

Achieving the safest balance between applied PEEP, inspired oxygen concentration, small tidal volumes and the maintenance of adequate cardiac output requires a good understanding of the interactions and effects that each of these may have. Impacting on this balance, the level of pneumoperitoneal pressure (see the next section), ventricular function and fat distribution will also play a role. There is, as ever, no 'one size fits all' approach to ventilation

Pneumoperitoneum

Fundamentals

Laparoscopic surgery is not new. In 1902, Georg Kelling from Dresden described 'Celioscopy' as he called it, in a dog. Eight years later the Swedish surgeon Hans Jacobeus reported a similar technique in humans. This was all performed without insufflation and before the advent of muscle relaxants, in the days when men were real men, and surgeons got on with it. The outcome of these patients and procedures is not known.

However today, in order for laparoscopic surgery to be performed safely, it is generally accepted that there is a need for a certain intra-abdominal volume of gas to provide the surgical workspace, usually in the order of 3–4 litres. In addition, there is also a requirement for a lack of movement, especially sudden straining, when considering upper gastro-intestinal (GI) surgery, particularly in minimising any diaphragmatic movement.

Surgical workspace is the increase in intra-abdominal volume following insufflation, which in the head-up posture allows the bowel to fall away into the pelvis, and the anterior abdominal wall to lift away; this combination giving optimal access to the surgical site when operating on the upper abdomen. The volume of workspace achieved is a function of insufflating pressure and abdominal compliance.

Abdominal Compliance

The determinants of the increase in intra-abdominal volume are complex, but basically follow the principles of La Place's law. The extent of the volume achieved is primarily a balance between abdominal wall tension or tone, external pressures and intra-abdominal pressure.

Tone in the abdominal wall has many contributing factors, including:

- muscle tone, throughout the various muscle groups of the abdominal wall;
- the laxity or otherwise of fibrous tissues, and particularly tension in the linea alba between xiphisternum and symphisis pubis; a small degree of flexion of the patient's lumbar spine, to de-tension the linea alba, may help and previous stretch, either through pregnancy and the gravid uterus, or through intra-abdominal fat subsequently lost, may create a natural laxity of the abdominal wall, improving compliance;
- the degree to which the diaphragm can move cephalad, which in turn relates to how much the chest can expand under anaesthesia, a function of the ventilatory settings and PEEP;
- the weight of anterior abdominal wall tissue bearing down; although not strictly affecting tone, this external fat will alter overall compliance of the abdomen;
- Degree of head-up versus head-down tilt; Trendelenburg (head-down) appears to improve compliance (although is unhelpful if performing upper GI surgery).

The interaction between these factors determines the compliance of the abdominal compartment and can be very different between individual patients. The anaesthetist and peri-operative team to some extent can modulate most of these factors, but in some patients there will still be a requirement for pressures in excess of 15 cmH$_2$O to achieve adequate workspace.

Complications of High Intra-abdominal Pressures

The risks of high intra-abdominal pressures during laparoscopy are exactly the factors that pre-dispose to intra-abdominal compartment syndrome. The combination of high intra-abdominal pressures, close to 20 mmHg, in association with low systemic blood pressures (typically a mean arterial pressure below 55–60 mmHg) is a recipe for splanchnic hypoperfusion and ischaemia of the kidney, liver and bowel. Prolonged bowel hypoperfusion following surgery will be associated with poor wound healing and by extension, anastomotic breakdown. Whilst the latter is rare in the younger patient undergoing bariatric surgery, the development of renal dysfunction in the immediate peri-operative period is a real risk.

Whilst considering intra-abdominal pressure, it almost goes without saying that in any patient placed in the prone position, scrupulous attention must be given to ensure that the patient's weight is supported through the chest and pelvis, and that the abdomen is minimally compressed. Failure to achieve this risks an abdominal pressure rise and subsequent abdominal compartment syndrome. In the obese patient undergoing spinal surgery there have been a number of reports of splanchnic organ failure with fatal sequelae.

Surgical Workspace

Returning to the need for an adequate workspace and optimal surgical operating conditions, diaphragmatic movement may be an issue. The diaphragm is very resistant to neuromuscular blockade, and movement may persist even with abdominal wall relaxation; this is influenced primarily by central respiratory drive. This drive can be ablated by high-dose opioids, which is one of the great benefits of remifentanil infusion techniques. Ventilating the patient to a greater minute volume to drive down arterial CO$_2$ levels, is widely recognised as an alternative technique to reduce respiratory drive, but hypocapnia tends to reduce cardiac output and blood flow and pressure. This reduction in flow may in turn mask bleeding points intra-operatively, and could be associated with increased post-operative bleeding rates. Hyperventilation in laparoscopic bariatric surgery is not recommended routinely.

There is a spectrum of sensitivity of different muscle groups to the effects of neuromuscular blocking agents, with the ocular muscles the most sensitive, oropharyngeal muscle groups the next most sensitive, then general skeletal muscle, such as the adductor pollicis muscle, and finally the diaphragm the most resistant of all; in order to achieve full paralysis of the diaphragm, very large doses of muscle relaxants must be administered.

Measurement of quality of workspace is subjective and very complex. There are several systems described, including the Leiden Surgical Rating Scale (L-SRS), which has a five-point grading:

5 Optimal

4 Good

3 Acceptable

2 Poor

1 Extremely Poor

The clinical reality is that patients frequently jump from good to poor grades, and without formal regular neuromuscular monitoring and maintaining an adequate level of neuromuscular blockade, it is very difficult to predict the point at which straining (coughing) may begin. The danger of overdosing neuromuscular blocking agents, with risk of subsequent post-operative residual curarisation (PORC) is very real, especially in the morbidly obese patient with limited reserve and a propensity for upper airway collapse, the situation typical in those with degrees of sleep apnoea. There is a complex balance of post-operative risk versus intra-operative benefits to be considered, which should probably be assessed on a case-by-case basis.

Practical Problems

Respiratory Compromise

Respiratory challenges of the pneumoperitoneum may be significant, especially with higher levels of intra-abdominal pressure, as may be needed in the morbidly obese. In the classic paper by Sprung et al., static lung compliance decreased by some 40% following insufflation, and in clinical practice when using pressure control ventilation one frequently sees a halving of tidal volumes as the pneumoperitoneum is established.

Reassuringly it is often a matter of increasing inspiratory peak pressures by only some 4–5 cmH$_2$O to re-establish baseline tidal volumes. However, in some patients, especially larger males with central fat distribution, these pressure changes may be inadequate and in some clearance of CO$_2$ may be truly problematic, and a degree of hypercapnia may have to be tolerated.

Cardiovascular Compromise

The impact of pneumoperitoneal insufflation on cardiovascular parameters can be negligible or massive, and is primarily dependant upon ventricular function and volume status, accentuated by a head-up patient posture. Stroke volume and cardiac output will on average fall by some 25–35%, but in some the fall

will be much greater. A degree of pre-loading and the use of modest amounts of vasopressor, and close monitoring of the blood pressure, particularly during changes in posture, are advisable. It is unclear whether it is of benefit to use deeper levels of neuromuscular blockade, in turn allowing lower intra-abdominal pressures and thus having a lesser effect on venous return, but the concept is attractive and potentially beneficial in patients vulnerable to such compromise. The key is pre-operative identification of the higher-risk patient, and utilisation of advanced and possibly invasive, i.e. arterial pressure and waveform, monitoring allowing early management of instability.

Sudden Massive CO$_2$ Absorption

Carbon dioxide has been the insufflation agent of choice for many years, and is considered the safest agent, partly because it is inert, but mostly because of its rapid solubility in the event of intravenous bolus. But with this solubility there is a down side, that transperitoneal absorption may become an issue, even during routine usage.

In uneventful procedures, the rate of absorption of insufflated CO$_2$ will be in the order of 20–50 ml/min, whilst the overall metabolic CO$_2$ production is in the order of 250–300 ml/min. Thus there will be a requirement for a small increase in minute alveolar ventilation rates in order to clear, perhaps in the order of around 20%.

However, if the peritoneum is breached such that pneumoperitoneal gas extravasates into the tissues, leading to marked surgical emphysema, these rates of gas escape and subsequent absorption can be massive. This is commonly seen to a modest level during laparoscopic inguinal hernia surgery, and operations around the oesophageal hiatus, but rarely massive CO$_2$ absorption can occur, particularly if there is an associated pneumomediastinum.

Concept of Deep NMB and Reversal

Patient movement during laparoscopic procedures, such as low-level diaphragmatic breathing, can be tolerated to a degree, depending on the experience of the surgeon and the difficulty of the case. Low levels of abdominal wall tone can also be tolerated, providing the intra-abdominal gas volume and workspace is adequate. However more marked inter-breathing and particularly the sudden onset of straining by the patient, causing a loss of optimal conditions during a critical phase of surgery, causes difficulty to the operating surgeon and is potentially dangerous to the patient. With the advent of enhanced recovery techniques and the desire to avoid deeper levels of anaesthesia and to minimise opioid usage, the risk of this occurring is increased.

Deep levels of neuromuscular blockade (that is, a level of block with a post-tetanic count of only one to two twitches) will prevent any sudden straining without the requirement for running depths of anaesthesia much in excess of 1 MAC.

The advent of cyclodextran agents that effectively bind and thus completely reverse the effect of the amino-steroidal muscle relaxants, has allowed deep levels of neuromuscular blockade to be achieved intra-operatively through the administration of considerably higher doses of relaxants, yet still allow safe and rapid recovery of muscle function at the end of surgery. Currently sugammadex is the only cyclodextran agent licensed for this use, but cost has precluded its routine use in most centres.

Studies so far have been small and few in numbers with some contradictions. However, there has now been a meta-analysis published that suggests that the use of deep levels of blockade is associated with both markedly improved operating conditions and improved patient recovery pain scores, although the authors fully accept that at this early stage publication bias may be behind this finding. Nonetheless, this seems an area of some promise.

Currently in selected patients there would seem to be a justification for profound levels of neuromuscular block, in order to make surgical access easier and hence to shorten the operative time, minimising the risk of complications. Once the price of these agents reduces to a level where they are no more expensive than the acetylcholinesterase inhibitors (as has already happened in the US), the use of cyclodextrans will become routine.

Pneumoperitoneum Summary

Laparoscopic and minimal access surgery undoubtedly has been one of the prime drivers of enhanced recovery, and there are very few procedures or patients where it is not indicated. An understanding of the factors involved in achieving an adequate surgical workspace and operating field is of vital importance for the anaesthetist. There is again a balance to be achieved, between preventing diaphragmatic movement through suppression of central respiratory drive using opioids, deep anaesthesia or driving down

$PaCO_2$, with the potential intra-operative risks and greater 'hangover' effects, versus the use of very deep levels of paralysis with the associated risks of residual paralysis, and/or the costs of routine aminosteroid agents and cyclodextran reversal. The precise balance in this risk-benefit equation, and in which patients one or the other should be preferred, will be elucidated over the coming years.

Further Reading

Aldenkortt M, Lysakowski C, Elia N, Brochard L, Tramèr MR. Ventilation strategies in obese patients undergoing surgery: a quantitative systematic review and meta-analysis. *Br J Anaesth.* 2012;**109**(4):493–502.

Bruintjes MH, van Helden EV, Braat AE, et al. Deep neuromuscular block to optimize surgical space conditions during laparoscopic surgery: a systematic review and meta-analysis. *Br J Anaesth.* 2017;**118**(6):834–42.

Duggan M, Kavanagh BP. Pulmonary atelectasis: a pathogenic peri-operative entity. *Anesthesiology.* 2005;**102**:838–54.

Gander S, Frascarolo P, Suter M, Spahn DR, Magnusson L. Positive end-expiratory pressure during induction of general anesthesia increases duration of nonhypoxic apnea in morbidly obese patients. *Anesth Analg.* 2005;**100**(2), 580–4.

Mulier JPJ, Dillemans B, Van Cauwenberge S. Impact of the patient's body position on the intra-abdominal workspace during laparoscopic surgery. *Surg Endosc.* 2010;**24**(6): 1398–402.

Popescu WM, Bell R, Duffy AJ, Katz KH, Perrino AC. A pilot study of patients with clinically severe obesity undergoing laparoscopic surgery: evidence for impaired cardiac performance. *J Cardiothor Vasc Anesth.* 2011;**25**(6): 943–9.

PROVE Network Investigators; Hemmes SNT, Gama de Abreu M, Pelosi P, Schultz MJ. High versus low positive end-expiratory pressure during general anaesthesia for open abdominal surgery (PROVHILO trial): a multicentre randomised controlled trial. *Lancet.* 2014;**384** (9942):495–503.

Sprung J, Whalley DG, Falcone T, et al. The impact of morbid obesity, pneumoperitoneum, and posture on respiratory system mechanics and oxygenation during laparoscopy. *Anesth Analg.* 2002;**94**(5):1345–50.

Tusman G, Groisman I, Fiolo FE, et al. Noninvasive monitoring of lung recruitment maneuvers in morbidly obese patients. *Anesth Analg.* 2014;**118**(1):137–44.

Watson RA, Pride NB, Thomas EL, Ind PW, Bell JD. Relation between trunk fat volume and reduction of total lung capacity in obese men. *J Appl Physiol.* 2011;**112**(1): 118–26.

Analgesic Techniques

Naveen Eipe and Adele S. Budiansky

Introduction

One of the basic principles of acute pain management is ensuring effective analgesia within the paradigm of improved patient safety and outcomes. In recent times, peri-operative pain management has witnessed considerable advances through innovative multimodal pharmacology, drug delivery systems, standardised protocol implementation and acute pain service organisation. These changes in pain management are now backed by extensive research in ERAS (enhanced recovery after surgery) where peri-operative outcomes are being measured with better-defined patient-centred goals. Clearly, patients enrolled in ERAS programmes are not just leaving hospital earlier after surgery; they are doing so with less pain, fewer side effects, and better recovery and satisfaction scores, with an earlier return to their baseline functional status.

Obese surgical patients are often excluded from the ERAS clinical trials. Obese patients are perceived as having co-morbidity burdens that require alternative post-operative care and need different recovery goals; both in turn can alter outcomes for these patients. Preceding chapters have well described the fact that MO is also unique because both the pharmacokinetics and pharmacodynamics of drugs can be altered and/or become unpredictable. In pain management, clinicians themselves are also likely to underestimate pain and overestimate the adverse effects of analgesics in these patients. This conundrum is probably largely due to the well-described association of MO with an increased prevalence of sleep disordered breathing (SDB). SDB itself, without acute pain or opioid analgesic use, can be associated with peri-operative respiratory adverse events (PRAE), especially in the early post-operative period. Despite these apparent lacunae in the evidence for pain management in MO, increasing cohorts of patients with MO are now undergoing bariatric or weight loss surgery (WLS). Here, similar

to the ERAS paradigm, the standardisation of care and measurement of clinically relevant outcomes is being both sought and implemented. Therefore, though indirectly, the evidence for pain management in MO is coming from experience with WLS protocols. It is only natural that in the near future, with appropriate knowledge translation, pain management in WLS will benefit the peri-operative care of all morbidly obese patients undergoing any surgical procedure.

Principles of Multimodal Analgesia in Morbid Obesity

In the late 1990s, the declaration of pain being the fifth vital clinical sign coupled with then prevailing clinical understanding that there was no ceiling to the dose of opioids, together (and probably equally) contributed to 'conventional' pain management being largely based on the opioid class of drugs. For acute pain, within this opioid-centric paradigm, other pharmacological agents were at-times 'added later' and often to 'supplement' the opioids. This practice has continued for decades and probably still continues in many areas, both geographically and across surgical sub-specialties. It is now well known that relying on opioids alone is not only ineffective for post-operative pain management, it can have significant immediate, intermediate and long-term adverse effects for the patient. The opioid-related adverse effects in the peri-operative period have more serious outcomes in vulnerable populations, notably the elderly and the morbidly obese. MO also predisposes patients to possible serious PRAE with further increased risk in those with undiagnosed or untreated SDB.

In MO, therefore, one of the foremost goals is to reduce opioid analgesic consumption with a particular focus on avoiding the side effects – sedation, respiratory depression, nausea, vomiting and mood changes, etc.

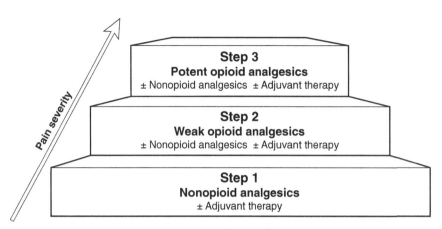

Figure 24.1 WHO step-ladder for pain management.

The cornerstone of pain management in MO is multimodal analgesia. Here multiple analgesics are concurrently used, not only to improve pain management, but also to reduce side effects of individual agents. To better appreciate and apply the multimodal analgesia rationale to clinical practice, we first require a structural and functional framework for acute pain management. This framework is essential to standardise our pain management protocols, implement consistently with our own colleagues (surgeons, recovery room and ward nurses, etc.) and most importantly, share with the patient. The well-established, time-tested and widely respected WHO step-ladder is one such pain management concept that is simple and useful to start with (Figure 24.1). Originally designed for management of cancer pain, the WHO step-ladder provides four principles: (1) severity based, (2) stepwise approach that aims to (3) minimise the use and/or need for opioids. This also (4) introduces and encourages the use of non-opioid adjuvants for acute pain at any level (or every step) of pain (or the ladder). These, for reasons mentioned previously, are especially applicable to post-operative pain in the morbidly obese surgical patient.

Recent consensus statements suggest that adherence to a stepwise approach can improve patient safety and outcome from acute pain management. Experts also strongly recommend the development of standardised protocols for post-operative pain. All these recommendations have come from good-quality research undertaken in acute pain management. The role of multimodal analgesia and individual components of non-opioid adjuvant therapy is also shown to be beneficial in a variety of procedure-specific post-operative pain management protocols. This has led to the widespread adoption and application of principles of ERAS. Understanding the appropriate acute pain pharmacology is considered one of the cornerstones of ERAS.

Acute Pain Pharmacology in Morbid Obesity

The physiological changes associated with MO affect the pharmacokinetics of anaesthetic and analgesic drugs. These are typically dosed on scalars related to the patient's weight. Changes in the distribution of lean and adipose mass, and increases in blood volume and cardiac output will affect the distribution and clearance of commonly used drugs. When calculating dosing based on weight, it is important to consider that using the patient's total body weight can result in overdosing medications, and that the lean body mass does not increase proportionally with fat mass in obesity. As a result, multiple dosing scalars have been proposed, and are described in detail, including their shortfalls, elsewhere in this book.

To facilitate a focused description of the pharmacology of acute pain management, only systemically acting analgesics will be discussed in this chapter. For systemic analgesia, the drugs will be described per the new Ottawa step-ladder approach (Figure 24.2). They will be described as anti-nociceptive modalities (foundational analgesics, weak and strong opioids) and anti-hyperalgesic modalities (non-opioid adjuvant analgesics).

Acute Nociceptive Pain

Tissue injury, secondary to trauma and surgery, usually has a major nociceptive component. But as

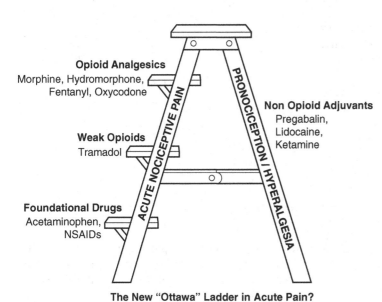

Figure 24.2 The new 'Ottowa' ladder in acute pain.

The New "Ottawa" Ladder in Acute Pain?

will be discussed further, acute hyperalgesia can present, co-exist and even predominate this presentation, irrespective of the intensity of the pain. For nociceptive pain alone, it is rational to follow the step-wise, severity-based opioid-sparing multimodal analgesia protocol previously described as the WHO step-ladder.

Foundational analgesics (paracetamol, NSAIDS) are named so that they are used as the 'foundation' of any standardised acute pain protocol. In the peri-operative protocol, these should be started first (possibly as routine oral pre-medication) and continued till the end ('first on–last off'). They can be used as the sole analgesics in mild to moderate nociceptive pain, especially where tissue inflammation predominates. These drugs are particularly useful in musculoskeletal trauma and in minimally invasive (laparoscopic) surgery, where their opioid-sparing effect (variably estimated at 30–60%) can be significant. The benefits of peri-operative foundational analgesia has been measured in terms of reduction of opioid-related side effects – decreased sedation, respiratory depression and nausea/vomiting. Unless contraindicated, they should be used in all morbidly obese surgical patients, started pre-operatively and administered regularly, especially in the early post-operative period.

The 'second step' on the nociceptive side of the ladder is 'reserved' for weak opioids. While codeine and 'low-dose' opioids were previously considered here, this remains rather contentious. The current consensus is that this position is best filled by tramadol and tapentadol. Tramadol is a unique agent as it is 'inherently multimodal' – weak mu-opioid receptor agonist with serotonergic and noradrenergic properties. These properties make tramadol especially effective, not only for moderate nociceptive pain; it is also a useful as an anti-hyperalgesic (see below). Peri-operative tramadol side effects in morbidly obese surgical patients include increased (and sometimes troublesome) nausea and vomiting, serotonin syndrome-inducing interactions (with anti-depressants) and intolerance. Despite these, this drug has been very useful in most models of post-operative pain management, as its use contributes an additional estimated 30% 'opioid-sparing' effect. Tapentadol is a newer molecule, approximately twice as potent as tramadol and devoid of the serotonin-related side-effect profile. Despite these promising advantages over tramadol, experience and evidence for tapentadol use in MO is currently limited. As with any other pure mu-opioid receptor agonist, these 'second-step' drugs also have the potential for sedation and respiratory depression, especially when used in MO and particularly in patients who have undiagnosed or untreated OSA. If encountered, these events should be treated with standard opioid reversal protocols.

The opioid class of drugs occupies the 'third step' of the nociceptive ladder. While an extensive review of their pharmacology and use in acute pain is beyond the scope of this chapter, the relationship of obesity, OSA and opioids is discussed in the last section of this chapter.

As in the non-obese population, pre-operative exposure to opioids may be an independent predictor of poorly controlled pain post-operatively. Opioid-naïve patients with MO should be given titrated doses of opioid analgesics for moderate to severe pain that is not adequately controlled with Step 1 and Step 2. The presence of hyperalgesia should ideally be sought (using the DN4 questionnaire) and appropriately treated, before initiating opioid analgesic therapy. In the post-operative period, if intermittent parenteral opioid therapy is required, the use of intravenous patient-controlled analgesia (IVPCA) with similar settings (as in non-obese patients) has been described. The use of continuous or basal infusions is contraindicated in morbidly obese surgical patients; intensive care units with intubated and ventilated patients may be the only exception to this rule.

Opioid-dependent and -tolerant morbidly obese surgical patients should continue to receive their baseline opioid drugs, possibly with reduced doses, throughout the peri-operative period. Opioid conversions and rotations may allow for improved analgesia with reduced doses, but these require both expertise and individualisation of care. Similarly, the peri-operative management of patients with methadone maintenance therapy (MMT), opioid antagonist therapy (OAT) and transdermal opioid therapy (TOT) should always involve consultations with specialists with expertise in their use. The risk of peri-operative opioid overdose and/or acute withdrawal reaction is amongst the highest in these sub-groups of patients with chronic opioid use. In MO, patients with chronic opioid use receive extended post-operative monitoring for PRAE and same-day discharge, ambulatory or outpatient surgery should be avoided.

Acute Pro-nociception and Hyperalgesia

The WHO step-ladder is the fundamental basis for pain management and recommends the use of non-opioid adjuvants. The original ladder does not clearly define why, when and how these drugs should be used. Ongoing research in acute pain is supporting the use of non-opioid adjuvants in the management of post-operative pain. This direction has also received momentum from the need to not only improve acute pain management, but also to prevent the long-

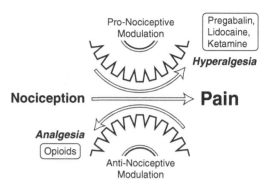

Figure 24.3 Four-dimensional pain model.

term consequences of opioid use and abuse in the community, with the goal to stem the socio-economic consequences of non-medical prescription opioid use.

Published evidence has described acute hyperalgesia or 'pro-nociception' occurring more frequently in some patients. This emerging concept is based on two inter-related acute pain management principles. Firstly, it is well established that opioids are not only ineffective in treating acute hyperalgesia and neuropathic pain; they can paradoxically worsen pain, producing opioid-induced hyperalgesia and contribute to the development of chronic post-surgical pain. Secondly, convincing evidence for non-opioid adjuvants (notably ketamine, lidocaine and pregabalin) has shown that they work effectively to prevent or treat acute hyperalgesia and also prevent the progression to chronic neuropathic pain. This concept is described in the four-dimensional pain model where opioids and non-opioid adjuvants act on opposing ends of the pain spectrum (Figure 24.3). The use of these non-opioid adjuvants should be based on the identification of pro-nociception or acute neuropathic pain, which presents as hyperalgesia. The diagnosis of acute neuropathic pain can be objectively made with the validated DN4 questionnaire. We believe that this understanding and explanation for the use of anti-hyperalgesic drugs (ketamine, lidocaine and pregabalin) in acute pain management improves patient safety and outcomes, especially in MO. The peri-operative use of ketamine, lidocaine and pregabalin has been demonstrated to significantly reduce pain scores, analgesic consumption and opioid-related side effects in the post-operative period.

Another important clinical caveat of using the 'new Ottawa pain ladder' and hyperalgesia as an indicator of pro-nociception is when a patient complains of increasing or poorly controlled pain in the post-operative setting. If the DN4 is positive, the decision should be to increase the anti-hyperalgesic drugs and not the opioids. Similarly, as the pain is improving, the weaning of analgesics and anti-hyperalgesics can be determined by the persistence of hyperalgesia. Another correlate of this concept is the patients with persistence of hyperalgesia will require continuation of these anti-hyperalgesic therapies and early referral to the chronic pain specialists – they are at high risk for developing persistent pain after surgery or chronic post-surgical pain (CPSP).

Individual Anti-hyperalgesic Agents in Morbid Obesity

Ketamine

Despite decades of use and other recent advances in pharmacotherapy of acute pain, the NMDA antagonist ketamine remains the most widely available, easily administered and relatively inexpensive non-opioid analgesic with a wide range of doses and applications. The peri-operative use of ketamine in patients with MO can be attributed to its analgesic, anti-hyperalgesic, opioid-sparing actions, with additional cardiorespiratory stability and relative lack of sedation and respiratory depression. The effects and side effects of ketamine are primarily dependent on the dose administered and these can be considered as 'high or anaesthetic', 'low or analgesic' and 'ultra-low or anti-hyperalgesic' doses.

A 'high or anaesthetic' dose of ketamine (bolus >1 mg/kg IBW and/or infusion of >1 mg/kg IBW/hour) will result in profound analgesia, but unpredictable loss of consciousness and very likely stormy emergence phenomena. This should be reserved for use in trauma and/or anaesthetic management where the patient's airway has been secured and prolonged controlled ventilation is planned. A 'low or analgesic' dose of ketamine (bolus 0.5 mg/kg IBW and/or infusion of 0.5 mg/kg IBW/hour) also provides excellent analgesia, but can often be accompanied by psychomimetic effects, emergence reactions and prolonged sedation. This dose range is widely used as an anaesthetic adjunct, especially when regional anaesthesia techniques and/or opioids have not been used. Ultra-low dose ketamine refers to the use of sub-analgesic doses (bolus <0.1 mg/kg IBW and/or infusion of

<0.1 mg/kg IBW/hour) and is almost always devoid of any neuropsychiatric effects. This is our recommended dose as a component of multimodal analgesia in the peri-operative period. While studies have reported the clinically relevant use of ketamine in patients with MO, it is almost always described in conjunction with other modalities.

One unique method of ketamine therapy in patients with MO is to combine it with morphine (1:1) for delivery via a standard IVPCA device. This combination has significant benefits – it not only decreases opioid consumption and pain scores, and improves the quality of analgesia (mood and patient satisfaction), but ketamine with morphine in the PCA also decreases the most prominent opioid side effects: sedation-respiratory depression and nausea/vomiting. The indications for the addition of ketamine to the IVPCA from our centre are:

- *Trauma* – multiple and/or major injuries; burns, de-gloving and crush injuries, rib fractures
- *Acute pain* – poorly controlled, acute on chronic pain, prevention of CPSP, opioid tolerance and/or dependence, substance abuse
- *Neuropathic pain* – acute hyperalgesia, opioid-induced or opioid-resistant, malignancy-related, vascular insufficiency and ischaemia, sickle cell crisis, etc.
- *Gastro-intestinal surgery* – with or without epidural analgesia, laparoscopic procedures and laparoscopic 'converted' to open, ERAS
- *Obese, OSA and elderly* – sensitive to opioids or having opioid side effects.

In our opinion, any patient with MO, with or without SDB, being considered for an IVPCA should be offered a solution containing morphine and ketamine.

Lidocaine

Lidocaine is an amide-type sodium channel blocker, which, when applied in close proximity to neural elements, disrupts impulse transmission. When administered intravenously, lidocaine is a very potent anti-hyperalgesic and anti-inflammatory agent with some analgesic and anti-stress effects. Through direct and indirect effects on the gut, it promotes motility and prevents the development of post-operative ileus.

Level I evidence in the general population has shown that intravenous (IV) lidocaine has a significant effect on improving post-operative pain control, especially in abdominal surgery. The most

Table 24.1 Summary of Indications for IV lidocaine

	Alternative to Regional Anesthesia	Acute Pain with Pro-nociception (hyperalgesia)
Intra-operative	Epidural – contraindicated or failed Laparoscopic Surgery Enhanced Recovery Protocols Trauma – multiple, significant injuries	Opioid dependence or tolerance Surgery at a site of chronic pain Previous experience of poorly controlled pain Substance abuse
Post-operative	Epidural – inadequate or failed Laparoscopic converted to open Trauma – burns, de-gloving, crush injury Rib, clavicle or sternal fractures Prevention or treatment of ileus	Acute neuropathic pain – DN4+ Opioid sparing technique – obese, OSA, elderly and those with opioid side effects Difficult to treat patients – chronic pain/opioid tolerance/substance abuse Neuropathic pain models – spine surgery and limb amputations

commonly reported dose is 1–2 mg/kg IBW given as a bolus at induction of anaesthesia and followed by an infusion of 1–2 mg/kg IBW/hour continued till emergence. We have continued the infusion of lidocaine for 3–4 days and, using pharmacokinetic simulation, predicted its safety in patients with MO. The indication for the peri-operative use of IV lidocaine has been described as an alternative to epidural analgesia and other regional analgesic techniques (Table 24.1). It is especially useful for thoracic, abdominal, pelvic or lower limb surgery where epidurals are contraindicated, refused by patient or have been attempted and/or have failed. It is also useful for patients with difficult to control acute pain – acute on chronic pain, chronic opioid use, abuse or dependence, and substance abuse. Others who are sensitive to the central nervous system (CNS) effects of opioids, notably the elderly and the obese, also benefit from the addition of IV lidocaine to their post-operative pain management strategy.

Evidence for IV lidocaine in patients with MO is limited to a single trial in laparoscopic WLS demonstrating significantly decreased opioid consumption in patients receiving lidocaine. Intravenous lidocaine has also been studied as part of a multimodal, opioid-free analgesia regimen. While these results are promising, there are no clear guidelines on IV lidocaine dosing in patients with MO at this time and the accumulating experience for the use of this modality needs to be converted to good-quality evidence.

Dexmedetomidine

Dexmedetomidine is a novel short-acting intravenous α2-agonist that is closely related to its predecessor,

clonidine. Clonidine was also used as an oral pre-medication in patients with MO and studied for the reduction of post-operative pain. The popularity and use of clonidine is limited by both intra-operative bradycardia and hypotension, and post-operative sedation. These cannot be adjusted for, within the small clinically relevant dose range, especially when given as a single oral dose before surgery.

Dexmedetomidine is highly selective for the α2-receptor with fewer cardiovascular and CNS side effects and was introduced as a 'sedative without respiratory depression'. Its approved use in the UK is in intensive care units as a sedative for mechanical ventilation; improved patient neurological assessment was concurrently possible with better haemodynamic stability and tolerance of mechanical ventilation. Elsewhere in the world approval has been obtained for use before, during and after general anaesthesia, both with and without controlled ventilation. This has led to wide use and description of significant anaesthetic and analgesic properties. This clinical profile of dexmedtomidine was thought to be uniquely beneficial for use in patients with MO. Though tempered by higher cost considerations, the perceived safety of dexmedetomidine in MO patients with SDB led to its current popularity and widespread use in WLS. Dexmedetomidine was found to decrease opioid consumption in patients undergoing laparoscopic gastric bypass and banding, earlier discharge from the recovery room and shorter lengths of stay. Another WLS study using the opioid-free anaesthesia concept demonstrated a significant decrease in both anti-emetic use and the risk of developing PONV. Compared to the then standard of care, intra-operative dexmedetomidine infusion was superior to fentanyl infusion in terms of pain scores and PCA morphine use in the early recovery period.

Pregabalin/Gabapentin

Pregabalin has been widely studied as an adjuvant to improve peri-operative pain management. Though related to its predecessor, gabapentin, the potency, clinical and more favourable side-effect profiles have made this the gabapentinoid of choice in the peri-operative period. In the non-obese surgical population, pregabalin has been found to significantly decrease opioid consumption, pain scores and certain opioid side effects (e.g. PONV), but can increase sedation and visual disturbances. In patients with MO, a single pre-operative dose of pregabalin demonstrated reductions in morphine consumption and pain scores that were significant during the recovery period. However, like gabapentin, pregabalin may be associated with increased sedation and post-operative respiratory depression. Since these drugs impact sleep architecture, their use in the peri-operative period require careful assessment of the risk-benefit in patients with MO and especially those with SDB.

Pre-operative Optimisation and Post-operative Follow-up

As in the general surgical population, there seem to be certain risk factors that can predispose patients with morbid obesity to poorly controlled peri-operative pain. Increased pain scores and opioid consumption have been described in surgical patients with MO who are: younger, of female gender, with chronic pain or chronic opioid use, and those with a history of hospitalisations for psychiatric illnesses.

In the non-obese surgical patient population, recent advances in pre-operative optimisation have led to the introduction of an innovative transitional pain service (TPS), primarily to identify and treat patients at risk of developing CPSP. These patients at risk are identified pre-operatively, their pain management is optimised and they are prepared for their surgery. As patients with MO are at higher risk for severe pain after surgery, it may be reasonable to predict that this patient population would also benefit from management with a TPS-like model, pre-operative evaluation and optimisation of their acute pain coupled with close follow-up after discharge.

Obesity, Obstructive Sleep Apnea and Opioids

One important clinical correlate to managing post-operative pain in morbidly obese surgical patients is the presence of obstructive sleep apnea (OSA). In the morbidly obese surgical patient, the major risk of using opioids during intra-operative and post-operative pain management is the well-known and often exaggerated CNS depressant response – somnolence, sedation and respiratory depression. Also as patients with MO and SDB have an increased sensitivity to sedative effects of pre-medication and anaesthetics, they also are at risk for respiratory insufficiency and the need for either respiratory support or re-intubation after opioid analgesic administration. It is therefore of vital importance to the pain management of the morbidly obese surgical patient that not only their pain be adequately and appropriately managed, but the presence of OSA be clearly determined and adequately treated before surgery.

A surgical patient with MO with an elevated serum bicarbonate level is at the highest risk for sedation and/or serious respiratory depression from opioids. We recommend avoiding or decreasing doses of opioids and increasing the frequency of (or continuous) monitoring be instituted. Early and prompt reversal of CNS depression with naloxone (40 μg IV bolus repeated every 5 mins, up to 10 doses) should be part of standard procedures and policy in the post-operative management of morbidly obese surgical patients with elevated serum bicarbonate levels. While post-operative monitoring in MO should be directed towards detecting hypoventilation, pulse oximetry alone will fail to detect brief apnoeic episodes, especially when supplemental oxygen is administered. Clinical respiratory rate monitoring should be standard, but can be unpredictable in MO, especially in patients with obesity hypoventilation syndrome (OHS). Some post-operative units equipped with continuous ECG monitoring can monitor respiratory rate as derived from trans-thoracic impedance or by ECG-derived respiration (EDR) monitoring. While artifacts are possible in patients with MO, these may still offer additional information that can serve as early warning systems. More accurate post-operative respiratory monitoring in MO can be achieved with measuring exhaled CO_2 (capnography) and newer monitors available have been adapted to nasal prongs and face masks. All these monitoring techniques will improve the safety of acute pain management in the morbidly obese surgical patient.

Conclusions

The current evidence confirms that the use of a stepwise, severity-based, opioid-sparing multimodal pharmacological approach in obese patients will improve acute pain management. The identification and treatment of acute hyperalgesia with non-opioid adjuvants (ketamine, lidocaine and pregabalin) can further improve the safety and efficacy of multimodal analgesia. The presence of OSA can affect the peri-operative pain management of the morbidly obese surgical patient.

As rapid advances and further improvements in the peri-operative pain management and general care of the entire surgical population continue, it is hoped that the morbidly obese surgical patient would benefit from being included in these processes, protocols and programmes.

Further Reading

Alimian M, Imani F, Faiz SH, et al. Effect of oral pregabalin premedication on post- operative pain in laparoscopic gastric bypass surgery. *Anesth Pain Med*. 2012;**2**:12–16.

Alvarez A, Singh PM, Sinha AC. Postoperative analgesia in morbid obesity. *Obes Surg*. 2014;**24**:652–9.

Awad S, Carter S, Purkayastha S, et al. Enhanced recovery after bariatric surgery (ERABS): clinical outcomes from a tertiary referral bariatric centre. *Obes Surg*. 2014;**24**:753–8.

Bell RF, Dahl JB, Moore RA, Kalso E. Perioperative ketamine for acute postoperative pain. *Cochrane Database Syst Rev*. 2006;25:CD004603.

Bouhassira D, Attal N, Alchaar H, Boureau F et al. Comparison of pain syndromes associated with nervous or somatic lesions and development of a new neuropathic pain diagnostic questionnaire (DN4). *Pain*. 2005;**114**:29–36.

Budiansky AS, Margarson MP, Eipe N. Acute pain management in morbid obesity – an evidence based clinical update. *Surg Obes Relat Dis*. 2017;**13**:523–32.

Cabrera Schulmeyer MC, de la Maza J, Ovalle C, Farias C, Vives I. Analgesic effects of a single preoperative dose of pregabalin after laparoscopic sleeve gastrectomy. *Obes Surg*. 2010;**20**:1678–81.

Chou R, Gordon DB, de Leon-Casasola OA, et al. Management of postoperative pain: a clinical practice guideline from the American Pain Society, the American Society of Regional Anesthesia and Pain Medicine, and the American Society of Anesthesiologists' Committee on Regional Anesthesia, Executive Committee, and Administrative Council. *J Pain*. 2016;**17**:131–57.

De Oliveira GS Jr., Duncan K, Fitzgerald P, et al. Systemic lidocaine to improve quality of recovery after laparoscopic bariatric surgery: a randomized double-blinded placebo-controlled trial. *Obes Surg*. 2014;**24**:212–8.

Eipe N, Penning J, Yazdi F, et al. Perioperative use of pregabalin for acute pain-a systematic review and meta-analysis. *Pain*. 2015;**156**:1284–300.

Feld JM, Laurito CE, Beckerman M, et al. Non-opioid analgesia improves pain relief and decreases sedation after gastric bypass surgery. *Can J Anaesth*. 2003;**50**:336–41.

Lemanu DP, Srinivasa S, Singh PP et al. Optimizing perioperative care in bariatric surgery patients. *Obes Surg*. 2012;**22**:979–90.

Morone NE, Weiner DK. Pain as the 5th vital sign: exposing the vital need for pain education. *Clin Therapeut*. 2013;**35**:1728–32.

Porhomayon J, Leissner KB, El-Solh AA, Nader ND. Strategies in postoperative analgesia in the obese obstructive sleep apnea patient. *Clin J Pain*. 2013;**29**:998–1005.

Radvansky BM, Puri S, Sifonios AN, et al. Ketamine: a narrative review of its uses in medicine. *Am J Ther*. 2016;**23**:e1414–26.

Raebel MA, Newcomer SR, Reifler LM, et al. Chronic use of opioid medications before and after bariatric surgery. *JAMA*. 2013;**310**:1369–76.

Schug SA, Raymann A. Postoperative pain management of the obese patient. *Best Pract Res Clin Anaesthesiol*. 2011;**25**:73–81.

Sollazzi L, Modesti C, Vitale F, et al. Preinductive use of clonidine and ketamine improves recovery and reduces postoperative pain after bariatric surgery. *Surg Obes Relat Dis*. 2009;**5**(1):67–71.

Sun Y, Li T, Wang N, et al. Perioperative systemic lidocaine for postoperative analgesia and recovery after abdominal surgery: a meta-analysis of randomized controlled trials. *Dis Colon Rectum*. 2012;**55**:1183–94.

Tawfic QA, Faris AS. Acute pain service: past, present and future. *Pain Manag*. 2015;**5**:47–58.

Weingarten TN, Sprung J, Flores A, et al. Opioid requirements after laparoscopic bariatric surgery. *Obes Surg*. 2011;**21**:1407–12.

Zeidan A, Al-Temyatt S, Mowafi H, Ghattas T. Gender-related difference in postoperative pain after laparoscopic Roux-En-Y gastric bypass in morbidly obese patients. *Obes Surg*. 2013;**23**:1880–4.

Chapter 25

Reversal and Emergence from Anaesthesia

Marcus Wood

Emergence from anaesthesia, for the obese population, is a complicated and risky undertaking. A suitably trained and experienced anaesthetist must be present, and the points below should be considered before commencing the process.

Past Medical History of Patient and Procedure Performed

The anaesthetic pre-assessment will have highlighted specific patient co-morbidities that may impact on the successful emergence from anaesthesia. General considerations are the procedure length and complexity, patient temperature and estimated blood loss. Specific to the obese population are the body mass index (BMI), distribution of fat (apple versus pear shape), obstructive sleep apnoea (OSA) and obesity hypoventilation syndrome (OHS).

Anaesthetic Agent Being Used

The inhalational agent used for maintenance of anaesthesia in the obese population will dictate the speed of emergence. The difference between lean body weight and total body weight is the amount of body fat present. Inhalational anaesthetic drugs that are more lipid soluble will have deposited in this compartment and therefore emergence from anaesthesia will be slower than inhalational compounds that are less lipid soluble. The least soluble inhalational agents in terms of blood/gas solubility co-efficients are desflurane (0.42) and sevoflurane (0.6).

Use of Opioids and Regional Anaesthesia

Wherever possible, the use of regional anaesthesia is recommended to minimise the administration of opioids. Of course, in the obese patient, the use of regional anaesthesia can be difficult or impossible.

When systemic opioids are used, it is important to realise that their use will impact on the emergence from anaesthesia and patient recovery in the immediate post-operative period. In particular, the effects on ventilation should be monitored closely, especially in those patients known to have sleep disordered breathing. Assessment of this using peripheral oxygen saturation alone is far from reliable. Indeed the delay in desaturation after apnoea can result in a catastrophic situation arising. Assessment of adequate ventilation should be through respiratory rate, pattern and volume. By far the better method is using end tidal carbon dioxide monitoring. Various systems are available to monitor this.

Reversal of Paralysis

Where muscle relaxant is administered as part of the anaesthetic technique, it is advisable to use a peripheral nerve stimulator to monitor the level of block. The most widely used mode is the train of four ratio (TOF), although the use of double-burst stimulation (DBS) is more sensitive in patients with a profound block. The TOF is a subjective assessment of the fourth twitch compared to the first. A ratio of at least 0.7 is suggested as being reversible. Being a subjective assessment, this is prone to error.

There is increasing evidence that residual neuromuscular block is common in patients in the recovery area, and also that it may adversely affect patient outcome (reduced ventilatory effort and increased risk of aspiration due to impaired pharyngeal and laryngeal function). Studies have demonstrated that as many as 47% of patients have residual curarisation in the recovery room. Spontaneous recovery of the first twitch (T1), in the TOF, to 25% has been found to take significantly longer in obese and overweight patients compared to normal weight patients.

Neostigmine/glycopyrrolate

The use of neostigmine/glycopyrrolate has long been the mainstay of neuromuscular paralysis reversal. Neostigmine is a reversible, acid-transferring cholinesterase inhibitor, which binds to the esteratic site of acetylcholinesterase. This causes acetylcholine levels to increase at the neuromuscular junction and competitively antagonises all neuromuscular blockers. The addition of glycopyrrolate counteracts the effects of increased acetylcholine levels at muscarinic sites. Reversal using neostigmine can cause adverse effects that include bradycardia and prolongation of the QT interval of the ECG, bronchoconstriction, salivary gland stimulation, increased gastro-intestinal tone and miosis.

The use of neostigmine as a reversal agent has its limitations. The onset of action at a dose of 0.04–0.07 µg/kg is within 1 minute, but peak effect takes 9 minutes. Its duration of action is between 20 and 30 minutes and it is metabolised by the liver with 80% excreted in the urine within 24 hours.

Cyclodextrins

Org 25969 or sugammadex (Merck, NJ, USA), as it is known, is a γ-cyclodextrin that was first discovered by Bom. The lipophilic core encapsulates the free aminosteroid neuromuscular blockers (rocuronium > vecuronium > pancuronium) in the plasma and prevents them from exerting an effect. This encapsulation of the aminosteroid blockers in the plasma creates a concentration gradient that promotes the movement of further aminosteroid blockers away from the neuromuscular junction. Given that acetylcholine levels are not affected, there are no associated muscarinic adverse effects.

Appropriate dosing of sugammadex as advised by the product literature is:

- Routine reversal following rocuronium- or vecuronium-induced block, 2–4 mg/kg (median time to T4/T1 = 0.9 is 2–3 minutes).
- Immediate reversal of rocuronium 1.2 mg/kg-induced block, 16 mg/kg (median time to T4/T1 = 0.9 is 1.5 minutes). Sugammadex to be given 3 minutes after rocuronium dose.

Sugammadex dose should be calculated using adjusted body weight.

Drugs in Development

Calabadion 2 (Isaacs laboratory, Maryland, USA) is a cucurbituril derivative, which the developers say is more potent than sugammadex, and will reverse the neuromuscular block caused by *cis*-atracurium as well as aminosteroid-induced block. Currently it is undergoing research.

Patient Position

Positioning of the patient is vitally important when considering emergence from anaesthesia. A supine patient will have the majority of the excess weight pressing down on the abdomen, raising intra-abdominal pressure and causing splinting of the diaphragm. This will lead to rapid, shallow, ineffective breathing, which in turn will cause atelectasis and less lung units available for efficient gas exchange. The raised intra-abdominal pressure may also increase the risk of gastric contents passing retrograde and the risk of aspiration.

In order to remove the endotracheal tube from a patient successfully, a ramped or sitting upright position is advised. This allows maximal unimpeded excursion of the diaphragm and reduces the force of the abdominal wall pressing down on the abdominal contents. In order to place the patient into this position, first we must consider the safe transfer of the patient from the operating table to the hospital bed. Obese patients represent a transfer risk, not only to themselves, but also to the staff moving them. Departmental moving and handling guidelines must be adhered to so that the risk of injury to patient and staff is minimised.

Equipment specific to the moving of obese patients are items such as a hover mattress, which utilises a cushion of air, to facilitate the movement of obese patients with relative ease. Slide sheets can be used but they must be removed once the patient has been transferred. If the slide sheet remains, then once the patient is sitting upright, they will slowly slide down the bed again.

Fully Awake

Rarely, if ever, is it appropriate to extubate an obese patient 'deep'. The patient should be in an appropriate sitting or ramped position and airway reflexes should be present to reduce the risk of aspiration. The respiratory pattern should be regular, with appropriate tidal volumes before attempting extubation. Once extubated, the patient's breathing pattern and tidal volume should be re-checked before transferring to recovery. The placement of a naso-pharyngeal airway can help maintain the airway, particularly in those with sleep disordered breathing. This can be a useful trick as the patient will tolerate this for some time in the recovery room and assist their airway patency.

Consider Extubation to CPAP

Once the patient has been successfully extubated, it might be appropriate to consider the application of continuous positive airway pressure (CPAP) in the recovery room. This is particularly important if the patient routinely uses CPAP for sleep disordered breathing. Other reasons to consider CPAP are use of opioids during surgery, prolonged procedure or a strong suspicion of unconfirmed OSA having scored >5 on a pre-operative STOP-BANG questionnaire.

If the patient suffers from decreased oxygen saturation levels or has observed hypopnoeas in recovery, then transfer to a high-dependency unit is indicated.

Other considerations in the immediate post-operative period are thromboprophylaxis and the need for potentially prolonged prescriptions. This may have implications, depending on the type of surgery undertaken, and discussion with the surgical team is advised.

Further Reading

Andersen B, Madsen JV, Schurizek BA, Juhl B. Residual curarisation: a comparative study of atracurium and pancuronium. *Acta Anaesthiol Scanda.* 1988;**32**:79–81.

Bom A, Cameron K, Clark JK et al. Chemical chelation as a novel method of NMB reversal: discoveryof Org 25969. *Eur J Anaesthesiol.* 2001;**18**:99.

Bom A, Clark JK, Palin R. New approaches to reversal of neuromuscular block. *Curr Opin Drug Discov Dev.* 2002;**5**:793–800.

Cammu G, De Witte J, De Veylder J et al. Postoperative residual paralysis in outpatients versus inpatients. *Anesth Analg.* 2006;**102**:426–9.

D'Honneur G, Lofaso F, Drummond GB, et al. Susceptibility to upper airway obstruction during partial neuromuscular block. *Anaesthesiology.* 1998;**88**:371–8.

Eriksson Ll, Sundman E, Olsson R, et al. Functional assessment of the pharynx at rest and during swallowing in partially paralysed humans: simultaneous videomanometry and mechanomyography of awake human volunteers. *Anaesthesiology.* 1997;**87**:1035–43.

Gottlieb JB, Sweet RB. The antagonism of curare: the cardiac effects of atropine and neostigmine. *Can Anaesth Soc J.* 1963;**10**:114–21.

Haerter F, Simons JC, Foerster U et al. Comparative effectiveness of calabadion and sugammadex to reverse non-depolarizing neuromuscular-blocking agents. *Anesthesiology.* 2015;**123**(6):1337–49.

Kirkegaard- Nielsen H, Helbo-Hansen HS, Lindholm P et al. Optimum time for neostigmine reversal of atracurium-induced neuromuscular blockade. *Can J Anaesth.* 1996;**43**:932–8.

Miller RD, Van Nyhuis LS, Eger El II et al. Comparative times to peak effect and duration of action of neostigmine and pyridostigmine. *Anaesthesiology.* 1974;**41**:27–33.

Pratt CI. Bronchospasm after neostigmine. *Anaesthesia.* 1988;**43**:248.

Suzuki T, Masaki G, Ogawa S. Neostigmine-induced reversal of vecuronium in normal weight, overweight and obese female patients. *Br J Anaesth* 2006;**97**:160–3.

Chapter 26

The Morbidly Obese Parturient

Elinor Wighton and Paul Sharpe

Introduction

There are approximately 11 million women of child-bearing age in the UK; around half are classified as overweight or obese. The rate of obesity in this population has doubled over the past two decades, with the prevalence of severe obesity (BMI $\geq$40 kg/m^2) increasing threefold. The CMACE (Centre for Maternal and Child Enquiries) National review found 5% of women who went on to deliver at 24-weeks' gestation or more had a BMI of $\geq$35 kg/m^2.

This represents a substantial burden on maternity services and the obstetric anaesthetist, with increasing co-morbidities and interventions required. In the 2011–2013 period of the MBRRACE-UK report, 30% of women who died were obese and 22% were overweight.

Thromboembolic disease remains the leading cause of direct deaths, with cardiac disease being the leading cause of indirect deaths. Obese women are at increased risk of venous thromboembolism and are more likely to have pre-existing cardiac disease. These factors should be taken into account in their anaesthetic management.

Weight Gain in Pregnancy

Weight gain throughout pregnancy consists of the fetus, placenta and amniotic fluid, as well as variable amounts of maternal fluid and fat deposits. The composition of weight gain is therefore different to that seen outside of pregnancy. Dieting during pregnancy is not recommended, but moderate exercise is encouraged and obese women should be offered professional dietary advice with vitamin supplementation as appropriate.

Maternal and Fetal Morbidity

Obese mothers are at risk of non-obstetric-related co-morbidities, including hypertension, type 2 diabetes, osteoarthritis and obstructive sleep apnoea. These can be worsened during pregnancy, and the mother has a higher chance of developing obstetric-related pathologies. During the antenatal period there is an increased incidence of thromboembolism, gestational diabetes, pre-eclampsia, miscarriage and pre-term labour. It is recommended that all women with BMI >30 at booking should be screened for gestational diabetes. Obese women have a higher

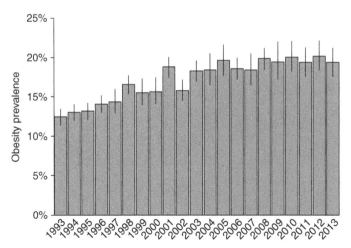

Figure 26.1 Prevalence of obesity in females aged 16-44 years between 1993 and 2013. (Source: Health Survey for England 1993–2013. Published with permission from Public Health England www.noo.org.uk/NOO_about_obesity/maternal_obesity_2015/prevalence. Accessed 11/07/2016.)

incidence of induction of labour, instrumental delivery, caesarean section, fetal distress, fetal meconium aspiration and stillbirth. Following delivery they are more likely to have post-partum haemorrhage, wound infection, breastfeeding problems and admission to intensive care. Fetal monitoring throughout pregnancy is technically challenging in these women, due to difficulty in ultrasonic imaging and fetal heart rate monitoring. A fetus that has been exposed to maternal obesity *in utero* has an increased risk of developing obesity and metabolic disorders itself in later life.

Physiological Changes and Anaesthetic Implications

The incidence of failed intubation in the obstetric population is estimated at 1 in 390 with obesity contributing to this. Airway engorgement, maternal habitus and external human factors all contribute to this. The functional residual capacity is reduced in the pregnant patient, as the gravid uterus pushes the abdominal contents upwards towards the diaphragm. Oxygen consumption is increased by combined fetal and maternal requirements, further compounded by obesity, leading to a rapid rate of desaturation at induction of anaesthesia.

Blood volume and cardiac output increase by up to 40% during pregnancy. This may not be well tolerated if the patient has pre-existing cardiovascular disease. Aortocaval compression is exacerbated by obesity; therefore the supine position should be avoided, with a 15–30° left lateral tilt applied to prevent cardiovascular instability. In some circumstances, especially maternal collapse, it may be more appropriate to apply manual uterine displacement of the uterus to the left, as this maximises the relief of aortocaval compression and optimises cardiac output. The uteroplacental unit does not autoregulate its blood flow, so any hypotension can have significant adverse fetal effects.

All pregnant women are felt to be at higher risk of gastric aspiration. This may be further increased in patients with hiatus herniae, commonly seen in the obese population.

Anaesthetic Pre-assessment and Maternal Information

All women should have their BMI calculated at their antenatal booking visit. A lack of resources or logistical problems may mean that values reported by the patient are used, leading to significant inaccuracies. Measurement of weight in the third trimester allows more detailed plans to be made for delivery, including specialist equipment, although many treatment guidelines are based on the weight recorded at first booking. Obesity is a significant risk factor in anaesthetic-related maternal mortality, therefore The Royal College of Obstetricians and Gynaecologists suggests that women with BMI ≥40 kg/m^2 should be referred to the obstetric anaesthetist for review during their antenatal care to plan for labour and delivery. The anaesthetist should be informed if a woman with a BMI ≥40 kg/m^2 is admitted to the labour ward.

Labour Analgesia

Obese women are at increased risk of dysfunctional labour and operative delivery and are encouraged to consider epidural anaesthesia early in their labour, as siting epidurals in this population can be technically difficult. The rate of re-siting them is often higher than in the non-obese populations too, therefore the epidural should be well fixed to prevent accidental dislodgement. If an epidural is sited, it is essential that it is checked regularly and ready to be used for anaesthesia if an emergency situation occurs.

When inserting the epidural needle it is commonplace to see the skin indented by at least a centimetre, leading to a potential underestimation of the epidural depth (Figure 26.2). This additional depth should be taken in to consideration when deciding the final measurement for the value of skin to epidural space. In addition, when moving from the flexed to the extended position, the catheter can be seen to be drawn in, as it is fixed by the ligamentum flavum, whilst the lumber spine moves away from the skin surface. If the catheter is fixed to the skin before this movement it may be pulled outwards and result in a non-functioning epidural. To account for this we would recommend asking the patient to sit up straight, the catheter will appear to be pulled further in relative to the skin, before final fixation of the catheter.

As previously noted, epidurals are more likely to fail in this population, requiring re-siting. In the case of inadvertent dural puncture they may be less likely to develop post-dural puncture headache, as the

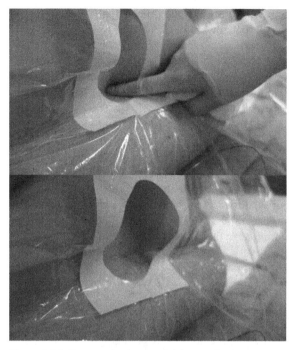

Figure 26.2 Photographs showing the degree of indentation possible while adjusting the epidural catheter. The upper picture shows the catheter markings at the skin to be 2.5 cm less than the lower one. The only difference being the release of pressure on the soft tissue.

transmitted intra-abdominal pressure engorges the lumbar veins, artificially reducing the impact of cerebrospinal fluid (CSF) volume loss.

Meticulous midwifery care is vital following epidural insertion. Positioning of these patients is very difficult and may be compounded by any iatrogenic motor block. The supine position must be avoided to prevent aortocaval compression. Regular position changes are needed to prevent pressure sores, and epidural checks should include the monitoring of vulnerable areas.

Intravenous access is mandatory prior to siting any neuraxial block. This again can be challenging and require anaesthetic input, with or without the aid of ultrasound.

Less invasive analgesic techniques may be appropriate in women in whom neuraxial block is contraindicated.

Non-opioid techniques, including deep breathing, transcutaneous electrical nerve stimulation (TENS), entonox and simple analgesia will not be discussed further in this chapter. Opioids, such as pethidine and diamorphine can be given intramuscularly. In many

cases, however, only subcutaneous injection may be achieved therefore the action of these interventions in this patient group may be unpredictable.

Intravenous opioids, especially via patient-controlled analgesia, may often be contraindicated in the obese parturient. They are at risk of obstructive sleep apnoea and opioid sensitivity, and such history should be sought prior to the commencement of any opioid treatment. A decrease in dose, increase time gap between administration of doses or both should be applied if opioids are used.

Operative Anaesthesia

Regional anaesthesia would be the anaesthetic of choice for most obese parturients. The enhanced cephalad spread of intrathecal drugs during spinal anaesthesia is debated. Many studies have found the required dose to be equivalent to that of non-obese parturients, while some older publications recommended reducing the volume of local anaesthetic used intrathecally by up to 25%; more recent evidence has shown this reduction may not be required. The cephalad spread of intrathecal injectate may be explained by injection at a higher than intended level in these patients. It should be noted, however, that any intercostal block can lead to dyspnoea, hypoxaemia and hypoventilation as the functional residual capacity in these patients is significantly reduced, especially in the supine position.

In morbidly obese patients, many would choose to site a combined spinal epidural (CSE) as the duration of surgery may be increased over the time covered by a spinal alone. The spread of spinal injectate can be extended by administration of aliquots of saline or local anaesthetic solution into the epidural space. The additional tactile feedback offered by the Tuohy needle, along with its structural rigidity compared with a spinal needle, means its use can be a real advantage for finding your direction. This can be useful in time-limited situations too as it can be quicker to find the epidural space with the Tuohy needle, through which a spinal needle can be quickly passed, rather than multiple attempts with spinal needles alone.

As in other specialties, surgery in these patients can be technically challenging. The abdominal 'apron' lies directly in the surgical field. This must be appropriately retracted, which may require more surgical assistants or mechanical means. Historically various makeshift arrangements have been devised to retract the panniculus. More recently specialised retractors, such as Traxi® and the Alexis O-ring® have revolutionised the quality of surgical access, often reducing the need for additional personnel. Once access to the peritoneum has been gained, the surgeon may choose to use a special retractor to keep the surgical field clear. The Alexis O-ring has revolutionised the quality of surgical access in the morbidly obese parturient, often reducing the need for additional personnel.

Positioning the patients on the theatre table is always troublesome, especially with a 15–30° left lateral tilt. Doing this safely may require table extensions or arm boards. A slight head-up position may be required to manage block height and improve ventilation. An elevation pillow can be used to optimise the patient's position during regional techniques and ensures favourable intubating conditions, should the need to convert to general anaesthesia arise. This can improve ventilation and patient comfort, but may affect regional anaesthetic spread, so a Trendelenberg tilt may need to be adopted with the operating table.

General Anaesthesia

Experience in obstetric general anaesthesia is decreasing, but skills in this area should be maintained and preparations for its conduct always be made.

Recent guidelines from the Obstetric Anaesthetists Association and Difficult Airway Society give advice on the safe conduct of obstetric general anaesthesia and plans for failed intubation.

Every woman should have an airway assessment prior to a surgical procedure. If a difficult airway is predicted, early referral to anaesthetic services allows a peri-partum plan to be made. In some morbidly obese women it may be recommended that a general anaesthetic should be avoided unless performed for maternal reasons.

Obese and high-risk women should be allowed clear fluids only during labour and receive 6-hourly oral H2 antagonists.

A multidisciplinary discussion should take place, timely and before induction, regarding the anaesthetic plan in the event of a failed intubation. Increasing BMI would sway the decision to wake in this circumstance, as safe ventilation via a facemask or second-generation supraglottic airway device cannot be guaranteed and the risk of hypoventilation, hypoxaemia, aspiration and maternal morbidity are greatly increased.

Pre-oxygenation should occur in a head-up position to free the area from the effects of large breasts or panniculus and increase the FRC and oxygen reserve. Further oxygenation can be achieved with nasal cannulae. An end tidal oxygen fraction of ≥90% is desirable prior to induction. The choice of induction agent has been under much discussion, with more anaesthetists choosing to use propofol instead of the traditional thiopentone, the use of which has been implicated in cases of awareness in the NAP5 study. Whichever agent is used, a dose based on ideal body weight should be administered. Likewise, rocuronium is gaining popularity in use in obstetric anaesthesia. If used, sugammadex should be readily available and the rescue dose pre-calculated before induction. Alternatively, suxamethonium may be used, but again, adequate doses should be given to ensure optimal intubating conditions. Plasma cholinesterase activity does decrease slightly in pregnancy, but this is not usually clinically significant.

Regardless of the anaesthetic, post-partum haemorrhage should be anticipated, with a plan for post-delivery uterotonics made, remembering that these women can have hypertensive disorders, which may contraindicate the use of ergometrine.

Extubation should occur in a fully reversed, co-operative patient. A head-up position ensures optimal respiratory mechanics at this time. Pressure support may be used until extubation to reduce de-recruitment of the lung tissue, and CPAP may be necessary following extubation to maintain oxygenation.

Positioning

As in many situations when caring for these patients, specialist equipment is often required with extra personnel available for manual handling requirements. The woman should be weighed close to the delivery date to ensure equipment used at delivery is adequately rated. It is important to remember that the maximum loads quoted may only be valid in the neutral position and may be less when the table is tilted. If the woman's weight is approaching the stated table limit, advice on safe tilting of the table should be gathered from the manufacturer. Where time does not permit this information to be gained quickly it may be safer to leave the table flat and reduce aortocaval compression by using manual uterine displacement. As previously mentioned, side extensions may be required for the theatre table and arm boards are often used to maintain alignment of the upper limbs. Non-invasive blood pressure monitoring is usually used with very frequent inflation rates and a straight arm may improve accuracy. Invasive arterial blood pressure monitoring or newer non-invasive methods, such as the Finapres®, may be indicated.

Post-operative Care

Post-operative care facilities should conform to published standards. The AAGBI recommend that two members of staff should be present when a patient is in recovery and does not fulfill criteria for discharge, with at least one trained in line with the UK National Core Competencies for post-anaesthesia care. Anaesthetic vigilance remains vital in these situations, as post-operative respiratory complications have resulted in anaesthetic-related maternal mortality. Patients with significant co-morbidities should be considered for critical care admission.

Ultrasound

Ultrasound is being used with increasing frequency on delivery suites for siting regional anaesthesia and vascular access in the obese population. Its use for the siting of lumbar epidurals has long been described and techniques have now been described to visualise insertion in real time, although this is rarely used outside of research projects. Image quality may be poor in obese patients so interested parties are encouraged to practice on slimmer individuals to gain experience in recognising the appropriate anatomy. A detailed knowledge of vertebral anatomy is essential. A curvilinear probe (2–5 MHz) is recommended for the purpose.

The lumbar spine can be imaged with the woman in the sitting or lateral position, but it is significantly easier in the former. The lumbar spine should be flexed in the position required for siting the epidural. The sacrum can be identified by a midline longitudinal view with the probe positioned just above the natal cleft. The L5–S1 interspace should be seen as a gap between the sacrum and the L5 facets. Taking a para-median longitudinal view, with the probe 1–2 cm lateral to the spinous process and the beam angled towards the midline, the classic saw tooth pattern, Figure 26.3), will be seen. The facet joints form the tips of the saw teeth and the base is made of the complex, formed by the ligamentum flavum and posterior dura. These can sometimes be identified as

separate structures, the gap between being the epidural space, but this is rarely, if ever, the case in obese patients. It is possible to move up the interspaces to the level of L3–4. It should be noted that this is often much lower than the level estimated by surface anatomy. Once at the desired level, the probe can be turned 90° to obtain a transverse image of the spinal interspace. The spinous process will appear as a hyperechoic structure with an anechoic shadow obscuring all neuraxial structures deep to it. On moving the probe cranially or caudally the interspace will be visualised. The classic image of the 'flying bat' should then be visible. The wings are formed from the transverse processes, the ears from the facet joints and the head from the ligamentum flavum/dura complex. Deep to this it is usually possible to see the posterior border of the vertebral body. In the obese parturient it may only be possible to identify the boney structures, which can lead to overestimation of the depth to the epidural space if there is confusion of the posterior body of the vertebra deep to the ligamentum complex. The depth of the epidural space can be measured and the interspace marked.

In an attempt to improve the view of the ultrasound structures, the skin may be indented by several centimetres, causing underestimation of measured depth. Relaxing the pressure on the skin before taking the measurement on the ultrasound screen can increase the accuracy of correlation between measurement and needle depth. The quality of the image on the screen will be reduced, but focusing on a fixed point whilst relaxing the skin pressure allows focus to be maintained on the area to be measured.

Indication of the interspace position can be done with a surgical marker, well away from the needle insertion point, or by indentation with the probe and then the blunt hub of a needle. The angle of the probe should be noted and a similar angle adopted on insertion of the neuraxial block. The back should be completely cleaned of ultrasound gel as this can be potentially neurotoxic prior to pre-procedural sterilisation.

The choice of appropriate needle length will be informed by a combination of BMI and measured depth. If the measured length is >7cm and the BMI is >40 kg/m^2, the 11 cm Tuohy needle can be most appropriate. The longer needle tends to be more flexible, with altered sensation to loss of resistance, so gaining experience in using it is incredibly valuable.

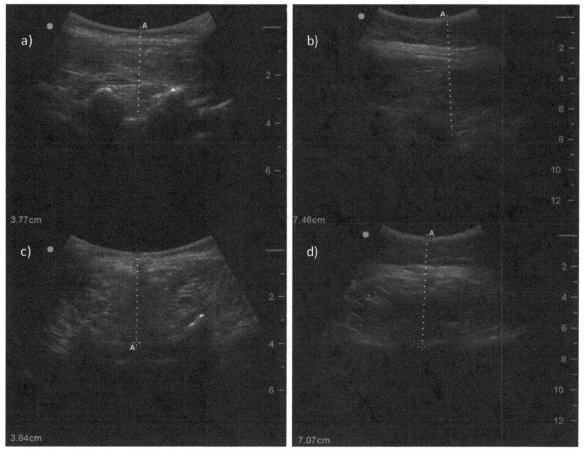

Figure 26.3 Comparison of image quality with (a) low BMI longitudinal view, (b) high BMI longitudinal view, (c) low BMI transverse view and (d) high BMI transverse view
.

Venous Thromboembolism Prophylaxis

Obese mothers are at a significant risk of venous thromboembolism (VTE). Women with booking BMI ≥30 kg/m^2 should be assessed for VTE prophylaxis during their antenatal care and in the post-natal period. It is recommended that those with BMI ≥30 kg/m^2 and two other risk factors should be considered for low molecular weight heparin for prophylaxis, beginning as early in pregnancy as possible and continuing for six weeks after delivery. Low molecular weight heparin (LMWH) is dosed according to maternal body weight, which may be the booking or most recent weight. As with all anti-coagulants, careful timing should be adhered to between dosing of the drug and neuraxial blockade. AAGBI guidelines state that neuraxial anaesthesia, or epidural catheter removal, should be performed 12 hours after administration of prophylactic dose of LMWH or 24 hours after therapeutic dose. Following the intervention, most LMWHs can be given after 4 hours, providing there are no contraindications.

New oral anti-coagulants have been used in pregnancy, which leads to difficulty in timing of neuraxial blockade. These drugs have no routinely available method of reversal and therefore haematological advice should be sought regarding their use.

Further Reading

Carvalho B, Collins J, Drover DR, Atkinson Ralls L, Riley ET. ED(50) and ED(95) of intrathecal bupivacaine in morbidly obese patients undergoing cesarean delivery. *Anesthesiology*. 2011;**114**(3):529–35.

Kinsella SM, Winton AL, Mushambi MC, et al. Failed tracheal intubation during obstetric general anaesthesia: a literature review. *Int J Obstet Anesth*. 2015;**24**(4):356–74.

Broadbent CR, Maxwell WB, Ferrie R, et al. Ability of anaesthetists to identify a marked lumbar interspace. *Anaesthesia.* 2000;**55**(11):1122–6.

Centre for Maternal and Child Enquiries (CMACE). *Maternal Obesity in the UK: Findings From a National Project.* London: CMACE; 2010.

Centre for Maternal and Child Enquiries and Royal College of Obstetricians and Gynaecologists. *Joint Guideline: Management of Women with Obesity in Pregnancy.* London: CMACE/RCOG; 2010.

Dresner M, Brocklesby J, Bamber J. Audit of the influence of body mass index on the performance of epidural analgesia in labour and the subsequent mode of delivery. *Br J Obstet Gynaecol.* 2006; **113**(10):1178–81.

Hodgkinson R, Husain FJ. Obesity and the cephalad spread of analgesia following epidural administration of bupivacaine for cesarean section. *Anesth Analg.* 1980;**59**:89–92.

Mushambi MC, Kinsella SM, Popat M, et al. Obstetric Anaesthetists' Association and Difficult Airway Society guidelines for the management of difficult and failed tracheal intubation in obstetrics. *Anaesthesia.* 2015;**70**(11):1286–306.

MBRRACE-UK: Mothers and Babies: Reducing Risk through Audit and Confidential Enquiry. *Saving Lives, Improving Mothers' Care Lessons Learned to Inform Future Maternity Care from the UK and Ireland Confidential Enquiries into Maternal Deaths and Morbidity 2009–2012.* Oxford: MBRACE-UK; 2014

MBRRACE-UK: Mothers and Babies: Reducing Risk through Audit and Confidential Enquiry. *Surveillance of maternal deaths in the UK 2011–13 and lessons learned to inform maternity care from the UK and Ireland Confidential Enquiries into Maternal Deaths and Morbidity 2009–13.* Oxford: MBRACE-UK; 2014

Peralta F, Higgins N, Lange E, Wong CA, McCarthy RJ. The relationship of body mass index with the incidence of postdural puncture headache in parturients. *Anesth Analg.* 2015;**121**(2):451–6.

Public Health England Obesity Knowledge and Intelligence. Maternal Obesity Prevalence. London: Public Health England; 2015.

Royal College of Obstetricians and Gynaecologists. *Reducing the Risk of Venous Thromboembolism during Pregnancy and the Puerperium.* Green-top Guideline No. 37a. London: RCOG; 2015.

www.rcog.org.uk/en/guidelines-research-services/guidelines/gtg37a/ (acessed May 2018).

Chapter 27

Day Case Surgery for Obese Patients

Mark Skues

Introduction

Day case, or ambulatory surgery, is defined as the admission, treatment and discharge of patients within the same calendar day, with planned management intent for admission as a daycase. While there has been progressive development in the concept of management, driven predominantly by advances in minimally invasive surgical techniques and developments in anaesthetic pharmacology, there remains significant variation between trusts within the United Kingdom for the management of such patients, irrespective of their body mass index. Within this chapter, day surgery will be evaluated as a concept worthy of engagement, before concentrating on the obese patient and their management in this environment.

Day Surgery: 'A good news story?'

Day surgery has its origins in a publication by James Nicoll in 1909, a Glaswegian surgeon who highlighted the potential benefits of ambulatory care for a paediatric population. Driven by financial considerations, bed shortfalls and concerns about a high cross-infection rate, Nicoll's solution was the early mobilisation of post-operative children and the organisation of home follow-up by a visiting nurse. Subsequent progress continued across the Atlantic with the opening of a downtown anaesthesia clinic in Sioux City, Iowa by Ralph Waters in 1916, followed by hospital-based day units in Grand Rapids, Michigan in 1951, and in Los Angeles in 1952. Progress in the United Kingdom was a little more constrained, as a result of lack of appreciation of the need for skilled consultants to perform surgery that was previously delegated to junior colleagues, and the need to review patients on the day of surgery, rather than the night before. In 1969, Professor James Calnan opened the first dedicated day unit at the Hammersmith Hospital in London, with the subsequent management of 10 000 patients treated from a variety of specialities without significant incident within the first 10 years. The further opening of additional day case units in England reporting success prompted the Royal College of Surgeons of England to publish *Guidelines for Day Case Surgery* in 1985. The report, which was revised in 1992, advocated that day surgery was the best management option for 50% of all patients undergoing elective surgery, at a time when the national average was less than 15%.

The British Association of Day Surgery was founded in 1989 as a multidisciplinary group of clinicians, nurses and managers to promote the new speciality and formulate guidelines and standards related to quality of care. Now in its 27th year, the association has developed a series of booklets covering every facet of day surgery care, promoted the concept of day surgery being an elective care pathway, and published a series of directories providing evidence-based guidelines for expected duration of stay for over 180 day surgery procedures, together with contemporary evidence of performance in England.

Appleby in 2015 cited the ongoing success of day surgery, calculating that if the historical transfer to day surgery had not occurred, the cost of managing the 6.96 million elective day and inpatients in 2013 would have been £11bn, but that savings of 22% had been made, reducing the sum to £8.9bn. Assuming a similar increase in the proportion of daycase surgery for the next decade, a further 1.5 million patients would be treated for no real increase in spending. This is further supplemented by the ongoing development of 'best practice tariffs' for day surgery, where for a number of procedures, admission and treatment on the same day with management intent, care is financially incentivised with an increase of payment compared with an inpatient cohort. There are now 15 procedures that benefit from best practice tariffs, with an average of £265 gained for every operation conducted as a day case. Given that the hypothesised cost

Table 27.1 WHO and other definitions of obesity

BMI range	Classification
25 ≤ BMI < 30	Overweight
30 ≤ BMI < 35	Obesity Class I
35 ≤ BMI < 40	Obesity Class II
40 ≤ BMI < 50	Obesity Class III/morbid obesity
50 ≥ BMI	Super morbid obesity
70 ≥ BMI	Ultra obesity

of an overnight bed is estimated at approximately £225, translocation of an inpatient operation to the day surgery environment should accrue close to £500, whilst freeing up the hospital bed for other patients.

Obesity and Day Surgery

The prevalence of obesity continues to rise within the United Kingdom, in common with the rest of the developed world. Defined as a body mass index of >30 kg/m, 25.6% of adults in England exceeded this threshold in 2014, with Scotland reaching 27.7% (2011), Wales, 22.1% (2011) and Northern Ireland 23% (2011). The World Health Organization (WHO) definition further classifies patients with varying levels of obesity into different groups, while there are a number of additional informal classifications defining morbid, super morbid and ultra obesity. (Table 27.1).

The aim of any pre-operative assessment exercise is to screen day surgery patients for potential co-morbidities, evaluate them with appropriate diagnostic investigations and then manage them with a view to reducing peri-operative risk for proposed surgery. Cardiovascular symptoms that may co-exist with obesity include a covariance with metabolic syndrome, a triad of hypertension, dyslipidaemia and dysglycaemia, believed to be produced by the endocrine and immunological components of adipose tissue. However, there may be a percentage of up to 30% of obese patients who are metabolically healthy as a result of differing depositions of adipose tissue, where higher amounts of visceral fat are more likely to be associated with an adverse association with the syndrome. Indices such as waist circumference and waist:hip ratio, together with assessment of functional capacity, may assist in the differentiation of the two groups. For morbidly obese patients with limited cardiovascular functional ability, an ECG should be obtained if there is more than one risk factor for heart disease. Signs of right ventricular hypertrophy predictive of pulmonary hypertension or left bundle branch block suggestive of occult cardiac disease are indicative of the need for further evaluation with chest radiography to evaluate heart chamber size, cardiopulmonary exercise testing to formalise functional ability and transfer to inpatient care.

Respiratory Pre-assessment Signs

One of the major co-morbidities associated with obesity is obstructive sleep apnoea (OSA), characterised by repetitive partial or complete collapse of the upper airway during sleep leading to hypoxaemia and/or hypercapnia, with associated signs of daytime sleepiness, loud snoring, witnessed breathing interruptions or awakenings because of gasping or choking in the presence of at least five respiratory obstructive events per hour of sleep. Most patients with OSA are undiagnosed, therefore all obese patients presenting for surgery should be assessed for presence using the STOP-BANG questionnaire (Table 27.2), with a score ≥5 providing a presumptive diagnosis. Both the Society for Ambulatory Anaesthesia and the American Society of Anesthesiologists have provided guidelines for management of OSA patients as a daycase, which rely upon optimisation of co-existing co-morbidities, utilising a peri-operative technique that avoids opioid analgesia, and the use and presence of a CPAP machine to provide post-operative respiratory care after discharge. On the premise that these conditions are fulfilled, there is no reason why daycase surgery cannot proceed on suitable patients.

Associated with OSA is the potential presence of obesity hypoventilation syndrome (OHS) that manifests as associated hypercapnia (arterial partial pressure of carbon dioxide ≥ 6 kPa) during wakeful daytime. OHS is associated with sleep disordered breathing such as sleep apnoea, but may co-exist with chronic obstructive pulmonary disease. OHS might also be associated with daytime hypoxaemia as a presumed consequence of loss of respiratory drive. If OHS is diagnosed by blood gas analysis (allowing for potential agitated hyperventilation during sampling) the patient is better managed in the inpatient environment.

Obese patients may also have asthma-like symptoms associated with poorer control and response to therapy, though it remains uncertain whether this is

Table 27.2 The STOP-BANG Questionnaire

Snoring	'Do you snore loudly' (louder than talking or heard through a closed door?)
Tired	'Do you often feel tired, fatigued or sleepy during the daytime? Do you fall asleep during the daytime?'
Observed	'Has anyone observed you stop breathing, or choking or gasping during your sleep?'
Blood **P**ressure	'Do you have, or are you being treated for high blood pressure?'
BMI	BMI ≥35 kg/m^2
Age	Age ≥50 years
Neck	Circumference (measured around Adam's apple) >43 cm (17 inches) for males, >41 cm (16 inches) for females
Gender	Male

allergic early onset symptoms complicated by concomitant obesity, or a non-allergic adult onset disease as a consequence of weight gain. The respiratory pathophysiology of loading of the chest wall by adipose tissue produces a reduction in lung volumes, and compression of distal airways with increased closing capacity at lower functional residual capacity, but the associated direct relationship between asthma and obesity remains unproven.

Airway Evaluation

Debate still remains about the ease of mask ventilation, direct laryngoscopy and intubation in the obese patient. The Fourth National Audit study (NAP4) on complications of airway management in the UK found airway problems to be twice as common in obese patients and four times as common with morbid obesity, while an observational study of over 130 000 patients found that a BMI ≥30 kg/m^2 was an independent risk factor for both difficult mask ventilation and difficult intubation. However, this finding has not been universally replicated, with prediction potentially challenging, as no one discriminating factor appears reliable. For day surgery therefore, anaesthetists should conduct a formal evaluation of the airway, making note of mouth opening, neck extension, thyromental distance and the Mallampati score, and ensure that adjuncts are available for ventilation and intubation in the event of potential difficulties.

Diabetes Mellitus

The prevalence of type 2 diabetes is increased in the obese population with theories of linkage matched to either the pro-inflammatory release of mediators from abdominal adipose tissue disrupting the function of insulin-responsive cells, or the effect of the release of factors involved in the development of insulin resistance, associated with pancreatic islet beta cell dysfunction. It is estimated that 63% of obese adults between the ages of 16 and 54 have concomitant type 2 diabetes, with 90% of adults who are either overweight or obese experiencing raised blood sugar levels. Given that a quarter of patients are unaware of their glycaemic status, the cited prevalence may be an underestimate of the true figure.

The management of diabetes in the daycase environment is the subject of a number of handbooks from the British Association of Day Surgery, to which the reader is recommended.

Thromboembolic Risk

Obesity is recognised as an independent risk factor for peri-operative venous thromboembolism, and it is recommended that all obese patients should receive VTE prophylaxis for all but minor surgery. One therefore has something of a dilemma in determining which procedures are regarded as 'minor' in day surgery practice and applying prophylaxis accordingly. One solution is to employ a point-scoring algorithm summating all possible risk factors and use prophylaxis in the event of four or more points being scored. Weight-corrected dosage regimens for pharmacological prophylaxis are shown in Table 27.3.

Intra-operative Care

After final checks on the day of surgery involving nursing, anaesthetic and surgical team members, preferential operating list scheduling should be facilitated to allow obese patients to have their day surgery operation early in the day. As most day surgery units now employ operating trolleys rather than tables, the operating theatre team should be informed so that they can organise a trolley suitable for the patient's weight. Similarly, appropriately sized blood pressure cuffs would be required for such patients. Consideration should be given to routine premedication of patients for aspiration risk with either H2 antagonists or metoclopramide. The pre-operative

Table 27.3 Venous thromboprophylaxis risk assessment for day surgery

Risk Factors	
Patient	**Surgical**
Pregnancy immediately post partum (<6 weeks)	Laparoscopic salpingectomy
Obesity (body mass index >30≤39 kg/m^2)	Laparoscopic excision of endometrioisis
Age over 60 years	Knee and ankle arthroscopy
Family history of DVT/PE	Ankle/foot ligament reconstruction
Travel >3 h approx. 4 weeks before or after surgery	Laparoscopic cholecystectomy/inguinal hernia repair
Use of hormonal replacement therapy or oestrogen-containing contraceptive therapy	Foot/toe/bunion surgery
Severe varicose veins or active phlebitis	Laparoscopic oophorectomy
Immobility (e.g. paralysis or limb in plaster)	Laparoscopic ovarian cystectomy
Known cancer or cancer treatment	Laparoscopic salpingectomy
Current anti-coagulant therapy	Laparoscopic excision of endometrioisis
Morbid obesity (body mass index >40 kg/m^2)	Knee and ankle arthroscopy
Personal history of DVT/PE	
Thrombophilia	
Specific surgical procedures planned	
Low risk – Score 0–3 TED stockings, adequate hydration, early mobilisation	
High risk – Score 4 and above: TED stockings, adequate hydration, early mobilisation, tinzaparin/enoxaparin to be commenced on day of surgery	
Weight	**Tinzaparin dose**
<50 kg	2500 units daily
50–70 kg	3500 units daily
71–90 kg	4500 units daily
>91 kg	50 units/kg

team brief should highlight the pre-operative issues involved with patient care, and the planned anaesthetic technique for the procedure. Consideration should be given to the benefits of regional blockade compared with general anaesthesia, as the former avoids the need for airway intervention, obviates the requirement for intra-operative opioids in the event of concomitant obstructive sleep apnoea and provides longer-lasting pain relief than would otherwise be achieved.

Patient position should be managed by 'ramping', ensuring that the external auditory meatus is at the same level as the sternum. On the premise that general anaesthesia is required, postural change from supine to the 20° head-up position during pre-oxygenaton displaces abdominal contents away from the diaphragm, improving functional residual capacity, and extends the safe apnoea period from 155 to

201 seconds. Preparations for potentially difficult mask ventilation, laryngoscopy and intubation should be made, and it is recommended that for all but the most brief of daycase procedures, airway control by intubation is facilitated.

Drug doses for anaesthesia are different in the obese patient, and doses should be based upon lean body weight, with the exception of suxamethonium (if used) where total body weight should be used in calculations and propofol infusions where adjusted body weight should be employed. Given the safety requirement for prompt recovery post-operatively, it is sensible to employ volatile agents with a rapid recovery phase. Consideration should be given to the employment of multimodal analgesic techniques, with routine administration of paracetamol, non-steroidal anti-inflammatory agents (or COX2 inhibitors) and local anaesthetic infiltration of wounds to reduce the requirement for opioids in the post-operative period. Establishment of full reversal of neuromuscular blockade should ensure prompt recovery after the operation, minimising effects of residual paralysis.

The anaesthetist should facilitate immediate recovery after anaesthesia, with extubation directly supervised by them. Compliance with advice to use CPAP machines after discharge is mandatory, given Chung and co-workers evaluated the nocturnal performance of OSA and non-OSA patients for 7 days after discharge and found that the apneoa/hypopnoea index (number of apnoeic/hypopnoeic episodes per hour) increased significantly on the thrid post-operative night for those with OSA, and lasted for up to a week.

Post-discharge analgesia should be prescribed as appropriate, ensuring that opioids (including codeine) are avoided in OSA patients, and venous thromboembolism prophylaxis is continued.

Caveats to Day Surgery in the Obese Patient

Day surgery has an enviable track record for safety and outcomes, predominantly due to the relative fitness of the population it serves. However, some authors have suggested limits on the suitability of obese patients for day surgery, limiting activity to those with BMIs <40 kg/m^2. Joshi conducted a systematic review of the evidence for selection of such patients for ambulatory surgery and concluded that while BMI should not be the only determinant of patient selection, the super obese (BMI >50 kg/m^2) may be at higher risk of peri-operative complications for day surgery, with adverse criteria suggested as an inability to walk more than 200 feet, history of deep vein thrombosis, history of OSA, co-existing medical disorders and the invasiveness of the proposed procedure. On this basis, it would seem sensible to consider the suitability of such patients with careful pre-operative assessment and optimisation of existing co-morbidities in this group to determine best outcome.

Further Reading

American Society of Anesthesiologists Task Force on Perioperative Management of Patients with Obstructive Sleep Apnea Practice guidelines for the perioperative management of patients with obstructive sleep apnea. *Anesthesiology*. 2014;**120**:268–86.

Appleby J. Day case surgery: a good news story for the NHS. *BMJ*. 2015;**351**:h4060.

British Association of Day Surgery. 2016. http://daysurgeryuk.net/en/shop/handbooks/ (accessed May 2018).

British Association of Day Surgery. 2016. http://daysurgeryuk.net/en/shop/handbooks/managing-diabetes-in-patients-having-day-and-short-stay-surgery-4th-edition/ (accessed May 2018).

Bluth T, Pelosi P, Gama de Abreu M. The obese patient undergoing nonbariatric surgery. *Curr Opin Anesthesiol*. 2016;**29**:421–9.

Chung F, Liao P, Yegneswaran B, et al. Postoperative changes in sleep-disordered breathing and sleep architecture in patients with obstructive sleep apnea. *Anesthesiology*. 2014;**120**:287–98.

Cook TM, Woodall N, Frerk C. Fourth National Audit Project. Major complications of airway management in the UK: results of the Fourth National Audit Project of the Royal College of Anaesthetists and the Difficult Airway Society. Part 1: Anaesthesia. *Br J Anaesth*. 2011;**106**:617–31.

De Baerdemaeker L, Margarson M. Best anaesthetic drug strategy for morbidly obese patients. *Curr Opin Anesthesiol*. 2016;**29**:119–28.

Dixit A, Kulshrestha M, Mathews JJ, et al. Are the obese difficult to intubate? *Br J Anaesth*. 2014;**112**:770–1.

Joshi GP, Ankichetty SP, Gan TJ, et al. Society for Ambulatory Anesthesia consensus statement on preoperative selection of adult patients with obstructive sleep apnea scheduled for ambulatory surgery. *Anesth Analg*. 2012;**115**:1060–8.

Joshi GP, Ahmad S, Riad W, Eckert S, Chung F. Selection of obese patients undergoing ambulatory surgery: a systematic review of the literature. *Anesth Analg*. 2013;**117**:1082–91.

Kheterpal S, Healy D, Aziz MF, et al. Incidence, predictors, and outcome of difficult mask ventilation combined with difficult laryngoscopy: a report from the multicenter perioperative outcomes group. *Anesthesiology*. 2013;**119**:1360–9.

Lam KL, Kunder S, Wong J, et al. Obstructive sleep apnea, pain and opioids: is the riddle solved? *Curr Opin Anesthesiol*. 2016;**29**:134–40.

Mahajan V, Hashmi J, Singh R, et al. Comparative evaluation of gastric pH and volume in morbidly obese and lean patients undergoing elective surgery and effect of aspiration prophylaxis. *J Clin Anesth*. 2015;**27**:396–400.

National Institute for Health and Clinical Excellence. *Venous Thromboembolism: Reducing the Risk*. NICE Clinical Guideline 92. London: NICE; 2010.

Nicoll JH. The surgery of infancy. *BMJ*. 1909;**2**:753–6.

Nightingale CE, Margarson MP, Shearer E, et al. Peri-operative management of the obese surgical patient 2015. *Anaesthesia*. 2015;**70**(7):859–76.

NHS Institute for Innovation and Improvement. Delivering quality and value. *Focus on: Cholecystectomy*. Coventry: NHS Institute for Innovation and Improvement; 2006.

Norskov AK, Rosenstock CV, Wetterslev J, et al. Diagnostic accuracy of anaesthesiologists' prediction of difficult airway management in daily clinical practice: a cohort study of 188064 patients registered in the Danish Anaesthesia Database. *Anaesthesia*. 2015;**70**:272–81.

Public Health England. Adult obesity and type 2 diabetes. 2014. www.gov.uk/government/uploads/system/uploads/attachment_data/file/338934/Adult_obesity_and_type_2_diabetes_.pdf (accessed May 2018).

Royal College of Surgeons of England *Commission on the Provision of Surgical Services. Report of the Working Party on Guidelines for Day Case Surgery*. London: Royal College of Surgeons;1992.

Shah U, Wong J, Wong DT, Chung F. Preoxygenation and intraoperative ventilation strategies in obese patients: a comprehensive review. *Curr Opin Anesthesiol*. 2016;**29**:109–18.

Skues M. *BADS Directory of Procedures – National Dataset for Calendar Year 2015*. London:British Association of Day Surgery; 2016. http://daysurgeryuk.net/en/shop/publications/national-dataset-(calendar-year-2015)/ (accessed May 2018).

Skues M, Montgomery J. *BADS Directory of Procedures, 5th Edn*. London: British Association of Day Surgery; 2016. http://daysurgeryuk.net/en/shop/publications/bads-directory-of-procedures-5th-edition/ (accessed May 2018).

Emergency Surgery and Trauma in the Obese

Peter Shirley and Neil MacDonald

Introduction

The increase in adult obesity in the developed world over the last decade is well documented and this is reflected in the emergency trauma and surgical patient population. These patients present a higher risk and currently there is no surgical scoring risk for emergency surgery that carries obesity as an individual risk factor. Obesity is associated with increased complications after emergency surgery; evidence demonstrates a direct correlation between the degree of obesity and development of post-operative complications. This concurs with data that reveals no difference in mortality, but increases in complications and intensive care admissions following non-planned surgery in the obese; in obese trauma patients undergoing emergency surgery, mortality is increased. Focused care starts at the first clinical encounter and the anaesthetist must anticipate the entire perioperative journey. The same factors under consideration for the obese patient undergoing elective surgery should also be considered in emergency surgery with the full understanding that the time frames may necessitate a modified assessment (Table 28.1). Chronic conditions are common in obese individuals, e.g. hypertension, diabetes mellitus and ischaemic heart disease. In the emergency situation it can be difficult (and often impossible) to identify the presence of these pathologies.

The Obese Trauma Patient

Obese patients are more likely to be involved in road traffic accidents, possibly due to the presence of obstructive sleep apnoea (OSA). They are more likely to suffer chest, pelvis and limb fractures, but mildly overweight patients are less prone to intra-abdominal injury because of the protective effect of the abdominal fat (also known as the cushion effect). BMI is an independent risk factor for morbidity and mortality after trauma and the trauma team needs to be aware of

Table 28.1 Peri-operative considerations in the obese patient requiring emergency surgery

1. Airway	Modified assessment done? Anticipated difficulty? Plan A/Plan B/Plan C Airway adjuncts identified?
2. Breathing	Modified assessment of function? Positioning for anaesthesia (Ramping) considered? Ventilation settings post-intubation Post-operative ventilation plan/need for CPAP
3. Circulation	Known cardiac dysfunction? ECG/previous ECHO studies reviewed Requirement for cardiac monitoring?
4. Disability	Pressure areas protected? Post-operative physiotherapy plan? Post-operative analgesia plan?
5. Everything else	Team brief Modified WHO checklist Post-operative care discussed with surgical team?

the logistical difficulties associated with some of these patients. Securing the airway and emergency venous access (central and peripheral) can be challenging. The use of bedside ultrasound (ECHO, FAST scanning) can be of limited use. Maintaining spinal precautions and logrolling can present difficulties due to the collar positioning, the effects on ventilation and the numbers of staff required for safe moving and positioning. Transit to CT scanning can also create major challenges and more staff may need to be involved than normal. In the extremely obese more than one anaesthetist will often be required to overcome the challenges presented in securing the airway, venous access and patient transfer.

Airway

The airway of the obese patient is generally considered to be more difficult to manage than in the non-obese. Features that should be noted in the history are: the presence of suspected or diagnosed OSA, problems with previous anaesthesia/airway management and the presence of treated or untreated gastro-oesophageal reflux disease (GORD).

The obese patient at risk of airway obstruction under general anaesthesia can be identified by having a short mental–hyoid distance, flattened, compressed anterior–posterior craniofacial architecture, retrognathism, relative macroglossia and a narrower, bulky oropharynx. Airway assessment on an obese patient about to undergo emergency surgery should therefore include: neck circumference, Mallampati (MP) score, thyromental distance, assessment of mouth opening and jaw protrusion, range of neck movement and general assessment of facial structure. The presence of a cervical fat pad or 'hump' should also be noted as this can lead to difficulty in positioning the patient optimally for intubation. An increased BMI along with the absence of teeth, limited jaw protrusion, MP 3 or 4, snoring and a beard help predict difficult mask ventilation. A high BMI >25 but <35 does not appear to correlate directly with a worse view on laryngoscopy in the absence of some of the features listed above. Certain traits associated with increased BMI, such as increased neck circumference can aid the prediction of a difficult airway, but there are no clear studies demonstrating any reliable predictive tools for a difficult airway in the obese patient. In emergency surgery these uncertainties compound the difficulties in managing the airway. Video laryngoscopy has been shown to improve the view of the larynx and reduce the time to tracheal intubation in obese patients undergoing elective surgery. Initial experience with video laryngoscopy for elective tracheal intubation of obese patients has been promising; its use in emergencies remains unproven. The most important aspect of managing the obese airway is to have a clear, communicated plan with a default in case of difficulty, in accordance with current Difficult Airway Society (DAS) guidelines. Front of neck access is likely to be more difficult in obese patients, both surgically and percutaneously.

Breathing

Physiological changes associated with obesity mean that a reduced functional residual capacity provides less time for establishing ventilation prior to desaturation. In the acutely unwell patient there is likely to be a higher metabolic rate through pain, illness or both, leading to an accelerated desaturation time. Pre-oxygenation is mandatory prior to inducing anaesthesia in the obese patient and 'ramping' to 25° is suggested. Continuous positive airway pressure (CPAP) has been shown to be of benefit in increasing the time to desaturation. Transnasal humidified rapid-insufflation ventilatory exchange (THRIVE technique), which employs high-flow nasal oxygen, may also be of benefit at the induction of anaesthesia. It has been shown to extend apnoea times at the induction of anaesthesia in obese patients with predicted difficult airways. Consideration must be given though to the additional risk in emergency patients whose time to desaturation may be further reduced due to their higher metabolic and pro-inflammatory state. Evidence suggests that PEEP alongside recruitment manoeuvres can improve intra-operative oxygenation and lung compliance. Ideal body weight should be used to guide correct tidal volume. There is no evidence of one ventilation mode being preferable to another. A higher PEEP (around 10 cmH$_2$O) is associated with improved intra-operative oxygenation and does not appear to cause haemodynamic compromise or result in barotrauma. Following extubation, CPAP may be required as part of the recovery process and admission to a critical care area may be necessary to facilitate this if it is required for a prolonged period.

Circulation

Hypertension is a recognised condition in 60% of obese patients; this may be due to a combination of activation of the renin–angiotensin system, increased adrenergic activity, alteration in intra-cellular calcium/sodium/potassium distribution, and elevated cardiac output (due to an expanded circulating and cardiopulmonary volume). It has implications when interpreting 'normal' blood pressures, particularly in emergency situations. Invasive cardiac output monitoring should be utilised to guide fluid and ionotropic therapy. The use of bedside transthoracic echocardiography is of limited value due to the interpretation of images, which often can be poor.

Table 28.2 Emergency drug dosing calculations in the obese patient

Emergency drug	Dosing schedule basis
Propofol	Ideal body weight 3–5mg/kg
Ketamine	Ideal body weight
Suxamethonium	Total body weight 1mg/kg
Rocuronium	Ideal body weight 0.5–1.2 mg/kg
Fentanyl	Ideal body weight 1–2 μg/kg
Thiopentone	Ideal body weight 5–7mg/kg
Noradrenaline	Ideal body weight 0–1 μg/kg/min
Adrenaline	Ideal body weight 0–1 μg/kg/min

IBW (kg) = Height (cm) – x (where x = 105 in males and x = 100 in females)

$$LBW\ (kg) = \frac{9270 \times TBW(KG)}{6680 + (216 \times BMI)(kg/m^2)} \quad \text{MALE}$$

$$LBW\ (kg) = \frac{9270 \times TBW(KG)}{8780 + (244 \times BMI)(kg/m^2)} \quad \text{FEMALE}$$

ABW (kg) = IBW (kg) + 0.4 (TBW – IBW) (kg)

IBW = ideal body weight; LBW = lean body weight; TBW = total body weight; ABW = actual body weight

Emergency Drugs

There is a lack of data concerning correct drug dosing in obesity and as a consequence the majority of drugs administered in obese patients undergoing emergency anaesthesia is based on theory and experience. Several factors related to obesity may influence the metabolism and elimination of medications commonly used during emergency airway management. Lipophilic drugs have an increased volume of distribution in obesity; there does not appear to be an increase in metabolism of drugs, despite an increase in liver enzyme abnormalities. There is an increase in renal blood flow and a corresponding increase in the clearance of certain drugs. The interaction of increased renal clearance, changes in volume of distribution, and other factors, such as abnormal protein binding, can make predicting pharmacokinetics in obesity difficult. As a general principle, hydrophilic drugs should be dosed according to ideal body weight, and lipophilic drugs, owing to an increased volume of distribution, should be administered based on total body weight. Unfortunately, the lack of published data on medication dosing in obesity precludes an evidence-based approach to pharmacokinetics in obesity in the acute setting, and dosing of many medications is often based on theoretical considerations (Table 28.2).

Intra-operative Considerations and Damage Control

In the mildly obese this often presents no additional challenge, but in the extremely obese, ventilation in the operating theatre can be very difficult. The use of high PEEP and head-up position are all standard techniques, along with permissive hypercapnoea. Patients with an initial acidosis are difficult to manage and damage control principles need to be utilised to minimise the physiological impact on the patient. There needs to be a very clear line of communication between the anaesthetist and operating surgeon. The accepted damage control principles (temperature >35.5 °C, operating time less than 90 minutes, pH >7.25) may need revision depending on the clinical situation at the time. There will be clear risk–benefit decisions about when surgery needs to be curtailed or conversely when it can be continued.

Critical Care

Studies looking at critical care outcomes for the extremely obese (BMI >40 kg/m^2) are mixed, but do consistently demonstrate worse outcomes in trauma surgical patients in relation to mortality and complications: multiorgan failure, severe acute lung injury, renal failure, myocardial infarction and pressure ulcers. There are also logistical issues associated with looking after this patient group in the intensive care unit (ICU), including adaptation of beds, hoists and imaging equipment to cope with the elevated BMI. In the survivor group, obese patients have longer critical care and hospital lengths of stay. Limited data exists, including randomised trials about the right clinical approach to obese trauma patients. Much of this evidence related to obese patients is generated from pooled observational data. It is necessary to rely on generalist knowledge about treating obese patients in the ICU.

Transfer and Admission to the ICU

Post-procedure transfer to the ICU requires planning, whether from the operating theatre or interventional radiology suite. This should be regarded as a high-risk transfer, particularly if the patient is ventilated. It is normal practice in the UK to move the patient to their designated ICU bed prior to transfer, with all the attendant risks of accidental extubation and line dislodgement. Transfer ventilators are often not sophisticated and ventilation modes simple. High airway pressures should be avoided where possible (even for short periods) and establishing the patient on a 'proper' ICU ventilator prior to transfer may be required. If the patient is ventilated, the ability to use higher PEEP should be available and recruitment manoeuvres should be considered following any ventilator disconnection. Oxygen requirements are higher than in non-obese patients, so additional oxygen cylinders will be required. Admission to ICU needs to be done in a systematic fashion to ensure continuity of care and clear planning for the next phase of treatment. This means that a formal medical and nursing handover needs to take place and ongoing treatment aims highlighted to the intensive care team. These are summarised in Table 28.3.

Breathing and Ventilation

Obese patients are more prone to hypoxaemia and hypercapnia. This is due to decreased chest wall and lung compliance, less respiratory muscle endurance

Table 28.3 Checklist for admission of the obese trauma patient to intensive care

1. Ensure safe transfer to appropriate bed and mattress and obtain direct medical handover
2. Establish actual and ideal body weights
3. Clear the cervical spine in a sedated and ventilated trauma patient
4. Establish ventilation and cardiorespiratory monitoring
5. Determine timing of any fracture fixation and further surgical interventions
6. Plan to achieve short- and medium-term resuscitation endpoints
7. Follow aseptic strategies for mitigation of central venous catheter bloodstream infections
8. Early feeding via enteral route
9. An early physiotherapy/rehabilitation assessment
10. Next of kin identified and aware

and increased demand on their diaphragm. This is associated with a reduction in functional residual capacity and alveolar hypoventilation results in ventilated obese trauma patients having longer periods of mechanical ventilation and higher failure rates for extubation. During mechanical ventilation, higher PEEP settings are usually required to improve compliance and offset ventilation–perfusion mismatch due to distal airway collapse. The use of protective lung ventilation strategies is recommended in the trauma population and should be instituted as early as practicable in the patient's pathway; in the emergency department or theatres if possible. For obese patients this should be based on their ideal body weight, but there may need to be early adjustments depending on airway pressure and PaCO$_2$ levels. The objective is to minimise the risk of acute lung injury (ALI). Management of this condition in obese patients is challenging. The use of prone positioning or extracorporeal membrane oxygenation (ECMO) is a major challenge.

Circulation

Obese patients have a greater left ventricular workload leading to left ventricular dilatation and hypertrophy. This has lead to the term 'obesity cardiomyopathy', evidenced by alterations in stroke volume and cardiac output related to the poor left ventricular compliance. Additionally, obesity decreases intra-thoracic volume and concurrently raises intra-thoracic pressure (from increased intra-abdominal pressure), which results in falsely elevated central venous pressure measurements. The interpretation of cardiovascular measurements, particularly when resuscitating obese patients can be difficult. The use of invasive cardiac output monitoring has its place, but must be linked to careful patient assessment.

Modulation of Systemic Inflammatory Response Syndrome

Evidence has emerged which shows that inflammation is an integral component of obesity-linked illness, including insulin resistance and type 2 diabetes mellitus. Clinical and research data has revealed a complex mechanism involving adipose tissue, chemokines and adipocytokines that link metabolic regulation and immune response. It is becoming clear that obesity is in itself a state of low-grade inflammation. Major trauma and emergency surgery are now known to provoke pro-inflammatory responses. Systemic inflammatory response syndrome (SIRS) is not inherently dangerous and is ultimately required for tissue repair, but an unregulated response in extreme conditions can compromise healthy tissue, distant end organs and further promote inflammation. SIRS in trauma is characterised by a three tier response: metabolic, immunological and haemodynamic. The chronic low-grade inflammatory effect of obesity may provide a protective effect in mildly obese individuals, whereas more severe obesity is linked to an increased rate of inflammatory complications and dysregulated immune responses.

Surgical Planning

Planning further surgical intervention for obese patients forms part of their intensive care management and needs to be undertaken as a multidisciplinary discussion. Effects on ventilation, circulation and nutrition can be severe and compromise longer-term recovery. Clear time frames need to be adhered to where possible and cases should be scheduled for daytime operating sessions unless the clinical situation dictates otherwise. Where more than one surgical team is involved, coordination to avoid multiple, separate operating theatre sessions is essential. There needs to be a risk–benefit discussion regarding the likely impact on the patient's physiology, even in the short term.

Nutrition

Compared with a lean population of patients, obese trauma patients in the catabolic phase of their critical illness will have increased protein loss as they are prone to muscle breakdown. Reduced calorie, high-protein feeding has been used to attempt to reduce protein catabolism and hyperglycaemia. The concept that these patients have plenty of fat reserves and feeding can therefore be delayed is incorrect. Feeding should be initiated as soon as possible, ideally via the enteral route; the use of prokinetics if full feeding is not established with 72 hours is recommended. Close liaison with dietetic staff is essential. Prolonged periods of starvation (prior to surgical procedures) should also be avoided.

Renal Failure

Obesity has been identified as a risk factor for acute kidney injury (AKI) in trauma. This may be linked to inflammatory cytokine release from adipose tissue potentiating AKI in this patient group. The difficulty in interpretation of blood pressure in the context of emergency therapy has been highlighted earlier; this can clearly have an impact on renal perfusion pressure targets. Renal vascular access in obese critical care patients further complicates provision of haemofiltration in the event of renal replacement therapy being required.

Traumatic Brain Injury

Obesity has a protective effect in certain injury patterns following major trauma. Whilst this may have some bearing on the severity of certain abdominal injuries, this is more than offset by the risk factors posed to the very obese from in-hospital complications and mortality following major trauma. There is mixed evidence for traumatic brain injury (TBI), but an increased frequency of severe head injury following blunt motor vehicle-related trauma in the obese is seen. The specific management of TBI in the obese is a major challenge due to the cardiorespiratory effects and their impact on the control of end tidal carbon dioxide, mean arterial pressure and consequently cerebral perfusion pressure. The use of intra-cranial pressure monitoring is relatively standard practice; this is imperative in the obese patient as changes in ventilation, positioning and fluctuations can have profound effects on the intra-cranial pressure, which may need urgent intervention to maintain cerebral perfusion. Early rehabilitation is the aim in TBI. However, in this group it can form a major challenge, particularly if early extubation is not possible. Early tracheostomy may facilitate weaning, as sedation can

Table 28.4 Modified care bundle for the obese trauma patient in intensive care

1. Admission targets	Traumatic brain injury guidelines followed if required?
	Tertiary survey completed?
	Surgical plan in place and being followed?
2. Infection control	Strict adherence to hand hygiene?
	Field-placed venous access lines changed?
	Assess need for current central venous access?
	Appropriate antibiotics?
3. Ventilated patients	Head-of-bed elevation?
	Low tidal volume ventilation protocol indicated/employed?
	pCO_2 targets necessary and achievable?
	Oral care protocol?
	Daily weaning attempt?
	Sedation and analgesia protocol?
	Is paralysis necessary?
	Pressure area protection?
4. Deep vein thrombosis prophylaxis optimised?	
5. Stress ulcer prophylaxis required?	
6. Glycaemic control best and safest for circumstance?	
7. Pain management	Pain well controlled?
	Candidate for regional anaesthesia?
8. Nutrition optimised	Candidate for early feeding?
9. Rehabilitation plan in place and being followed?	

often be reduced more quickly enabling better assessment of underlying neurological function. Recovery from TBI encompasses physical and cognitive rehabilitation in tandem; in the very obese physical rehabilitation may need to be modified.

Infection Control and Venous Thromboembolic Disease

Obesity is a predisposing factor for deep vein thrombosis. The impact of trauma on the coagulation system is better understood. There is evidence that patients move to a pro-coagulation state following major trauma. This combined with prolonged mechanical ventilation and lack of early mobility put these patients in a high-risk group for thromboembolic disease. Inadequate dosing of prophylactic anticoagulants and difficulties in applying thromboembolic stockings are compounding factors. Obese trauma patients are at increased risk of nosocomial infections for a number of reasons: difficulties in peripheral venous access (meaning prolonged use of central venous catheters), weight-related skin

breakdown and prolonged mechanical ventilation are all linked to this phenomenon. The use of care bundles can lessen some of these risks (Table 28.4)

Tracheostomy

Due to the incidence of prolonged mechanical ventilation and extubation failure, a high proportion of ventilated obese patients will progress to tracheostomy to aid ventilatory weaning. The commonplace use of percutaneous tracheostomy in the ICU is associated with higher complication rates in obese patients. Adequate access, positioning and the relative lack of surgical competencies if complications occur (amongst intensive care clinicians) are all important considerations. Surgical tracheostomy placement in the operating theatre is advisable, as the use of a long flange tracheostomy tube may be required and is often not part of a percutaneous technique. The treatment planning for tracheostomy needs to be done carefully, ideally during normal working hours with enough skilled assistance available.

Summary

Obesity prevalence in the adult population is increasing. Obese emergency surgical and trauma patients provide particular challenges for theatre and intensive care teams. Some of these are directly related to the increased body mass, but others are due to the alteration in physiology as a result of the obese state. Physiological parameters that are abnormal to start with can be compounded when acute pathology presents.

Complication rates are higher in the obese after emergency surgery, with intensive care and hospital stays longer compared to lean individuals. Ensuring basic aspects of care and continual re-assessment will alleviate some of these risks.

Further Reading

Aldenkortt M, Lysakowski C, Elia N, Brochard L, Tramer MR. Ventilation strategies in obese patients undergoing surgery: a quantitative systematic review and meta-analysis *Br J Anaesth*. 2012;**109**:493–502.

Brown CVR, Rhee P, Neville AL, et al. Obesity and traumatic brain injury. *J Trauma*. 2006;**61**:572–6.

Cheah MH, Kam PCA. Obesity: basic science and medical aspects relevant to anaesthetists. *Anaesthesia*. 2005;**60**: 1009–21.

Ditillo M, Pandit V, Rhee P, et al. Morbid obesity predisposes trauma patients to worse outcomes: a national trauma data bank analysis. *J Trauma Acute Care Surg*. 2014;**76**:176–9.

Elamin EM. Nutritional care of the obese intensive care unit patient. *Curr Opin Crit Care*. 2005;**11**:300–3.

Fernandez-Bustamante A, Hashimoto S, Neto AS, et al. Perioperative lung protective ventilation in obese patients. *BMC Anesthesiol*. 2015;**15**:56–68.

Glance LG, Li Y, Osler TM, Mukamel DB, Dick AW. Impact of obesity on mortality and complications in trauma patients. *Ann Surg*. 2014;**259**:576–81.

Joffe A, Wood K. Obesity in critical care. *Curr Opin Anaesthesiol*. 2007;**20**:113–18.

Küpper S, Karvellas CJ, Khadaroo RG, Widder SL; on behalf of the Acute Care and Emergency Surgery (ACES) Group. Increased health services use by severely obese patients undergoing emergency surgery: a retrospective cohort study *Canadian J Surg*. 2015;**58**:41–7.

Lagrand WK, van Slobbe-Bijlsma ER, Schultz MJ. Haemodynamic monitoring of morbidly obese intensive care unit patients. *Neth J Med*.2013;**71**:234–42.

Le D, Shafi S, Gwirtz P, et al. Effect of obesity on motor functional outcome of rehabilitating traumatic braininjury patients. *Am J Phys Med Rehabil*. 2015;**94**:627–32.

National Institute for Health and Care Excellence. Rehabilitation after Critical Illness in Adults. Clinical Guideline 83. Manchester: NICE; 2009.

Norton L, Harrison JE, Pointer S, Lathlean T. Obesity and Injury: A Review of the Literature. Injury research and statistics series no. 60. Canberra: Australian Institute of Health and Welfare; 2011.

Quante M, Ditrich A, ElKhal A, Tullius SG. Obesity-related immune responses and their impact on surgical outcomes. *Int J Obes*. 2015;**39**:877–83.

Patel A, Nouraei SA. Transnasal humidified rapid-insufflation ventilatory exchange (THRIVE): a physiological method of increasing apnoea time in patients with difficult airways. *Anaesthesia*. 2015;**70**: 323–9.

Pirrone M, Fisher D, Chipman D, et al. Recruitment maneuvers and positive end-expiratory pressure titration in morbidly obese ICU patients. *Crit Care Med*. 2016;**44**: 300–7.

Shashaty MGS, Stapleton RD. Physiological and management implications of obesity in critical illness. *Ann Am Thorac Soc*.2014;**11**:1286–97.

Tagliaferri F, Compagnone C, Yoganandan N, Gennarelli TA. Traumatic brain injury after frontal crashes: relationship with body mass index. *J Trauma*. 2009;**66**: 727–9.

Winfield RD, Delano MJ, Dixon DJ, et al. Differences in outcome between obese and non-obese patients following severe blunt trauma are not consistent with an early inflammatory genomic response. *Crit Care Med*. 2010;**38**: 51–8.

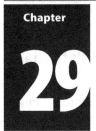

Chapter

29

Post-operative Recovery: Location and Potential Complications

Michele Carron and Francesco Zarantonello

Introduction

Over the last three decades, the incidence and prevalence of obesity has increased worldwide. Accordingly, anaesthetists will care for an increasing number of obese patients in their clinical practice.

Obese individuals appear to have a higher risk of peri-operative complications involving all organ systems and worse long-term mortality at higher body mass index (BMI) values (>40 kg/m^2). Their risk may further increase in the presence of obstructive sleep apnoea (OSA) and metabolic syndrome (MetS). Meta-analysis has revealed that severe, but not mild to moderate, OSA is significantly associated with increased risk of all-cause mortality (pooled hazard ratios (HR) 1.6, 95% confidence interval (CI) 1.2–1.9). Obese patients with MetS undergoing surgery have a greater risk of stroke and cardiac incidents, respiratory and renal failure, and venous thromboembolic events. They also have 2.5-fold increased peri-operative mortality after cardiac surgery compared to patients without MetS.

To predict the risk of mortality for obese patients undergoing surgery, the Obesity Surgery Mortality Risk Score (OS-MRS) was developed. This system considers five variables that have been correlated with mortality: BMI ≥50 kg/m^2, age ≥45 years, male sex, hypertension and pulmonary embolus susceptibility (i.e. previous thrombosis, pulmonary embolus, inferior vena cava filter, right heart failure or obesity hypoventilation). Based on the OS-MRS, the mortality risk is low (0.31%) in the presence of one variable, intermediate (1.90%) with two or three variables and high (7.56%) with four or five variables.

Obese patients should be carefully managed in the peri-operative period, and an optimal anaesthetic approach is required to minimise peri-operative complications contributing to morbidity and mortality.

Intra-operative Management to Reduce Risk of Post-operative Complications

The choice of anaesthesia may influence the post-operative course of obese patients. When appropriate, regional anaesthesia offers substantial advantages over general anaesthesia, including a reduced need for airway intervention, fewer drugs with less cardiopulmonary depression, decreased need for opioids and other sedatives, greater post-operative pain control, decreased post-operative nausea and vomiting (PONV), and reduced post-anaesthesia care unit (PACU) and overall hospital length of stay. Nevertheless, difficulties with performing regional techniques must be considered.

The majority of surgical procedures are performed under general anaesthesia. Although the superiority of an inhalational or total intravenous technique for maintenance of anaesthesia has not been clearly established for obese patients, inhalational anaesthesia continues to be favoured by many bariatric anaesthetists. Evidence reveals that post-operative recovery is significantly faster after desflurane than after sevoflurane, isoflurane or propofol anaesthesia in obese patients, without clinically relevant differences in the incidence of PONV or post-operative pain. Other benefits of desflurane include a reduced incidence of desaturation, faster recovery of protective airway reflexes and improved patient mobility in the post-operative period. These effects were most marked in obese patients and after prolonged procedures. Anaesthetic effects can persist after surgery, and the more rapidly an anaesthetic is eliminated, the more quickly its inhibitory effects on respiratory function, the hypoxic–ventilatory response and genioglossus muscle activity will dissipate. This should shorten the period during which the patient is at risk for post-operative hypoventilation, hypoxaemia and upper airway collapsibility. Furthermore, desflurane, as well as sevoflurane, may confer organ protection. In cardiac surgery, when compared to total intravenous anaesthesia, general anaesthesia with these volatile anaesthetics is associated with reduced likelihood of mortality, pulmonary complications and other complications.

For intra-operative analgesia, predominant use of short-acting opioids (i.e. remifentanil) and sparing use of long-acting opioids are recommended to reduce the risk of post-operative upper airway obstruction, hypoxaemia, hypoventilation and respiratory failure. There is growing interest in multimodal non-opioid anaesthetic methods to reduce the necessity for intra-operative and post-operative opioids. Non-steroidal anti-inflammatory drugs (NSAIDs), local anaesthetics (e.g. intra-peritoneal, transversus abdominis plane blocks), dexmedetomidine, and ketamine have all demonstrated efficacy when used as part of a multimodal approach.

Neuromuscular blockade (NMB) must be carefully managed in obese patients, and full reversal should be verified before tracheal extubation. A train-of-four ratio ≥1.0 is useful for confirming complete recovery from NMB. Sugammadex should be considered for safe and complete reversal of rocuronium-induced NMB in obese patients. A recent meta-analysis demonstrated that sugammadex is superior to neostigmine, as it reverses NMB faster and more reliably, with a lower likelihood of post-operative weakness and adverse events, particularly respiratory and cardiovascular events.

Prophylactic intra-operative lung protective mechanical ventilation, using lower tidal volumes, moderate positive end expiratory pressure (PEEP) and recruitment manoeuvres (RMs), should be considered to improve post-operative outcomes in obese patients. General anaesthesia promotes reduced lung volumes, which are a key determinant of atelectasis formation, regardless of whether inhalational or intravenous agents are used. Atelectasis persists into the post-operative period, and alterations in both oxygenation and lung compliance are correlated with the degree of atelectasis. Published evidence reveals that morbidly obese patients have more atelectasis on computed tomography scans (expressed as percentage of the total lung area) than non-obese patients immediately after tracheal extubation (7.6% versus 2.8%) and 24 hours later (9.7% versus 1.9%). Repeated RMs followed by application of PEEP during surgery and before tracheal extubation, aim to keep the alveoli open and reduce the incidence of intra-operative and post-operative atelectasis.

Post-operative Course and Potential Complications

The invasiveness of the surgical procedure, severity of obesity and OSA, and requirement for post-operative analgesics (particularly opioids) should be considered when determining whether a patient has an increased risk of post-operative complications.

Role of Surgery

Obesity, particularly a BMI >40 kg/m^2, represents a risk factor for surgical complications (e.g. longer operative times, possibly increased blood loss, increased re-intervention and infection rates). Conversely, the type and duration of surgery may influence the post-operative course of obese patients.

In a study of obese patients undergoing bariatric surgery, overall post-operative complication rates, including both medical and surgical complications, were lower after laparoscopic than after open surgery. Laparoscopic surgery was also associated with a lower likelihood of pulmonary complications (e.g. aspiration, pneumonia, acute lung injury, respiratory arrest, re-intubation, ventilatory support beyond PACU, need for non-invasive ventilation (NIV)) and 'other' complications (e.g. myocardial infarction, dysrhythmia, stroke, thromboembolism, severe sepsis, and liver and renal failure).

Not only minimally invasive, but also short-lasting surgical procedures reduce the incidence of post-operative pulmonary complications (e.g. atelectasis, pneumonia, pleural effusion, respiratory failure, acute respiratory distress syndrome) compared with longer surgery. Furthermore, in a study of 12 062 patients undergoing bariatric surgery, open or revision surgery was among the strongest factors associated with unplanned intensive care unit (ICU) admission.

Role of Obesity

Obesity is a risk factor for post-operative complications. In one major study by Weingarten, the likelihood of overall complications increased with increasing BMI. A higher BMI was also associated with an increased likelihood of pulmonary complications and other complications. In addition, increasing age was linked with significantly increased odds of overall, pulmonary and other complications. Surprisingly, OSA severity was not associated with the likelihood of peri-operative complications, probably because the majority of patients with OSA were treated with NIV during sleep and monitored throughout the peri-operative period. However, chronic untreated OSA has been identified as an independent risk factor for post-operative adverse events in bariatric surgical patients. Data demonstrates that the presence of OSA increases the likelihood of respiratory failure, desaturation, tracheal re-intubation, post-operative cardiac events (including myocardial infarction, cardiac arrest and arrhythmias) and ICU transfers. OSA should, thus, be identified and treated before surgery.

Although the risk of post-operative complications among obese patients is significantly higher than in non-obese patients, these risks are substantially higher when accompanied by MetS. A large study of peri-operative outcomes of patients undergoing non-cardiac surgery, reported that compared to normal-weight patients, those with modified MetS (presence of obesity, hypertension and diabetes) had an approximately 1.5- to 2.8-fold higher likelihood of pulmonary adverse events (e.g. pneumonia, ventilatory support for >48 h, unplanned intubation), 1.7- to 2.7-fold higher odds of cardiac adverse events (e.g. acute myocardial infarction, cardiac arrest), 1.6- to 2.3-fold higher odds of central nervous system adverse events (e.g. cerebrovascular accident, coma lasting >24 h) and 3.3- to 7.3-fold higher odds of acute kidney injury. The likelihood increased as BMI increased, with the lower number of each range representing patients with a BMI 30–39 kg/m^2 and the higher number representing those with a BMI ≥50 kg/m^2.

Extra precautions should thus be taken peri-operatively to reduce complications in morbidly obese patients with unrecognised (and untreated) OSA, MetS, age >45 years and BMI ≥50 kg/m^2, and/or those undergoing open, long or revision surgery.

Role of Post-operative Analgesia

Opioids affect respiration and upper airway patency by depressing ventilatory drive and pharyngeal tone. Therefore, opioids administered systemically or neuraxially (affecting respiration by rostral spread) increase the risk of respiratory depression (bradypnoea, hypoventilation, hypoxaemia, hypercapnia) and upper airway obstruction, which may lead to respiratory arrest, particularly in morbidly obese patients and/or those with OSA. In undisturbed subjects receiving patient-controlled intravenous morphine analgesia post-operatively, abnormal breathing patterns are extremely common and cyclical airway obstruction is frequent. If patient-controlled systemic opioids are used in obese patients, continuous background infusions should be avoided or used with extreme caution.

Multimodal analgesic techniques, including local and regional anaesthesia, enable opioid-sparing and are strongly recommended. NSAIDs are effective as part of a multimodal regimen, particularly in patients with OSA. Early NIV after surgery improves sleep disordered breathing and ameliorates the respiratory-depressant effects of opioids without undue haemodynamic effects. Patients receiving 30% oxygen via continuous positive airway pressure (CPAP; 8–10 cmH$_2$O) have been demonstrated to have a lower apnoea–hypopnoea index, fewer episodes of oxygen desaturation and 3% higher mean oxygen saturation than patients receiving standard care.

Post-operative Recovery

Immediate Recovery Period

Obesity, particularly in the presence of OSA, significantly increases the risk of tracheal extubation failure and difficult airway management. Extubation of the trachea should be planned in accordance with the Difficult Airway Society guidelines. Full monitoring should be maintained throughout the recovery process and in the recovery room. Surgery permitting, the patient should be managed in the reverse Trendelenburg position/sitting position with a 45° head-up tilt. Supplemental oxygen should be administered continuously to obese patients, particularly those with OSA, until they are able to maintain their baseline oxygen saturation while breathing room air. Caution is required, however, because supplemental oxygen may increase the duration of apnoeic episodes and hinder the detection of hypoventilation, transient apnoea and atelectasis by pulse oximetry.

If frequent or severe airway obstruction or hypoxaemia occurs after extubation, initiation of NIV should be considered. NIV strategies include CPAP, bi-level positive airway pressure (BiPAP), or pressure support ventilation (PSV). A recent meta-analysis showed that NIV is well tolerated and effective in improving peri-operative care in obese patients. Benefits including oxygenation, carbon dioxide clearance and improved

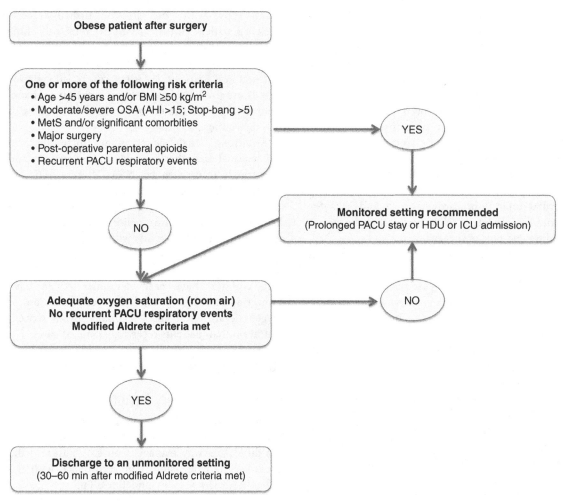

Figure 29.1 Post-operative management of the obese patient after general anaesthesia. BMI: body mass index; OSA: obstructive sleep apnoea; AHI: Apnoea–hypopnoea Index; MetS: metabolic syndrome; PACU: post-anaesthesia care unit: HDU: high-dependency unit; ICU: intensive care unit; recurrent PACU respiratory events: apnoea for ≥10 seconds (one episode needed), bradypnoea of <8 breaths/min (three episodes needed), pain–sedation mismatch, and desaturations to <90% (three episodes needed).

pulmonary function testing after general anaesthesia were observed with NIV application compared with standard care.

Recovery Room Discharge

All obese patients should aim to be discharged from the recovery room to an unmonitored hospital bed when routine discharge criteria are met; ability to maintain adequate oxygen saturation while breathing room air and exhibit adequate ventilatory function, without episodes of apnoea or hypopnoea with associated oxygen desaturation. Respiratory function should be determined by observing patients in an unstimulated environment, preferably while asleep, and these criteria maintained for at least 1 hour before confirming discharge suitability. It has been suggested that monitoring in the recovery room specifically record: no apnoea for ≥10 seconds (one episode needed); bradypnoea of <8 breaths/min (three episodes needed); pain–sedation mismatch and oxygen saturation <90% (three episodes needed). Pain–sedation mismatch refers to simultaneously high pain scores and sedation levels. If any one of these recurrent recovery room respiratory events occurs in two separate 30-min time blocks, an extended period of monitoring is recommended. Considering that obese patients who develop recurrent recovery respiratory events and/or meet high-risk criteria (i.e. age >45 years, BMI ≥ 50 kg/m^2, severe OSA, MetS) have an increased likelihood of post-operative respiratory complications, it is advocated that continuous monitoring with oximetry occurs in recovery, high-dependency unit, ICU, or ward equipped with remote telemetry and oximetry monitoring. This should be continued as long as the patient remains at increased risk (Figure 29.1). When feasible, NIV (with or without supplemental oxygen) should be administered to high-risk obese patients, unless contraindicated by the surgical procedure. Compliance with NIV may be improved if patients bring their own equipment to the hospital. Patients at increased peri-operative risk should not be discharged from the recovery area to an unmonitored setting (i.e. unmonitored hospital bed or home) until they are no longer deemed at risk of post-operative respiratory depression and complications.

Conclusions

All obese patients undergoing surgery should have a comprehensive pre-operative evaluation, particularly looking for the presence of OSA, MetS and significant co-morbidities. The preference should be for anaesthetic agents with a short half-life and rapid elimination. Neuromuscular blockade should be carefully managed. Prophylactic intra-operative lung protective mechanical ventilation should be considered, as well as post-operative NIV. Adequate post-operative monitoring is recommended for all obese patients, particularly those with OSA, MetS or another condition predisposing to a high risk of respiratory complications. Full recovery of respiratory function is mandatory and routine discharge criteria must be met before discharging obese patients from the recovery area to an unmonitored setting.

Further Reading

Adesanya AO, Lee W, Greilich NB, et al. Perioperative management of obstructive sleep apnea. *Chest*. 2010;138: 1489–98.

American Society of Anesthesiologists Task Force on Perioperative Management of Patients with Obstructive Sleep Apnea. Practice guidelines for the perioperative management of patients with obstructive sleep apnea: an updated report by the American Society of Anesthesiologists Task Force on Perioperative Management

of patients with obstructive sleep apnea. *Anesthesiology*. 2014;120:268–86.

Bellamy MC, Margarson MP. Designing intelligent anesthesia for a changing patient demographic: a consensus statement to provide guidance for specialist and non-specialist anesthetists written by members of and endorsed by the Society for Obesity and Bariatric Anaesthesia (SOBA). *Periop Med*. 2013;2:12.

Carron M, Parotto E, Ori C. The use of sugammadex in obese patients. *Canadian Journal of Anesthesia*. 2012;59:321–2.

Carron M, Zarantonello F, Tellaroli P, et al. Efficacy and safety of sugammadex compared to neostigmine for reversal of neuromuscular blockade: a meta-analysis of randomized controlled trials. *J Clin Anesth*. 2016;35:1–12.

Carron M, Zarantonello F, Tellaroli P, et al. Perioperative noninvasive ventilation in obese patients: a qualitative review and meta-analysis. *Surg Obes Rel Dis*. 2016;12:681–91.

Cavallone LF, Vannucci A. Review article: Extubation of the difficult airway and extubation failure. *Anesth Analg*. 2013;116:368–83.

Dahan A, Aarts L, Smith TW. Incidence, reversal, and prevention of opioid-induced respiratory depression. *Anesthesiology*. 2010;112:226–38.

DeMaria EJ, Portenier D, Wolfe L. Obesity surgery mortality risk score: proposal for a clinically useful score to predict mortality risk in patients undergoing gastric bypass. *Surg Obes Rel Dis*. 2007;3:134–40.

Drummond GB, Bates A, Mann J, et al. Characterization of breathing patterns during patient-controlled opioid analgesia. *Br J Anaesth*. 2013;111:971–8.

Ehsan Z, Mahmoud M, Shott SR, et al. The effects of anesthesia and opioids on the upper airway: A systematic review. *Laryngoscope*. 2016;126:270–84.

Eichenberger A, Proietti S, Wicky S, et al. Morbid obesity and postoperative pulmonary atelectasis: an underestimated problem. *Anesth Analg*. 2002;95: 1788–92.

Futier E, Marret E, Jaber S. Perioperative positive pressure ventilation: an integrated approach to improve pulmonary care. *Anesthesiology*. 2014;121:400–8.

Glance LG, Wissler R, Mukamel DB, et al. Perioperative outcomes among patients with the modified metabolic syndrome who are undergoing noncardiac surgery. *Anesthesiology*. 2010;113:859–72.

Ingrande J, Brodsky JB, Lemmens HJ. Regional anesthesia and obesity. *Curr Opin Anaesthesiol*. 2009;22:683–6.

Kaw R, Chung F, Pasupuleti V, et al. Meta-analysis of the association between obstructive sleep apnoea and postoperative outcome. *Br J Anaesth*. 2012;109:897–906.

La Colla L, Albertin A, La Colla G, et al. Faster wash-out and recovery for desflurane vs sevoflurane in morbidly obese patients when no premedication is used. *Br J Anaesth*. 2007;99:353–8.

Liu FL, Cherng YG, Chen SY, et al. Postoperative recovery after anesthesia in morbidly obese patients: a systematic review and meta-analysis of randomized controlled trials. *Can J Anesth*. 2015;62:907–17.

McKay RE, Malhotra A, Cakmakkaya OS, et al. Effect of increased body mass index and anaesthetic duration on recovery of protective airway reflexes after sevoflurane vs desflurane. *Br J Anaesth*. 2010;104:175–82.

Morgan DJ, Ho KM, Armstrong J, et al. Incidence and risk factors for intensive care unit admission after bariatric surgery: a multicentre population-based cohort study. *Br J Anaesth*. 2015;115:873–82.

Mulier JP. Perioperative opioids aggravate obstructive breathing in sleep apnea syndrome: mechanisms and alternative anesthesia strategies. *Curr Opin Anaesthesiol*. 2016;29:129–33.

Ng M, Fleming T, Robinson M, et al. Global, regional, and national prevalence of overweight and obesity in children and adults during 1980–2013: a systematic analysis for the Global Burden of Disease Study 2013. *Lancet*. 2014;384:766–81.

Nightingale CE, Margarson MP, Shearer E, et al.; Association of Anaesthetists of Great Britain; Ireland Society for Obesity and Bariatric Anaesthesia. Peri-operative management of the obese surgical patient 2015: Association of Anaesthetists of Great Britain and Ireland Society for Obesity and Bariatric Anaesthesia. *Anaesthesia*. 2015;70:859–76.

Pan L, Xie X, Liu D, et al. Obstructive sleep apnoea and risks of all-cause mortality: preliminary evidence from prospective cohort studies. *Sleep Breathing*. 2016;20:345–53.

Schumann R, Shikora SA, Sigl JC, et al. Association of metabolic syndrome and surgical factors with pulmonary adverse events, and longitudinal mortality in bariatric surgery. *Br J Anaesth*. 2015;114:83–90.

Seet E, Chung F. Management of sleep apnea in adults – functional algorithms for the perioperative period: continuing professional development. *Can J Anesth*. 2010;57:849–64.

Tsai A, Schumann R. Morbid obesity and perioperative complications. *Curr Opin Anaesthesiol*. 2016;29:103–8.

Tung A. Anaesthetic considerations with the metabolic syndrome. *Br J Anaesth*. 2010;105:i24–i33.

Uhlig C, Bluth T, Schwarz K, et al. Effects of volatile anesthetics on mortality and postoperative pulmonary and other complications in patients undergoing surgery: a systematic review and meta-analysis. *Anesthesiology*. 2016;124:1230–45.

Weingarten TN, Flores AS, McKenzie JA, et al. Obstructive sleep apnoea and perioperative complications in bariatric patients. *Br J Anaesth*. 2011;106:31–9.

Zaremba S, Shin CH, Hutter MM, et al. Continuous positive airway pressure mitigates opioid-induced worsening of sleep-disordered breathing early after bariatric surgery. *Anesthesiology*. 2016;**125**(1):92–104.

Enhanced Recovery for the Obese Patient

Khaleel Fareed and Sherif Awad

Introduction

Enhanced recovery after surgery (ERAS, also known as fast-track, multimodal, rapid or accelerated recovery) pathways were first pioneered in the late 1990s for patients undergoing colorectal surgery. Traditional anaesthetic and surgical practices (such as pre- and post-operative nil by mouth regimens, bowel preparation, etc.) were challenged and instead multimodal interventions were utilised to facilitate early recovery and discharge for patients undergoing colonic surgery. Over two decades later, ERAS pathways are now well established and considered standard of care across numerous surgical disciplines, including colorectal, oesophagogastric, hepatobiliary, vascular, urological, orthopaedic and bariatric surgery.

Worldwide, the prevalence of obesity among adults has increased. In the United Kingdom, direct costs attributable to treating overweight and obese individuals are projected to reach £9.7 billion (approx. 10% of the UK health budget) per year by 2050. Coupled with an ageing population, increasingly complex anaesthetic and surgical practices, and financially constrained healthcare systems, this has highlighted the need for optimised, streamlined and clinically safe surgical pathways.

The Morbidly Obese Surgical Patient

Morbidly obese (Class III severe obesity, body mass index (BMI) ≥40 kg/m^2) patients are a complex group presenting a unique set of peri-operative challenges to anaesthetists and surgeons alike. Obesity is associated with numerous pathophysiological changes and impairment in cardiac, pulmonary and immunological function. This may be associated with the presence of numerous chronic co-morbidities, such as type 2 diabetes, hypertension, sleep apnoea syndromes, ischaemic heart disease and fatty liver disease, as well as mobility problems.

There is evidence of an increased risk of wound infections in various types of surgery performed in the morbidly obese. Obesity results in reduced functional residual lung capacity, significant atelectasis and shunting in dependent lung regions, predisposing patients to increased risk of pneumonia. The management of post-operative pain relief presents difficulties, with problems of intravenous access and a higher chance of failure of regional anaesthesia techniques. Another rare but serious complication is development of rhabdomyolysis, which if not recognised early can lead to significant acute kidney injury. Despite the aforementioned, it is of note that obesity per se was not identified as a risk factor for post-operative complications in a large prospective cohort study of 6336 patients undergoing general elective surgery. Although there was an increased risk of wound infections after open surgery, multivariate analysis did not identify obesity as a risk factor for development of post-operative complications. A recent study of patients who underwent both elective and emergency general surgical procedures with median follow-up of 6.3 years showed obese patients had more concomitant disease (diabetes, hypertension, cardiovascular disease and pulmonary disease) than normal weight patients, with increased risk of wound infections, greater intra-operative blood loss and longer operating times. Being underweight was associated with a higher risk of complications, although this was not significant in adjusted analysis. However, multivariate analysis showed underweight patients had worse survival, whereas being overweight and obese were associated with improved survival. Other studies have identified an obesity paradox, with moderate obesity safeguarding against adverse outcomes, while underweight patients being at greater risk. A regressive attitude towards obese patients undergoing surgery is therefore unjustified.

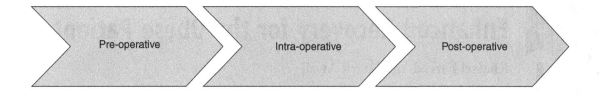

Pre-operative	Intra-operative	Post-operative

Pre-operative counselling & training	Standardised anaesthetic practice	Avoidance of opiods
Shortened pre-operative fasts	Surgical approach	Early mobilisation
Pre-operative metabolic conditioning	Avoidance of intra-operative hypothermia	Incentive spirometry
Thromboprophylaxis	Avoidance of drains & nasogastric tubes	Early post-operative nutrition
	Reducing post-operative nausea & vomiting	Avoidance of post-operative fluid overload
		Discharge & follow up advice

Figure 30.1 Multimodal interventions within ERAS pathways.

Components of ERAS

Multimodal interventions within ERAS pathways are traditionally classified into pre-, intra- and post-operative components (Figure 30.1). Whilst individual components of ERAS may not have been validated by data from randomised studies, when applied together they have been clearly shown to result in clinical benefit. A meta-analysis of six randomised controlled trials looking at the differences in outcomes in patients undergoing major elective open colorectal surgery within an ERAS pathway and those treated with conventional peri-operative care found the number of individual ERAS elements used ranged from 4 to 12, with a mean of 9. Both duration of hospital stay and complication rates were significantly reduced in the enhanced recovery group.

Overall, these interventions have not been individually examined in randomised studies in morbidly obese patients. Of importance in the delivery of ERAS pathways is compliance with individual interventions, which is variable within the real-life clinical setting. A previous study demonstrated better compliance to an evidence-based ERAS protocol led to better outcomes in colorectal cancer patients undergoing surgery. ERAS patients with less than 50% compliance were shown to have a complication rate of almost 50%, while those who adhered more closely to the protocol (90% compliance) had fewer than 20% complications.

Pre-operative

- *Pre-operative counselling and training*: Pre-operative information and education have been shown to improve patient satisfaction, allay anxiety and facilitate post-operative pain relief and recovery. The pre-operative counselling process involves input from physiotherapists, dieticians and specialist nurses. Use of ERAS information leaflets or videos is coupled with patient-specific assessments to identify issues that may delay discharge, such as lack of social support or need for specialist equipment at home.
- *Shortened pre-operative fasts*: Modern shortened pre-operative fasting regimens that permit a light meal (dry toast and clear liquid) up to 6 hours and clear liquids 2 hours pre-anaesthesia are now established clinical practice. There is Grade A evidence suggesting shortened fluid fasts do not result in an increased risk of aspiration, regurgitation or related morbidity compared with standard 'nil by mouth from midnight' regimens. There is no evidence of delayed gastric emptying in obese patients undergoing elective surgical procedures.
- *Pre-operative metabolic conditioning*: A key feature of ERAS pathways is utilising interventions that reduce metabolic stress and attenuate development of post-operative insulin resistance. Pre-operative administration of oral carbohydrates up to 2 hours before surgery

aims to replicate the normal metabolic response to eating breakfast. In patients undergoing major abdominal surgery, pre-operative conditioning with carbohydrate-based drinks is associated with a reduction in length of hospital stay of 1 day. It is worth noting that this meta-analysis did not include patients with BMI greater than 35, thus highlighting the limited data in obese patients. To date, there has only been one randomised study comparing ERAS versus standard care in morbidly obese patients undergoing laparoscopic sleeve gastrectomy. Amongst the interventions used in the protocol was pre-operative carbohydrate conditioning. Results showed no difference in overall complications between the two groups, although only 15% of ERAS patients were compliant with pre-operative carbohydrate conditioning. Further data on the constituents and effects of pre-operative carbohydrate drinks are therefore needed in obese patients.

- *Thromboprophylaxis*: Obesity is considered a pro-thrombotic state. Both chemical and mechanical measures should be employed to reduce risk of venous thromboembolism. Chemical thromboprophylaxis using low molecular weight heparin (LMWH) is preferred to unfractionated heparin due to the ease of once-daily dosing and lower risk of heparin-induced thrombocytopenia. In the obese population, the doses may need to be weight adjusted, although there is paucity of Level 1 data to inform practitioners and worldwide no consensus to date has been reached to date. Mechanical measures using anti-embolism stockings and intermittent pneumatic compression foot/calf pumps are advised, although there is no consensus on duration of use post-operatively.

Intra-operative

- *Standardised anaesthetic practice*: Guidelines have been published on the peri-operative management of the morbidly obese patient by AAGBI and SOBA. An enhanced recovery protocol is essential and an optimised bariatric anaesthetic protocol should be adhered to. This includes 30° head-up tilt during tracheal intubation and extubation, avoidance of long-acting sedatives and opioids, and multimodal analgesia (IV paracetamol, diclofenac and tramadol). Neuromuscular blockade should be monitored, volume-controlled ventilation with high PEEP (6–8 cmH_2O) and permissive hypercapnea (end tidal CO_2 >6.5kPa) may be used. Permissive hypercapnia results in abdominal vasodilatation enabling detection of bleeding intra-operatively. If epidural analgesia is to be used, mid-thoracic epidurals are more effective for pain relief and result in fewer respiratory complications when compared to intravenous opioids.

- *Surgical approach*: Minimal access surgery is now the preferred approach in numerous specialties and is associated with reduced post-operative pain, wound infections and intra-abdominal adhesion formation. If not possible, transverse incisions are favoured as they result in less post-operative pain. Previous studies that proved efficacy of ERAS pathways were undertaken in patients undergoing open surgery. The benefits of ERAS pathways in patients undergoing laparoscopic abdominal surgery remain unclear, but there is evidence that laparoscopic colorectal surgery performed within ERAS programmes can reduce length of hospital stay and reduce complications compared with open surgery within such programmes.

- *Avoidance of intra-operative hypothermia*: General anaesthesia can disrupt the normal thermoregulatory processes (e.g. reduced shivering, loss of sympathetic-induced vasoconstriction) leading to hypothermia. An oesophageal probe or urinary catheter with temperature probe may be used to monitor core temperature intra-operatively. Hypothermia (core temperature <36 °C) can lead to increased wound infection rates resultant from peripheral vasoconstriction and tissue hypoxia. Warm air blankets may be used to actively prevent hypothermia. In laparoscopic surgery, the humidification and warming of insufflated CO_2 may reduce post-operative hypothermia and pain, and result in lower analgesic requirements. Warming should be continued in the post-anaesthesia care unit (PACU) or ward using hot air blankets or warmed intravenous fluids following long procedures.

- *Avoidance of drains and nasogastric tubes*: Abdominal drains can cause increased risk of infections, local discomfort and hinder mobilisation. Numerous meta-analyses have shown routine abdominal drainage not to confer advantage. Grade A evidence supports avoidance of routine nasogastric tube placement, as this results in fewer pulmonary complications and earlier return of gut function.

- *Reducing post-operative nausea and vomiting (PONV)*: PONV is not only distressing to patients, but results in interruption of intake of oral analgesics, leading to reduced mobility and possible increased risk of atelectasis and respiratory infections. Risk stratification and scoring systems such as Apfel may identify patients at increased risk of PONV. Apfel factors include females, history of motion sickness, non-smokers and patients who receive opioids. Two risk factors constitute a moderate risk of PONV and three or more constitute high risk. Patients at moderate risk should receive prophylaxis with dexamethasone at induction or a serotonin receptor antagonist at the end of surgery.

Post-operative

- *Avoidance of opioids*: Up to a third of obese patients have a diagnosis of obstructive sleep apnoea. Opiates should be avoided to reduce harmful side effects on the respiratory system and delay in return of gut function. Patients should be prescribed multimodal analgesia regimens (such as paracetamol and non-steroidal analgesics) provided there are no contraindications. Opioid analgesia should be reserved for breakthrough analgesia.
- *Early mobilisation*: Early mobilisation should be actively encouraged and facilitated, ideally by dedicated ward ERAS nurses or physiotherapists. Obese patients should be encouraged to sit out of bed 3–4 hours after surgery and mobilise on the evening of surgery. Longer periods of immobilisation could have detrimental effects, resulting in pulmonary atelectasis and infection, thromboembolism, development of pressure sores and rhabdomyolysis.
- *Incentive spirometry*: This is a low-cost intervention that encourages deep breathing exercises, resulting in reduced atelectasis and pulmonary infection. It is recommended that incentive spirometry be used with deep-breathing techniques, directed coughing, early mobilisation

and optimal analgesia to prevent post-operative pulmonary complications.

- *Early post-operative nutrition*: The recommendation that patients commence early oral nutrition relates to bowel surgery. As yet there are no studies that have examined the association between return of gut function and early post-operative nutrition in obese patients per se. Traditionally, oral diet and fluids were re-introduced cautiously. There is Grade A evidence supporting the implementation of early enteral nutrition within the first 5 days of gastro-intestinal surgery. Data demonstrated a lower risk of infection, reduced mean length of hospital stay and reduced rates of anastomotic dehiscence. Commencing oral intake on the first post-operative day following upper gastro-intestinal anastomoses in bariatric surgery has been shown to be safe in numerous clinical series.
- *Avoidance of post-operative fluid overload*: There is little data from randomised trials to guide peri-operative fluid therapy in morbidly obese patients. The accurate assessment of fluid status in morbidly obese patients is challenging, due to the presence of multiple co-morbidities, poly-pharmacy and erroneous readings from non-invasive monitoring. In the elective setting, administration of excessive quantities of intravenous maintenance fluids should be avoided. There is Grade A evidence that a 'zero-balance' regimen is associated with earlier return of gut function, improved tissue healing, reduced post-operative complications and decreased length of stay in non-obese subjects. Conversely, data from non-randomised studies support 'liberal' fluid regimens in morbidly obese patients, as these are associated with reduced post-operative nausea and vomiting, acute renal failure and shortened hospital stay.
- *Discharge and follow-up*: In the pre-operative counselling phase, patients should be informed of the forthcoming discharge criteria, which may help alleviate their fears and anxieties. Appropriate 'safety-netting' and emergency contact numbers should be issued to patients as part of the ERAS discharge process in view of the relatively high re-admission rates reported in some series (0–20.1%).

Challenges of Using ERAS Pathways in Morbidly Obese Patients

High demands on nursing care can make compliance with ERAS pathways challenging; a dedicated ERAS nurse is needed to ensure compliance with the numerous components of ERAS pathways. Some early studies suggested high re-admission rates, but others have refuted this. There is little data on re-admission rates in morbidly obese patients who are part of ERAS pathways. Compliance with ERAS interventions may also be reduced due to resource limitations and out of hours weekend staff being unfamiliar with such pathways.

Although the implementation of ERAS may be sub-optimal in an emergency setting, particularly in terms of pre-operative education, evidence from studies of emergency colorectal and abdominal surgery supports the application of ERAS principles in emergency patients. There is emphasis on reducing use of urinary catheterisation and rates of urinary tract infection, patient-controlled analgesia usage and overall length of stay. Further studies are required to determine whether such benefits apply to morbidly obese emergency patients.

Conclusions

ERAS pathways integrate multimodal interventions designed to reduce metabolic stress and facilitate rapid recovery after surgery.

There is a lack of Level 1 evidence for application of ERAS pathways in morbidly obese patients. However, numerous case series have supported the applicability and safety of ERAS pathways in morbidly obese patients.

The application of ERAS in the morbidly obese encourages shortened pre-operative fasts, use of laparoscopic techniques, early post-operative mobilisation, use of incentive spirometry, early enteral feeding, avoidance of opiates and use of multimodal thromboprophylaxis as key to achieving good clinical outcomes.

Further Reading

Andersen HK,Lewis SJ, Thomas S. Early enteral nutrition within 24 h of colorectal surgery versus later commencement of feeding for postoperative complications. *Cochr Database Syst Rev.* 2006;4:CD004080.

Andersen J, Hjort-Jakobsen D, Christiansen PS, Kehlet H. Readmission rates after a planned hospital stay of 2 versus 3 days in fast-track colonic surgery. *Br J Surg.* 2007;94(7):890–3.

Apfel CC, Korttila K, Abdalla M, et al. A factorial trial of six interventions for the prevention of postoperative nausea and vomiting. *N Engl J Med.* 2004;350(24):2441–51.

Awad S, Carter S, Purkayastha S, et al. Enhanced recovery after bariatric surgery (ERABS): clinical outcomes from a tertiary referral bariatric centre. *Obes Surg.* 2014;24(5):753–8.

Awad S, Lobo DN. Metabolic conditioning to attenuate the adverse effects of perioperative fasting and improve patient outcomes. *Curr Opin Clin Nutr Metab Care.* 2012;15 (2):194–200.

Awad S, Varadhan KK, Ljungqvist O, Lobo DN. A meta-analysis of randomised controlled trials on preoperative oral carbohydrate treatment in elective surgery. *Clin Nutr.* 2013;32(1):34–44.

Azhar RA, Bochner B, Catto J, et al. Enhanced recovery after urological surgery: a contemporary systematic review of outcomes, key elements, and research needs. *Eur Urol.* 2016;70(1):176–87.

Domi R, Laho H. Anesthetic challenges in the obese patient. *J Anesth* 2012;26(5):758–65.

Ford SJ, Adams D, Dudnikov S, et al. The implementation and effectiveness of an enhanced recovery programme after oesophago-gastrectomy: a prospective cohort study. *Int J Surg.* 2014;12(4):320–4.

Gotlib Conn L, Rotstein OD, Greco E, et al. Enhanced recovery after vascular surgery: protocol for a systematic review. *Syst Rev.* 2012;1:52.

Greco M, Capretti G, Beretta L, et al. Enhanced recovery program in colorectal surgery: a meta-analysis of randomized controlled trials. *World J Surg.* 2014;38(6):1531–41.

Gustafsson UO, Hausel J, Thorell A, et al.; Enhanced Recovery After Surgery Study Group. Adherence to the enhanced recovery after surgery protocol and outcomes after colorectal cancer surgery. *Arch Surg.* 2011;146(5): 571–7.

Ingrande J, Brodsky JB, Lemmens HJ.Regional anesthesia and obesity. *Curr Opin Anaesthesiol.* 2009;22(5):683–6.

Kahokehr A, Sammour T, Zargar-Shoshtari K, Thompson L, Hill AG. Implementation of ERAS and how to overcome the barriers. *Int J Surg.* 2009;7(1):16–19.

Kehlet H, Slim K. The future of fast-track surgery. *Br J Surg.* 2012;99(8):1025–6.

Kiyohara LY, Kayano LK, Oliveira LM, et al. Surgery information reduces anxiety in the pre-operative period. *Rev Hosp Clin Fac Med Sao Paulo.* 2004;59(2):51–6.

Lee A, Gin T. Educating patients about anaesthesia: effect of various modes on patients' knowledge, anxiety and satisfaction. *Curr Opin Anaesthesiol.* 2005;18(2):205–8.

Lemanu DP, Singh PP, Berridge K, et al. Randomized clinical trial of enhanced recovery versus standard care after laparoscopic sleeve gastrectomy. *Br J Surg.* 2013;100(4):482–9.

Ljungqvist O, Soreide E. Preoperative fasting. *Br J Surg.* 2003;90(4):400–6.

Lobo DN, Bostock KA, Neal KR, et al. Effect of salt and water balance on recovery of gastrointestinal function after elective colonic resection: a randomised controlled trial. *Lancet.* 2002;359(9320):1812–18.

Melling AC, Ali B, Scott EM, Leaper DJ. Effects of preoperative warming on the incidence of wound infection after clean surgery: a randomised controlled trial. *Lancet* 2001;358(9285):876–80.

Members of the Working Party; Nightingale CE, Margarson MP, Shearer E, et al. Peri-operative management of the obese surgical patient 2015: Association of Anaesthetists of Great Britain and Ireland Society for Obesity and Bariatric Anaesthesia. *Anaesthesia.* 2015;70(7):859–76.

Mullen JT, Moorman DW, Davenport DL The obesity paradox: body mass index and outcomes in patients undergoing nonbariatric general surgery. *Ann Surg.* 2009;250(1):166–72.

Nossaman VE, Richardson WS, 3rd, Wooldridge JB, Jr., Nossaman BD. Role of intraoperative fluids on hospital length of stay in laparoscopic bariatric surgery: a retrospective study in 224 consecutive patients *Surg Endosc.* 2015;29(10):2960–9.

Ogunnaike BO, Jones SB, Jones DB, Provost D, Whitten CW.Anesthetic considerations for bariatric surgery. *Anesth Analg.* 2002;95(6):1793–805.

Restrepo RD, Wettstein R, Wittnebel L, Tracy M. Incentive spirometry: 2011. *Respir Care.* 2011;56(10):1600–4.

Sajid MS, Mallick AS, Rimpel J, et al. Effect of heated and humidified carbon dioxide on patients after laparoscopic procedures: a meta-analysis. *Surg Laparosc Endosc Percutan Tech.* 2008;18(6):539–46.

Schuster R, Alami RS, Curet MJ, et al. Intra-operative fluid volume influences postoperative nausea and vomiting after laparoscopic gastric bypass surgery. *Obes Surg.* 2006;16(7): 848–51.

Thorell A, MacCormick AD, Awad S, et al. Guidelines for perioperative care in bariatric surgery: Enhanced Recovery After Surgery (ERAS) Society recommendations. *World J Surg.* 2016;40(9):2065–83.

Tjeertes EK, Hoeks SE, Beks SB, et al. Obesity: a risk factor for postoperative complications in general surgery? *BMC Anesthesiol.* 2015;15:112.

Varadhan KK, Neal KR, Dejong CH, et al. The enhanced recovery after surgery (ERAS) pathway for patients undergoing major elective open colorectal surgery: a meta-analysis of randomized controlled trials. *Clin Nutr.* 2010;29(4):434–40.

Wisely JC, Barclay KL. Effects of an Enhanced Recovery After Surgery programme on emergency surgical patients. *ANZ J Surg.* 2016;**86**(11):883–8.

31 Thromboprophylaxis for the Obese Surgical Patient

Ben Bailiff and Will Lester

Introduction

Venous thromboembolism (VTE), primarily lower limb deep vein thrombosis (DVT) and their propagation and embolisation to the lungs, are one of the greatest risks to patients admitted to hospital. It is estimated that between 5 and 10% of all in-hospital deaths are as a direct result of thromboembolism. Although this data is based upon necropsy findings and may lead to an overestimate of direct causality, it demonstrates that VTE is a major concern for patients and doctors alike. Effective introduction of VTE risk assessment for a hospitalised patient has been shown to reduce the rate of hospital-associated VTE and also reduces avoidable deaths.

Identifying the Risk

Obesity has been estimated to increase the relative risk of post-operative VTE by 1.5–2.0-fold. Literature demonstrates a 37% increase in VTE risk for every 10-unit increment in BMI. How obesity interacts with other risk factors for post-operative VTE is unclear. The reported incidence of VTE in bariatric surgery ranges from 0–5.4%, although most large series and registries report symptomatic VTE rates of <1%. In the International Bariatric Surgery Registry, VTE was the most common cause of post-operative death, accounting for 30% of all mortality events.

Table 31.1 lists identified risk factors for VTE associated with bariatric surgery. It is important to note that over two-thirds of post-operative VTE events occur after discharge when thromboprophylaxis is completed, mostly within the first 30 days.

Thromboprophylaxis

In addition to standard advice regarding early mobilisation of patients, thromboprophylaxis falls into two main types: mechanical and pharmacological.

Table 31.1 Risk factors for venous thromboembolism following bariatric surgery

Patient-related risk factors
Age
Male sex
Patient weight or BMI
Patient history of venous thromboembolism
Smoking

Procedure-related risk factors
Open versus laparoscopic
Operative time greater than 3 hours
Post-operative anastomotic leak
Procedure type: <ul><li>Gastric bypass versus other bariatric surgery</li><li>Revision bariatric surgery</li><li>Sleeve gastrectomy, laparoscopic gastric bypass, open gastric bypass and duodenal switch procedures versus adjustable gastric band procedures</li></ul>

(Adapted from: Bartlett MA, Mauck KF, Daniels PR. Prevention of venous thromboembolism in patients undergoing bariatric surgery. *Vasc Health Risk Manag.* 2015;**11**:461–77.)

Mechanical Thromboprophlyaxis

Mechanical thromboprophylaxis for surgical patients can be 'passive', e.g. grade 1 graduated compression stockings (also referred to as anti-embolism stockings) or 'active', e.g. intermittent pneumatic compression devices/foot impulse devices.

Anti-embolism stockings (AES) have been assessed extensively in the surgical population and found to be of benefit in the reduction of DVT and PE by 4% and 3%, respectively, in a Cochrane review, although the majority of studies used a radioactive isotope uptake test rather than clinically diagnosed VTE. These studies cover a range of BMIs, but whether the data can be extrapolated to morbidly obese patients is presumptive as there are no randomised controlled trials in bariatric patients. One practical issue is that appropriately sized stockings may not always be available and if badly fitted, may increase the risk of complications, including skin damage. AES can be washed regularly and should ideally be worn until the patient is back to their usual mobility. Intermittent pneumatic compression devices have also been identified to reduce rates of thrombosis in the general population, but the same issues apply regarding appropriate fitting. Active mechanical thromboprophylaxis is often recommended for high-risk patients during surgery and there is some retrospective cohort evidence for a favourable VTE rate using sequential compression devices in combination with early mobilisation in bariatric patients.

Pharmacological Thromboprophylaxis

The most commonly used agents for pharmacological thromboprophylaxis are the low molecular weight heparins (LMWHs). LMWH works as an indirect inhibitor, primarily of factor Xa, by potentiating the effect of anti-thrombin and therefore reducing thrombin production necessary for clot formation. LMWHs are smaller fractions of heparin, preferred to unfractionated heparin (UFH) owing to their reproducible pharmacokinetics, ease of use, simple once-daily dosing and that they do not routinely require monitoring.

Compared with no prophylaxis, both UFH and LMWH have been shown to reduce the risk of VTE in general surgery patients by at least 60%. Higher doses of LMWH yielded slightly superior efficacy to standard dose UFH, but at the cost of increased haemorrhage. LMWH had favourable efficacy over UFH in one large study comparing different pharmacological regimes for bariatric surgery with no increase in bleeding rates, but in another study, LMWH had higher bleeding rates than UFH in bariatric patients, although higher doses were used.

It should be noted that although many published regimens for pharmacological prophylaxis include pre-operative doses, there is no clear evidence of superior outcomes compared to initiation 6–12 hours post surgery.

Direct oral anti-coagulants (DOACs) are now licensed for use after elective hip and knee arthroplasty, but not for other types of surgery to date. Large studies have demonstrated that DOACs have lower VTE rates than LMWH, with a variable comparative rate of bleeding in orthopaedic patients.

Pivotal trials in both surgical and medical patients have used fixed doses of pharmacological prophylaxis and patients with extremes of weight are not well represented. As such, appropriate dosing of pharmacological thromboprophylaxis is a key concern in obese patients undergoing surgery. Another consideration is that the potential risk of bleeding in bariatric surgery may be higher, e.g. because of poor laparoscopic views.

Special Considerations for Pharmacological Thromboprophylaxis in the Obese Surgical Patient

There is a lot of discussion regarding the appropriate dosing for obese patients. General concerns are that we may be underdosing the very obese patients, particularly as this group was under-represented in large clinical trials of LMWHs and manufacturers have produced less pharmacokinetic data in this population.

There are theoretical reasons to measure the effectiveness of LMWH in obese patients. Concerns that there may be prolonged absorption times due to increased subcutaneous fat may lead to subtherapeutic levels. Alternatively, the increased renal clearance in obese patients may also reduce levels. It is also worth considering whether the dosing strategy we use in obesity is valid, given that LMWH is mainly distributed intra-vascularly and adipose tissue is less vascular, yet we routinely dose using total body weight. Pharmacokinetic modelling in one study suggests that dosing of LMWH correlates more strongly with lean body weight as opposed to total body weight, however this is not currently recommended in practice.

Literature review identifies a number of varied outcomes. Authors have recommended increasing prophylactic doses of LMWH for obese patients on mainly pharmacological assumptions. Interpretation of studies comparing different doses of LMWH for bariatric surgery is difficult as they are either non-randomised and/or of insufficient power to detect a difference in efficacy and safety. One small randomised study of two doses of the LMWH nadropan showed no benefit from the higher dose and a larger study comparing two doses of parnaparin showed no statistical difference in VTE or bleeding rates.

Another sequential cohort non-randomised study identified a reduction in thromboses in obese patients utilising a higher prophylactic dosing regime of enoxaparin 40 mg versus 30 mg bd without increased bleeding. In contrast, a systematic review and meta-analysis of laparoscopic bariatric surgery concluded that the incidence of major bleeding seemed to increase using weight-adjusted doses of heparin with no advantage in terms of VTE reduction.

It has been postulated that obese patients should have routine monitoring of their anti-coagulant effect. To measure the degree of anti-coagulation with LMWH the simplest method is to test the anti-Xa level. Manufacturers of the various LMWH produce both therapeutic and prophylactic anti-Xa ranges. The correlation between anti-Xa levels and thrombosis and bleeding is poor, however. One study identified that over half of patients (mean BMI 48) had anti-Xa levels below target while receiving 40 mg enoxaparin twice daily and this has been echoed in other observational pharmacodynamic studies, concluding that patients with excessive body weight may not be adequately treated with fixed-dose enoxaparin thromboprophylaxis. One clinical study with no control arm used adjusted dose enoxaparin according to BMI with monitoring of anti-Xa levels for further dose adjustment. There was no clear increased risk in bleeding with the higher dosages levels, and equally, relatively low risk of thrombosis.

In conclusion, it is difficult to make a strong recommendation about dosing prophylactic LMWH in obese patients as the literature reviewed is too limited to make such a recommendation, with a paucity of randomised controlled trials and a predominance of retrospective data. All the studies use different obesity cut-offs, different methods of quantifying obesity, different LMWHs and varied dosing strategies. It is clear that more robust large randomised controlled trials in this area would be beneficial. However, the numbers needed to power significant results in regards to thrombosis and bleeding would be very large and potentially require international cooperation. There is currently no definitive supportive evidence correlating anti-Xa levels and post-operative VTE and bleeding risk for bariatric surgery patients.

Proposed Enoxaparin Dosing Schedule for High-risk Patients

<120 kg: 40 mg enoxaparin OD

120–150 kg: consider 40 mg enoxaparin BD

150–190 kg: 40 mg enoxaparin BD +/– measurement of anti-Xa post third dose with dose modification. If anti-Xa unavailable consider 60 mg enoxaparin BD – monitor carefully for bleeding.

>190 kg: Consider 60mg BD +/– measurement of anti-Xa post third dose with dose modification.

Proposed Dalteparin Dosing Schedule for High-risk Patients

<120 kg: 5000 units OD

120–150 kg: 5000 units BD

150–190 kg: 7500 units BD

>190 kg: consider 7500 units BD and measure anti-Xa levels after third dose with dose modification.

Other Issues

Extended Prophylaxis

Extended thromboprophylaxis is recommended in certain high-risk groups post-operatively (e.g. post-arthroplasty and after abdominal cancer surgery). Extended prophylaxis infers that anti-coagulation continues upon discharge from hospital. But should obesity be recognised as a great enough risk in isolation to recommend extended prophylaxis? A retrospective comparison concluded that extension of prophylaxis for 10 days post-discharge was safe and effective in reducing VTE compared to hospital-only prophylaxis, with no statistical increase in bleeding rates. Although there is insufficient data in this area to make a firm recommendation, extended prophylaxis should certainly be considered, especially in high-risk patients such as those with a history of previous VTE.

Inferior Vena Cava (IVC) Filters

There is no clear justification for the routine use of IVC filters in patients solely owing to their obesity. IVC filters are usually indicated in patients with high risk of thrombosis propagation who are temporarily unable to receive systemic anti-coagulation. Currently, all available data is observational in nature. One study in bariatric patients suggested worse outcomes for patients with IVC filters following propensity adjustment.

Bridging

Bridging anti-coagulation is the peri-operative management of anti-coagulation, a process with the aim of managing the risks of both thrombosis and haemorrhage in patients routinely taking anti-coagulants. We do not foresee any extra complications for the management of obese patients but recommend a formalised bridging plan is created in consultation with a haematologist with an interest in haemostasis. There are guidelines by Keeling on this area (see Further Reading).

DOACs

Obese patients only make up relatively small proportions of the large international trials and none of the phase III clinical trials reported the number of patients enrolled with BMI >40 kg/m^2, nor their clinical outcomes. Recent guidance would suggest DOACs could be used as prophylactic anticoagulants with a degree of confidence up to a BMI of 40 kg/m^2 or 120 kg. For patients with a BMI >40 or TBW greater than 120 kg, standard prophylaxis with LMWH is recommended. If DOACs are used in this larger weight category then a routine DOAC calibrated test to check drug level would be appropriate.

Conclusions

All hospitalised patients should be assessed for VTE risk. Obesity is a risk factor in isolation, but risks increase further with other patient- and procedure-related factors. In addition to early mobilisation, obese surgical patients should be considered for both mechanical and pharmacological thromboprophylaxis unless contraindicated.

It is difficult to give advice on dose and duration of LMWH based on current evidence; however, adjusted doses and a longer duration of treatment should be considered for patients at very high risk (e.g. with a history of previous VTE).

Use of IVC filters is not recommended in the perioperative management of obese surgical patients.

For patients with a BMI >40 kg/m^2 or weight >120 kg, LMWH is preferred over a DOAC due to the lack of data from trials.

Further Reading

Alikhan R, Peters F, Wilott R, Cohen AT. Fatal pulmonary embolism in hospitalised patients: anecropsy review. *J Clin Pathol*. 2004;**54**:1254-7.

Bartlett MA, Mauck KF, Daniels PR. Prevention of venous thromboembolism in patients undergoing bariatric surgery. *Vasc Health Risk Manag*. 2015;**11**:461-77.

Becattini C, Agnelli G, Manina G, Noya G, Rondelli F. Venous thromboembolism after laparoscopic bariatric surgery for morbid obesity: clinical burden and prevention. *Surg Obes Relat Dis*. 2012;**8**:108-15.

Birkmeyer NJ, Share D, Baser O, et al.; Michigan Bariatric Surgery Collaborative. Preoperative placement of inferior vena cava filters and outcomes after gastric bypass surgery. *Ann Surg*. 2010;**252**:313-18.

Birkmeyer NJ, Finks JF, Carlin AM, et al.; Michigan Bariatric Surgery Collaborative. Comparative effectiveness of unfractionated and low-molecular-weight heparin for prevention of venous thromboembolism following bariatric surgery. *Arch Surg*. 2012;**147**(11):994-8.

Borkgren-Okonek MJ, Hart RW, Pantano JE, et al. Enoxaparin thromboprophylaxis in gastric bypass patients: extended duration, dose stratification, and antifactor Xa activity. *Surg Obes Relat Dis*. 2008;**4**:625-31.

Celik F, Huitema A, Hooijberg J, et al. Fixed dose enoxaparin after bariatric surgery: the influence of body weight on peak anti-Xa levels. *Obes Surg*. 2015;**25**:628-34.

Diepstraten J, Janssen EJ, Hackeng CM, et al. Population pharmacodynamic model for low molecular weight heparin nadroparin in morbidly obese and non-obese patients using anti-Xa levels as endpoint. *Eur J Clin Pharmacol*. 2015;**71** (1):25-34.

Edmonds MJ, Crichton TJ, Runciman WB, Pradhan M. Evidence-based risk factors for postoperative deep vein thrombosis. *ANZ J Surg*. 2004;**74**:1082-97.

Finks JF, English WJ, Carlin AM, et al.; Michigan Bariatric Surgery Collaborative Center for Healthcare Outcomes and Policy. Predicting risk for venous thromboembolism with bariatric surgery: results from the Michigan Bariatric Surgery Collaborative. *Ann Surg*. 2012;**255**:1100-4.

Frantzides CT, Welle SN, Ruff TM, Frantzides AT. Routine anticoagulation for venous thromboembolism prevention following laparoscopic gastric bypass. *JSLS*. 2012;**16**:33-7.

Gould MK, Garcia DA, Wren SM, et al.; American College of Chest Physicians. Prevention of VTE in nonorthopedic surgical patients: antithrombotic therapy and prevention of thrombosis, 9th ed: American College of Chest Physicians evidence-based clinical practice guidelines. *Chest*. 2012;**141**: e227S-77S

Hamad GG, Choban PS. Enoxaparin for thromboprophylaxis in morbidly obese patients undergoing bariatric surgery: findings of the prophylaxis against VTE outcomes in bariatric surgery patients receiving enoxaparin (PROBE) study. *Obes Surg*. 2005;**15**:1368-74.

Ho KM, Tan JA. Stratified meta-analysis of intermittent pneumatic compression of the lower limbs to prevent thromboembolism in hospitalised patients. *Circulation*. 2013;**128**:1003-20.

Imberti D, Baldini E, Pierfranceschi MG, et al. Prophylaxis of venous thromboembolism with low molecular weight heparin in bariatric surgery: a prospective, randomized pilot study evaluating two doses of parnaparin (BAFLUX Study). *Obes Surg.* 2014;**24**:284–91.

Kalfarentzos F, Stavropoulou F, Yarmenitis S, et al. Prophylaxis of venous thromboembolism using two different doses of low-molecular-weight heparin (nadroparin) in bariatric surgery: a prospective randomized trial. *Obes Surg.* 2001;**11**:670–6.

Keeling D, Campbell Tait R, Watson H. Peri-operative management of anticoagulation and antiplatelet therapy. 2016. www.bcshguidelines.com/documents/BSH_periop_g uideline_for_editor.pdf (accessed May 2018).

Kothari SN, Lambert PJ, Mathiason MA. A comparison of thromboembolic and bleeding events following laparoscopic gastric bypass in patients treated with prophylactic regimens of unfractionated heparin or enoxaparin. *Am J Surg.* 2007;**194**(6):709–11.

Lester W, Freemantle N, Begaj I, et al. Fatal venous thromboembolism associated with hospital admission: a cohort study to assess the impact of a national risk assessment target. *Heart.* 2013;**99**:1734–9.

Martin K, Beyer-Westendorf J, Davidson BL, et al. Use of the direct oral anticoagulants in obese patients: guidance from the SSC of the ISTH. *J Thromb Haemost* 2016;**14**: 1308–13.

Mismetti P, Laporte S, Darmon JY, Buchmüller A, Decousus H. Meta-analysis of low molecular weight heparin in the prevention of venous thromboembolism in general surgery. *Br J Surg.* 2001;**88**:913–30.

NICE. Clinical guideline CG92: *Venous Thromboembolism: Reducing the Risk of Venous Thromboembolism in Patients Admitted to Hospital.* http://guidance.nice.org.uk/CG92 (accessed May 2018).

Nutescu EA, Spinler SA, Wittkowsky A, Dager WE. Low-molecular-weight heparins in renal impairment and obesity: available evidence and clinical practice recommendations across medical and surgical settings. *Ann Pharmacother.* 2009;**43**:1064–83.

Roberts LN, Porter G, Barjer RD et al. Comprehensive VTE prevention programme incorporating mandatory risk assessment reduces the incidence of hospital-associated thrombosis. *Chest.* 2013.;**144**:1276–81.

Rocha AT, de Vasconcellos AG, da Luz Neto ER, et al. Risk of venous thromboembolism and efficacy of thromboprophylaxis in hospitalized obese medical patients and in obese patients undergoing bariatric surgery. *Obes Surg.* 2006;**16**:1645–55.

Roftopoulous I, Martindale C, Cronin A et al. The effect of extended post-discharge chemical thromboprophylaxis on venous thromboembolism rates after bariatric surgery: a prospective comparison trial. *Surg Endosc.* 2008;**22**: 2384–91.

Rowan BO, Kuhl DA, Lee MD, Tichansky DS, Madan AK. Anti-Xa levels in bariatric surgery patients receiving prophylactic enoxaparin. *Obes Surg.* 2008;**18**:162–6.

Sachdeva A, Dalton M, Amaragiri SV et al. Graduated compression stockings for prevention of deep vein thrombosis. *Cochr Database Syst Rev.* 2014;**12**:CD001484.

Scholten D, Hoedema R, Scholten S. A comparison of two different prophylactic dose regimens of low molecular weight heparin in bariatric surgery. *Obes Surg.* 2002;**12**:19–24.

Simoneau MD, Vachon A, Picard F. Effect of prophylactic dalteparin on anti-factor Xa levels in morbidly obese patients after bariatric surgery. *Obes Surg.* 2010;**20**: 487–91.

Diepstraten J, Hackeng C, van Kralingen S et al. Anti-Xa levels 4 h after subcutaneous administration of 5,700 units IU nadroparin strongly correlate with lean body weight in morbidly obese patients. *Obes Surg.* 2012;**22**:791–6.

Winegar DA, Sherif B, Pate V, DeMaria EJ. Venous thromboembolism after bariatric surgery performed by Bariatric Surgery Center of Excellence Participants: analysis of the Bariatric Outcomes Longitudinal Database. *Surg Obes Relat Dis.* 2011;**7**:181–8.

Peri-operative Management of the Obese Diabetic Patient

Alexander Miras, Belén Pérez-Pevida and Nicolas Varela

Admission and Pre-operative Assessment

Glycaemic Control before Surgery

Glycaemic control before surgery is an important determinant of glycaemic behaviour after surgery in type 1 and type 2 diabetes (T2DM) patients. Therefore, diabetes treatment needs optimisation to proceed to surgery. On patient admission, staff should identify high-risk patients (long-term diabetes, poor glycaemic control, microvascular complication, history of severe hypoglycaemic episodes) and inform the medical team. Due to the complexity of T2DM patients, ideally every hospital should have written guidelines for hospital staff for the modification of diabetes treatment regimens on the day prior to and day of surgery. In hospitalised patients, hyperglycaemia has been defined as blood glucose >7.8 mmol/l (140 mg/dl), hypoglycaemia defined as blood glucose <3.9 mmol/l (70 mg/dl) and severe hypoglycaemia as <2.2 mmol/l (40 mg/dl). Due to the associated mortality associated with hypoglycaemia, a glucose target between 4.4 and 10.0 mmol/l (80–180 mg/dl) in the peri-operative period should be maintained. Table 32.1 summarises peri-operative care standards.

Table 32.1 Peri-operative care standards

Peri-operative period target glucose should be 4.4–10.0 mmol/l (80–180 mg/dl)

Pre-operative risk assessment for patients at high risk for ischaemic heart disease and those with autonomic neuropathy or renal failure

The morning of surgery or procedure, hold any oral hypoglycaemic agents and give half of intermediate or full doses of a long-acting or pump basal insulin.

Monitor blood glucose every 4–6 h while nil by mouth and dose with short-acting insulin as needed.

Surgery and Anaesthetic Influence

Major surgical procedures require a period of fasting during which oral glucose-lowering drugs cannot be used. This fact, combined with the peri-operative neuroendocrine stress response results in altered glycaemic control. The surgical stress itself may result in metabolic perturbations, endothelial dysfunction and post-operative complications (e.g. wound healing, sepsis). Furthermore, during surgery, anaesthetic technique also affects blood glucose readings, as induction, tracheal intubation and invasive monitoring are known to cause catecholamine discharge. Therefore, blood glucose should be monitored frequently in all patients to manage these possible glucose variations.

Post-operative Glycaemic Management

Glycaemic Targets

The management of hyperglycaemia in the hospital setting presents difficulty not only due to previously mentioned factors, but also those related to hospitalisation itself. These can include changes in nutritional status or level of consciousness. Therefore, reasonable glucose targets in the hospital setting after surgery are modestly higher than may be routinely advised for the outpatient setting. A glucose target between 7.8 and 10.0 mmol/l (140–180 mg/dl) is recommended for most patients in non-critical care units in the post-operative period. Conversely, due to the increased mortality associated with hypoglycaemia, higher glucose ranges may be acceptable in vulnerable patients, i.e. terminally ill patients or patients with severe co-morbidities. Clinical judgement combined with ongoing assessment of the clinical status of patients, including changes in the trajectory of glucose measures, illness severity, nutritional status or concomitant medications that might affect glucose levels (e.g. glucocorticoids), should be incorporated into the day-to-day decisions regarding insulin doses. Treatment recommendations for a given patient should be individualised, based on patient characteristics such as previous diabetes regimen, grade of glycaemic control, nature and extent of surgical procedure.

Post-operative Management of T2DM after Obesity Surgery

Effects of Obesity Surgery on Glycaemic Control

Remission of diabetes can be defined as a fasting plasma glucose level of less than 5.6 mmol/l (100 mg/dl) and a glycated haemoglobin level of less than 6.5% for at least 1 year without active pharmacologic therapy. In 2011, the American College of Surgeons Obesity Surgery Center Network (ACS-BSCN) found that, for diabetic patients undergoing bariatric surgery, the remission or improvement of diabetes at 12 months was achieved in 83% of those undergoing a Roux-en-Y gastric bypass (RYGB), 55% undergoing laparoscopic sleeve gastrectomy and 44% undergoing laparoscopic adjustable gastric band. Originally developed solely as a weight reduction therapy, obesity surgery not only improves glycaemia, but also reduces the rates of cardiovascular disease and death. Surgical treatment of obesity with diabetes results in the largest degree of sustained weight loss and largest improvements in blood glucose control compared to non-surgical approaches.

The Underlying Physiological Mechanisms

Following obesity surgery, several peripheral and/or central nervous system pathways lead to a reduction in hepatic glucose production, increase in tissue glucose uptake, improvement in insulin sensitivity and an enhanced pancreatic β-cell function. Depending on the obesity/metabolic intervention, these pathways are different, which explains the differences in diabetes remission and weight loss. Remission or improvement of diabetes is multifactorial, and can result both from weight-loss-dependent and weight-loss-independent mechanisms. The possible mediators maybe: caloric restriction with simple weight loss, gut hormone modulation, e.g. glucagon-like peptide 1 (GLP-1) and gastric inhibitory polypeptide (GIP), changes in bile acid metabolism and the intestinal microbiome, gastro-intestinal tract nutrient sensing and glucose utilisation, surgery-induced reductions in lipotoxicity and/or changes in adipose tissue hormone secretion.

Immediate Post-operative Glycaemic Management

Glycaemic Control and Possible Complications

Glycaemic control immediately after obesity surgery is different to other surgical procedures. Patients have unique glycaemic needs that are often not met with existing inpatient glucose protocols. Normoglycaemia can be achieved within hours and before weight loss, thus increasing the risk of a hypoglycaemic event. Hypoglycaemia is associated with increased morbidity as it causes deleterious effects, including tachycardia, diaphoresis, confusion, lethargy and syncope. Another infrequent complication that may occur is diabetic ketoacidosis (DKA), which is a life-threatening complication of diabetes and mainly occurs in patients with T1DM, but can present in patients with advanced T2DM under stressful conditions, such as surgery. The Endocrine Society generally recommends a post-operative fasting glucose goal <6.11 mmol/l and post-prandial glucose <9.9 mmol/l after bariatric surgery, which are similar to those stabilised for the post-operative management of diabetes in inpatient care. However, despite the possible complications, neither standardised protocols nor international validated guidelines addressing glycaemic control for this group exist. This may be because the hospitalisation period is often brief and differences exist in post-operative nutritional intake, making a definitive glucose management protocol difficult.

The advantages of these protocols are that they are readily followed and can be predominantly nurse-run. In addition, insulin dosing is conservative to account for rapid changes to insulin resistance and insulin secretion following obesity surgery, which reduces the risk of significant hypoglycaemia. However, due to this conservative insulin titration, those with severe insulin resistance requiring high doses of insulin may need higher dosing.

Post-discharge Recommendations

Metformin appears to have the safest profile immediately after obesity surgery. Initiation of therapy is normally held until the 2–4-week follow-up visit due to concerns with associated gastro-intestinal side effects, risk of dehydration and resultant renal dysfunction. If long-acting insulin is needed, calculation of the discharge dose is based on a patient's total insulin requirements during the 24 hours prior to discharge. It is vital that patients have an appointment in the endocrinology clinic, 2–6 weeks after discharge.

Summary

Obesity surgery achieves better glycaemic control and larger reductions in cardiovascular risk compared with non-surgical weight loss treatments. During the peri-operative period, several algorithms have been proposed to achieve glycaemic control. For inpatient care, physicians advocate the use of combined therapy; long-acting and short-acting insulin administered as an insulin sliding scale to maintain glucose levels within target ranges. Close monitoring by a specialist endocrinology team after discharge is recommended. Post-discharge recommendations include the use of oral glucose-lowering medications and long-acting insulin, equivalent to the patient's total insulin requirements during the 24 hours prior to discharge.

Further Reading

Aminian A, Kashyap SR, Burguera B, et al. Incidence and clinical features of diabetic ketoacidosis after bariatric and metabolic surgery. *Diabet Care*. 2016;39(4):e50–3.

Batterham RL, Cummings DE. Mechanisms of diabetes improvement following bariatric/metabolic surgery. *Diabet Care* 2016;39(6):893–901.

Chuah LL, Miras AD, Papamargaritis D, et al. Impact of perioperative management of glycemia in severely obese diabetic patients undergoing gastric bypass surgery. *Surg Obes Relat Dis*. 2015;11(3):578–84.

Cruijsen M, Koehestani P, Huttjes S, et al. Perioperative glycaemic control in insulin-treated type 2 diabetes patients undergoing gastric bypass surgery. *Neth J Med*. 2014;72(4): 202–9.

Fenske WK, Pournaras DJ, Aasheim ET, et al. Can a protocol for glycaemic control improve type 2 diabetes outcomes after gastric bypass? *Obes Surg*. 2012;22(1):90–6.

Golden SH, Peart-Vigilance C, Kao WH, Brancati FL. Perioperative glycemic control and the risk of infectious complications in a cohort of adults with diabetes. *Diabet Care* 1999;22(9):1408–14.

Heber D, Greenway FL, Kaplan LM, et al. Endocrine and nutritional management of the post-bariatric surgery patient: an Endocrine Society Clinical Practice Guideline. *J Clin Endocrinol Metab.*, 2010;95(11):4823–43.

Hutter MM, Schirmer BD, Jones DB, et al. First report from the American College of Surgeons Bariatric Surgery Center Network: laparoscopic sleeve gastrectomy has morbidity and effectiveness positioned between the band and the bypass. *Ann Surg*. 2011;254(3):410–20.

Lee CJ, Clark JM, Schweitzer M, et al. Prevalence of and risk factors for hypoglycemic symptoms after gastric bypass and sleeve gastrectomy. *Obesity (Silver Spring)*. 2015;23(5): 1079–84.

Lee WJ, Hur KY, Lakadawala M, et al. Gastrointestinal metabolic surgery for the treatment of diabetic patients: a multi-institutional international study. *J Gastrointest Surg* 2012;16(1):45–51; discussion 51–2.

Machnica K, Pannain S, Schulwolf E, Bartfield B, Emanuele MA. inpatient glycemic protocol for patients with diabetes undergoing bariatric surgery. *Obes Surg* 2015;25 (11):2200–4.

Mechanick JI, Youdim A, Jones DB, et al. Clinical practice guidelines for the perioperative nutritional, metabolic, and nonsurgical support of the bariatric surgery patient–2013 update: cosponsored by American Association of Clinical Endocrinologists, The Obesity Society, and American Society for Metabolic & Bariatric Surgery. *Obesity (Silver Spring)*. 2013;21(Suppl 1):S1–27.

Mingrone G, Panunzi S, De Gaetano A, et al. Bariatric surgery versus conventional medical therapy for type 2 diabetes. *N Engl J Med*. 2012;366(17):1577–85.

Mingrone G, Panunzi S, De Gaetano A, et al. Bariatric-metabolic surgery versus conventional medical treatment in obese patients with type 2 diabetes: 5 year follow-up of an open-label, single-centre, randomised controlled trial. *Lancet*. 2015;386(9997):964–73.

Miras AD, Risstad H, Baqai N, et al. Application of the International Diabetes Federation and American Diabetes Association criteria in the assessment of metabolic control after bariatric surgery. *Diabet Obes Metab*. 2014;16(1): 86–9.

Rometo D, Korytkowski M. Perioperative glycemic management of patients undergoing bariatric surgery. *Curr Diab Rep*. 2016;16(4):23.

Chapter 33

Nutritional Management of the Obese Surgical Patient

Gail Pinnock and Mary O'Kane

Introduction

Obesity is a major public health problem estimated to be the fourth largest risk factor for mortality in England. It is associated with a range of co-morbidities, notably type 2 diabetes mellitus, obstructive sleep apnoea (OSA), hypertension and cardiovascular disease, hyperlipidaemia, some cancers and osteoarthritis. These have a negative impact on health and psychosocial functioning, resulting in reduced quality of life.

The UK has the 10th highest rate of obesity amongst 45 developed nations. Prevalence increased from 15% in 1993 to 26% in 2014. Currently, 58% of women are classified as overweight or obese (27% obese) compared to 65% of men (24% obese). For those individuals classed as obese, the risk of associated poor health increases significantly with increasing BMI.

During 2014–2015, 440 288 patients were admitted to hospital in England with a primary or secondary diagnosis of obesity.

It is therefore inevitable that healthcare professionals in all specialties will encounter these individuals in their daily practice, either as general surgical patients or bariatric (weight loss) surgery patients.

Limitations of BMI as an Indicator of Metabolic Risk

BMI is commonly used to define obesity. The risk of ill health increases along with BMI (Table 33.1.). However, it fails to distinguish between lean body mass (LBM) and fat mass (FM). NICE recommends using waist circumference in addition to BMI to determine obesity-related health risks. Abdominal adiposity is a more sensitive indicator of potential health problems.

The use of BMI in non-White European populations has been debated for some time. Individuals from South Asian, Chinese, Black African and African-Caribbean communities have an equivalent risk of obesity-related co-morbidities such as diabetes at a lower BMI than White-European populations.

NICE therefore recommends the following for these populations:

- BMI of 23 kg/m^2 indicates increased risk
- BMI of 27.5 kg/m^2 indicates high risk.

The Obesity Paradox

This is a term used to describe the observed improvement in survival rates of overweight and obese patients compared to those of a normal body weight. It has been reported in numerous medical conditions such as coronary heart disease, heart failure, peripheral arterial disease, hypertension, stroke and renal failure. The idea is controversial and counter-intuitive; obese individuals have more co-morbidities and are therefore less likely to be able to compensate for the metabolic stress associated with critical illness. However, a recent systematic review and meta-analysis of cardiovascular interventions concluded that mortality was significantly lower in the overweight and obese groups compared to normal-weight groups; the reasons for this are unclear.

Opinion is divided, with critics claiming that the majority of evidence is based on observational data, with confounding factors not being taken into consideration. The use of BMI in these studies has also been criticised; there is insufficient evidence to support its use as a predictor of mortality in critically ill patients, and waist circumference may be a better measure of obesity in the peri-operative setting.

Malnutrition in the Obese

It is a common misconception that obese patients are well nourished. However, the prevalence of micronutrient deficiencies, in particular iron, vitamin D, folate and zinc, has been found to be higher in overweight and obese individuals. Many factors influence nutritional

Table 33.1 Association of BMI with co-morbidity and excess weight

	BMI	Excess weight (kg)	Risk of co-morbidities
Normal range	18.5–24.9		Average
Overweight	25–29.9	5–15	Increased
Obese class I	30–34.9	15–20	Moderate
Obese class II	35–39.9	20–25	Severe
Obese class III	>40	>25	Very severe

status, such as the systemic or pathological state of the individual as well as an unbalanced dietary intake.

An observational study of 6500 intensive care unit (ICU) patients concluded that the association between obesity and mortality is compounded by poor nutritional status; critically ill obese patients with malnutrition have worse outcomes than well-nourished obese patients.

Consequences of Surgery on Nutritional Status

Any surgical procedure produces changes in metabolic function and host defence mechanisms. The extent of these physiological changes depends on the nature of the surgery, whether it is elective or emergency, laparoscopic or open, and duration of the procedure.

Initially, there is a decline in body temperature, oxygen consumption and metabolic activity, despite the mobilisation of readily available energy reserves such as liver glycogen and adipose stores.

The subsequent acute phase is associated with hyper-metabolism, catabolism and increased energy expenditure mediated by counter-regulatory hormones and cytokines. Hyperglycaemia and insulin resistance are frequently seen during this phase. Mobilisation of stored protein provides amino acids for synthesis of acute-phase proteins and hepatic gluconeogenesis. This increased skeletal and visceral muscle catabolism together with a negative nitrogen balance leads to the depletion of LBM.

The acute phase also has an impact on micronutrients. Increased uptake of iron by iron-binding proteins results in low levels, which may continue for several weeks. Zinc, which is a co-factor for several enzymatic functions required during injury, is taken up by the liver, resulting in low zinc levels. Selenium levels are also known to decrease.

Obesity and its associated co-morbidities compound the metabolic response to surgery or critical illness. Malnutrition, whether from anorexia, poor diet or pre-operative fasting, exacerbates this response, putting the patient at greater risk of immunosupression, delayed wound healing and reduced muscle strength during the catabolic phase, prolonging hospital stay and increasing morbidity.

Nutritional Support

The aim of nutritional support is to preserve LBM, promote recovery and avoid complications associated with overfeeding.

There is considerable debate over the most appropriate method of predicting energy expenditure in obese patients. Indirect calorimetry (IC) is considered the gold standard, but is not readily available in all clinical settings. Dietitians therefore have to rely on the use of predictive equations to calculate energy expenditure. Unfortunately, these are inaccurate when used in the obese population, tending to over- or underestimate energy and protein requirements. Overfeeding the critically ill patient results in hyperglycaemia, insulin resistance, hepatic steatosis, prolonged mechanical ventilation and mortality. The American Society for Parenteral and Enteral Nutrition (ASPEN) recommends nutrition support should provide 65–70% of energy requirements in obese patients. This should encourage steady weight loss and may improve clinical outcomes, providing protein needs are met. Consideration should also be given to non-nutrient energy sources such as propofol infusions.

Dieticians need to use their clinical judgement when deciding which predictive equation to use, in accordance with local or national guidelines such as ASPEN or BAPEN (British Association for Parenteral and Enteral Nutrition). Regular monitoring should include standard nutritional parameters, blood glucose levels and respiratory function.

For those patients who have had bariatric surgery, additional thought must be given to the following: the type of bariatric procedure and corresponding changes in gut anatomy, the time since surgery, the diet tolerated prior to surgery and the reason for surgery, such as post-operative complication or non-bariatric-related surgery. Some bariatric procedures affect absorption in the long term and patients who have had surgery in the past may present with possible deficiencies of protein, iron, copper, zinc, selenium, thiamine, folate, vitamin B12 and vitamin D. In addition, those who have undergone a duodenal switch (DS) may be at risk of deficiencies in fat-soluble vitamins. These potential pre-existing deficiencies need to be taken into consideration.

Re-feeding Syndrome

Patients are at risk of re-feeding if they have had little or no food intake for >5–10 days, if they are malnourished (BMI 16–18.5) or have experienced unintentional weight loss of 10–15% within the previous 3–6 months. Patients should be assessed before starting nutritional support and managed according to local guidelines.

Routes of Feeding

The general consensus is that enteral nutrition (EN) should be prioritised providing there is a functioning gastro-intestinal tract. EN has a protective effect on gut barrier function and a positive influence on gut-associated lymphoid tissue (GALT), and maintains blood flow and peristalsis. Commencing EN within 24–48 hours is associated with decreased mortality and improved outcomes.

There is no contraindication to the use of EN in bariatric surgery patients, with nasojejunal feeding being the preferred route. For longer-term use, a surgical jejunostomy can be considered or a gastrostomy placed in the stomach remnant; however, there is an increased risk of leakage in the obese patient.

The accepted approach is to provide a hypocaloric feed in order to avoid the consequences of overfeeding, together with adequate protein to promote positive nitrogen balance. A peptide feed may be more appropriate if malabsorption is evident.

The use of parenteral nutrition (PN) is indicated when feeding via the gastro-intestinal tract is impossible, because of poor access, malabsorption or the patient's nutritional requirements not being met (because of, for example, low feeding rates or poorly tolerated feed). Bariatric surgery complications such as anastomotic leaks or obstructions may limit EN access. Patients who have had a malabsorptive procedure such as a DS may struggle to meet their requirements through EN alone.

Whichever method is used, the aim is to meet fluid requirements, and ensure adequate calories and protein, while preventing overfeeding. Regular monitoring is essential in order to assess the patient's response to nutritional support.

Bariatric Surgery

Bariatric surgery is a treatment option for people with severe and complex obesity, facilitating weight loss and improvements in co-morbidities. According to the National Bariatric Surgery Registry (NBSR), in addition to clinically significant weight loss, 61% of patients with OSA stopped treatment in the first year after surgery and 65% of patients with type 2 diabetes stopped hypoglycaemic medication within 2 years of surgery.

The most common surgical procedures are the gastric band, gastric bypass and sleeve gastrectomy (Figures 33.1–33.4). The DS is not commonly performed. The majority of procedures are performed laparoscopically. Assessment is carried out in tier 3 obesity services. Co-morbidities such as type 2 diabetes or OSA should be medically optimised and any nutritional deficiencies corrected. Some patients may require psychological and psychiatric assessments. Smoking cessation is encouraged. If surgery is considered appropriate, the patient is referred to a tier 4 surgical service, providing they understand and are motivated for surgery, and there is no medical, surgical, nutritional, psychological, psychiatric or social contraindication.

Within the tier 4 service, the multidisciplinary team consider potential benefits, associated risks, peri-operative mortality and longer-term implications of surgery. The decision about the type of procedure is made with the patient, taking account of co-morbidities and past surgical history.

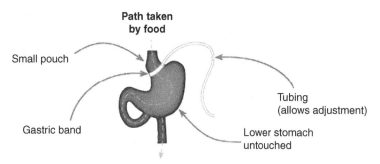

Figure 33.1 Adjustable gastric band. (Reprinted with kind permission of Dendrite Clinical Systems and the National Bariatric Surgery Registry (NBSR) Committee.)

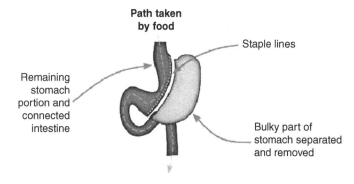

Figure 33.2 Sleeve gastrectomy. (Reprinted with kind permission of Dendrite Clinical Systems and the National Bariatric Surgery Registry (NBSR) Committee.)

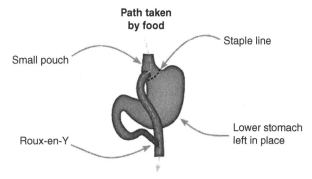

Figure 33.3 Roux-en-Y gastric bypass. (Reprinted with kind permission of Dendrite Clinical Systems and the National Bariatric Surgery Registry (NBSR) Committee.)

Pre-operative Liver Shrinkage Diet

Patients usually follow a strict low calorie/low carbohydrate diet to reduce liver volume and make surgery easier. The recommended time period for following the pre-operative diet varies between centres, but the decrease in liver size is within the first 2 weeks. Patients with type 2 diabetes may need to reduce oral hypoglycaemic medications whilst on the diet.

Nutritional Complications

Short Term

Post surgery, patients follow a phased approach to introduction of fluids and textures into their diet. They may struggle to achieve an adequate fluid intake initially, leaving them at risk of dehydration. Nausea, vomiting or regurgitation of food may occur in the

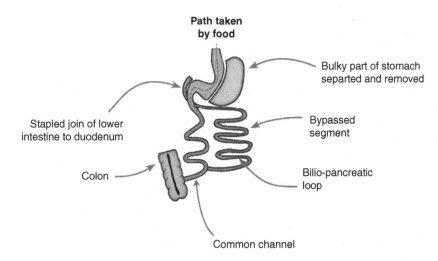

Path taken by food

Bulky part of stomach separated and removed

Stapled join of lower intestine to duodenum

Bypassed segment

Colon

Bilio-pancreatic loop

Common channel

Figure 33.4 Duodenal switch. (Reprinted with kind permission of Dendrite Clinical Systems and the National Bariatric Surgery Registry (NBSR) Committee.)

early stages. If this is prolonged, there is a high risk of thiamine deficiency, which may require emergency admission. Additional thiamine and vitamin B co strong should be given immediately (thiamine 200–300 mg daily, vitamin B co strong 1 or 2 tablets, three times a day) or intravenous thiamine. Oral or IV glucose must not be given to patients at risk of or with suspected thiamine deficiency, as it can precipitate Wernicke–Korsakoff syndrome.

Long term

Patients often find it difficult to achieve an adequate protein intake and need guidance on how to do so. A few may struggle with the introduction of some textures staying on a semi-solid, 'sloppy', nutritionally inadequate diet. Good specialist dietetic support of the patient is essential.

Those who have undergone sleeve gastrectomy, gastric bypass and DS procedures have an increased risk of nutritional deficiencies. These procedures affect absorption of iron, calcium, vitamin D and vitamin B12. In addition, the DS affects the absorption of protein, fat and fat-soluble vitamins. Patients are encouraged to consume 60–80 g protein/day after sleeve and gastric bypass and 80–120 g protein/day after DS. They need to take a complete multivitamin and mineral supplement lifelong.

UK bariatric surgery centres are generally commissioned to provide 2 years' follow-up and then transfer patients' care to the GP. Unfortunately, many primary care staff have no training in this

area. Patients should have access to long-term annual reviews as part of a shared care model. Guidelines on the long-term follow-up of bariatric surgery patients contain recommendations about this follow-up and guidance to GPs about when to refer back to specialist services and proposed shared care models.

Acknowledgements

Briony Robinson, Specialist Dietitian UGI/OG Surgery, Portsmouth Hospitals NHS Trust and Dr Denise Thomas, Chief of Service for Clinical Support, Portsmouth Hospitals NHS Trust.

Further Reading

Aasheim ET. Wernicke encephalopathy after bariatric surgery. *Ann Surg.* 2008;**248**:714–20.

Baker M, Harbottle L. *Parenteral Nutrition. Manual of Dietetic Practice, 5th edn.* Birmingham: The British Dietetic Assocation; 2014.

Baldry EL, Leeder PC, Idris IR. Pre-operative dietary restriction for patients undergoing bariatric surgery in the UK: observational study of current practice and dietary effects. *Obes Surg.* 2014;**24**:416–21.

Blackburn GL. Metabolic considerations in the management of surgical patients. *Surg Clin N Am.* 2011;**91**: 467–80.

Bundhan PK, Li N, Chen MH. Does an obesity paradox really exist after cardiovascular interventions?: a systematic review and meta-analysis of randomized controlled trials and observational studies. *Medicine (Baltimore).* 2015;**94** (44):e1910.

Colles S, Dixon JB, Marks P, et al. Preoperative weight loss with a very-low-energy diet: quantitation of changes in liver and abdominal fat by serial imaging. *Am J Clin Nutr.* 2006;**84**:304–11.

Galloway P, McMillan DC, Sattar N. Effect of the inflammatory response on trace element and vitamin status. *Ann Clin Biochem.* 2000;**37**:289–97.

Gerlach AT, Murphy C. An update on nutrition support in the critically ill. *J Pharm Practice.* 2011;**24**:70–7.

Gurunathan U, Myles PS. Limitations of body mass index as an obesity measure of perioperative risk. *Br J Anaesth* 2016;**116**(3):319–21.

McClave SA, Taylor BE, Martindale RG, et al. Guidelines for the Provision and Assessment of Nutrition Support Therapy in the Adult Critically Ill Patients: Society of Critical Care Medicine (SCCM) and American Society for Parenteral and Enteral Nutrition (ASPEN). *J Parenteral Enteral Nutr.* 2016;**40**(2):159–211.

Mechanick JI, Youdim A, Jones DB, et al. Clinical practice guidelines for the perioperative nutritional, metabolic, and nonsurgical support of the bariatric surgery patient 2013 update: cosponsored by the American Association of Clinical Endocrinologist, The Obesity Society, and American Society for Metabolic and Bariatric Surgery. *Surg Obes Relat Dis.*2013;**9**:159–91.

National Institute for Health and Care Excellence. *Nutrition support for adults: oral nutrition support, enteral feeding and parenteral nutrition.* NICE CG 32. 2006. www.nice.org.uk/guidance/cg32 (accessed May 2018).

National Institute for Health and Care Excellence. *BMI: preventing ill health and premature death in black, Asian and other minority ethnic groups.* 2013. www.nice.org.uk/guidance/ph46 (accessed May 2018).

National Institute for Health and Care Excellence. *Obesity: identification, assessment and management of overweight and obesity in children, young people and adults 2014 .* NICE CG 189. www.nice.org.uk/guidance/cg189 (accessed May 2018).

O'Kane M, Parretti HM, Hughes CA, et al. Guidelines for the follow-up of patients undergoing bariatric surgery. *Clin Obes.* 2016;**6**:210–24.

O'Kane M, Pinkney J, Aasheim ET et al. BOMSS guidelines on perioperative and postoperative biochemical monitoring and micronutrient replacement for patients undergoing bariatric surgery adults. 2014. www.bomss.org.uk/wp-content/uploads/2014/09/BOMSSguidelines.Final-version1Oct14.pdf (accessed May 2018).

Oliveros H, Villamor E. Obesity and mortality in critically ill adults: a systematic review and meta-analysis. *Obesity.* 2008;**16**:515–21.

Parrott, J, Frank, L, Rabena, R, et al. American Society for Metabolic and Bariatric Surgery Integrated Health Nutritional Guidelines for the Surgical Weight Loss Patient 2016 Update: Micronutrients. *Surg Obes Relat Dis.* 2017;**13**: 727–41.

Pinnock G, O'Kane M, Walker N. *Bariatric Surgery. A Pocket Guide to Clinical Nutrition.* Birmingham: PEN Group (Parenteral and Enteral Nutrition Group of the British Dietetic Association; 2013.

Preiser J-C, van Zanten ARH, Berger MM, et al. Metabolic and nutritional support of critically ill patients: consensus and controversies. *Crit Care.* 2015;**19**:35.

Robinson MK, Mogensen KM, Casey JD, et al. The relationship among obesity, nutritional status and mortality in the critcally ill. *Crit Care Med.* 2015;**43** (1):87–100.

Sakr Y, Alhussami I, Nanchal R, et al. Being overweight is associated with greater survival in ICU patients: Results from the Intensive Care Over Nations Audit. *Crit Care Med.* 2015;**43**:2626–32.

Van Zanten ARH. Full or hypocaloric nutritional support for the critically ill patient: is less really more? *J Thorac Dis.* 2015;**7**(7):1086–91.

Weimann A, Braga M, Carli F, et al. ESPEN guideline: clinical nutrition in surgery. *Clin Nutr.* 2017;**36**:623–50.

Critical Care Management of the Obese Patient

Matt Charlton and Christopher Bouch

Introduction

In recent years the prevalence of obesity has steadily increased, with 25% of the UK population classed as obese in 2014. Consequently, obese patients are increasingly encountered on the intensive care unit (ICU), with prevalence ranging from 5–25% (depending on the populations studied), this being highest on general medical/surgical intensive care units. Obese patients present for a myriad of reasons including in the post-operative period for both elective and emergent surgery, decompensated severe cardiorespiratory co-morbidity, and reasons unrelated to their obesity.

The high incidence of obese patients presenting to the general intensive care unit, and therefore being managed by non-specialist intensivists, necessitates a good understanding of the underlying pathophysiological consequences of obesity, specific problems encountered and general principles of their management.

Obesity in itself is not an indication for post-operative high dependency care. The majority of patients presenting for elective weight-loss surgery do not require intensive care management in the post-operative period, provided appropriate protocols are in place for their care in the post-anaesthetic recovery area and subsequent ward-based environment. Suggested criteria warranting consideration for ICU admission are highlighted in Table 34.1, although clearly, local guidelines should be followed if present.

General Principles of ICU Management of the Obese Patient

The obese patient presenting to the intensive care unit provides a unique set of challenges related to co-morbidity, altered underlying physiology and the obese body habitus. Simple procedures taken for granted amongst general intensive care patients such

Table 34.1 Factors warranting consideration of post-operative ICU care in the obese patient

Pre-existing co-morbidites
Indicated as high risk (OS-MRS 4–5 or limited functional capacity)
Surgical procedure
Untreated OSA plus a requirement for post-operative opioids
Local factors, including the skill mix of ward staff

OS-MRS: The Obesity Surgery Mortality Risk Stratification Score

as intravenous access and invasive monitoring, can be incredibly challenging in the obese population. Successful management involves the anticipation and prevention of predictable complications.

Obesity is an independent risk factor for the development of venous thromboembolism (VTE), with decreased mobility and thrombophilia recognised as contributing factors. Classical signs of deep vein thrombosis may be difficult to identify in this patient population and a high index of suspicion should be maintained. Venous thromboembolism has been implicated as the commonest cause of mortality following weight-loss surgery and particular attention should be given to the appropriate dosing of low molecular weight heparin thromboprophylaxis, based on actual body weight, alongside the use of intermittent pneumatic compression devices. Enoxaparin is the most extensively studied low molecular-weight heparin in obese patients.

Conflicting evidence exists on the risk of pressure ulcers in the obese population, with increased adiposity *potentially* providing a protective mechanism to their development. Critically unwell obese patients are, however, at increased risk of skin breakdown and soft tissue infections secondary to decreased perfusion of adipose tissue and overlying skin. Obese patients can provide considerable challenges to nursing staff with regards positioning, with increased size and weight making routine position changes difficult. Patients expected to require longer periods of immobility should be nursed on specialised bariatric beds with pressure-relieving air mattresses, with significant attention paid to pressure areas and skinfolds. Urinary and rectal catheters in the incontinent patient may provide some protection to the skin, reducing the need for turns associated with washing and the inherent risks associated with these manoeuvres (to both patient and staff). Early mobilisation is beneficial to reduce the risk of skin lesions and VTE.

Airway Management

Endotracheal Intubation

Formal assessment of the airway has been discussed in depth in Chapter 11. In summary, previous difficult intubation, neck circumference and high Mallampati grade (III/IV) are the strongest predictors of difficult intubation in the obese population. One in four of the major airway events reported in the 4th National Audit Project of the Royal College of Anaesthetists (NAP4) took place in the ICU or emergency department. The proportion of obese patients featured twice that in the general population. Obese patients were found to be at an increased risk of tracheal tube displacement and subsequent adverse outcome.

Of significant importance in the intensive care environment is the risk of rapid oxygen desaturation at induction/tracheal intubation, with intensive care patients at increased risk of severe hypoxaemia (SpO_2 <80%) when compared to the theatre population. Increased abdominal pressure causes a reduction in functional residual capacity (FRC), with closing volume encroaching on tidal volume breathing, leading to atelectasis. The consequence is considerable V/Q mismatch, with a decreased oxygen reservoir from which to maintain arterial oxygen saturations. This, coupled with increased oxygen utilisation in the critically unwell patient leads to dramatically reduced safe apnoea time, with a strong negative correlation being present between time to hypoxia and BMI.

Strategies for management of the obese airway in ICUs are the same as those in the theatre environment. The patient should be placed in the ramped position (25° head elevation), 30° reverse Trendelenburg and pre-oxygenated with an appropriate level of continuous positive airway pressure (CPAP). Non-invasive ventilation has been shown to be a potentially useful adjunct to standard pre-oxygenation techniques in the obese population, and can be applied in the ICU environment, although data is limited. In a small-randomised control trial of 33 patients with class III obesity, high-flow nasal oxygenation (HFNCO) were shown to be superior to standard facemask pre-oxygenation and comparable to CPAP with regards to PaO_2 in the pre-operative induction period and may have a role in the pre-oxygenation of intensive care patients.

Tracheostomy Management

Tracheostomy is a relatively common procedure in the management of the critically unwell adult. Approximately 7–19% of all patients admitted to ICU are managed with a tracheostomy. Critical care physicians perform the majority of these procedures percutaneously. Absolute and relative contraindications are a matter of debate, but it is generally accepted that obesity is a relative contraindication to percutaneous tracheostomy. The 2014 NCEPOD (National Confidential Enquiry into Patient Outcome and Death) study 'On the Right Trach?' prospectively collected data on tracheostomy insertions in UK hospitals over an 11-week period. Two thousand four hundred and fifty-six patients were included, 29.6% of which were obese, with an overall complication rate in ICU of 23.6%. Class III obesity is independently associated with an increased risk of tracheostomy complications.

Tracheostomy tube dislodgement is recognised as a significant issue in the obese population, with the NAP4 study identifying 14 cases of accidental tracheostomy tube dislodgement (11 leading to death or severe hypoxic brain injury), with over half of these being in obese patients. Standard length tracheostomy tubes are generally too short for the obese patient, due to an increased distance between the skin and trachea, reducing the intra-tracheal length of the tube and therefore predisposing dislodgement. A study of 40 obese patients (BMI 30–70 kg/m^2) demonstrated a combination of arm and neck circumference measurements could be used to reliably predict skin to trachea soft tissue distance when compared to ultrasound measurement (r = 0.82), with an error of 0.4 cm. Extra-long tracheostomy tubes with an inner tube should be used where possible. Adjustable flange tracheostomy tubes, allowing proximal and distal length adjustment, are a potential alternative, although flange malfunction (leading to dislodgement/endobronchial intubation) is a potential complication.

Respiratory Failure, Acute Respiratory Distress Syndrome and Ventilation

Pathophysiology

Respiratory function is markedly impaired in obesity. Extrinsic compression by fat deposition of the thoracic cavity with decreased chest wall and lung compliance lead to a restrictive ventilatory pattern, with reduced forced expiratory volume in 1 second (FEV_1) and forced vital capacity (FVC). Cephalad displacement of the diaphragm due to increased abdominal adiposity leads to a reduction in FRC. Closing volume, the volume of lung inflated when small airways begin to collapse, begins to encroach on FRC, meaning airway closure occurs during normal tidal ventilation. This leads to significant atelectasis and V/Q mismatch. Obesity is associated with a significantly increased work of breathing (and therefore basal oxygen consumption), brought about as a compensatory mechanism. Given the vastly reduced respiratory reserve, obese patients are at significant risk of acute respiratory failure due to mechanisms that may seem innocuous to the normal-weight individual.

Ventilatory Strategies

Non-invasive ventilation is safe and efficient to use in the obese patient. CPAP ventilation has a number of beneficial effects. Increased intra-thoracic pressure throughout the ventilatory cycle will result in alveolar recruitment and improved compliance, improving FRC and decreasing the work of breathing. Alveolar ventilation can be improved by the addition of bi-level pressure ventilation (such as BiPAP), although care must be taken to avoid gastric insufflation. Trials have suggested that the early implementation of non-invasive ventilation (NIV) can negate the requirement for invasive ventilation in this patient group.

Obese patients with respiratory failure managed with NIV should be monitored in a high-dependency area for signs of deterioration necessitating invasive ventilation.

A lung-protective ventilatory strategy should be employed when using invasive methods of ventilation. Tidal volume (Vt) should be based on ideal body weight, aiming for approximately 5–7ml/kg.

Positive end expiratory pressure (PEEP) facilitates alveolar recruitment and therefore improved oxygenation. There are no agreed upon methods of optimal PEEP determination, which may include the use of staircase recruitment manoeuvres and settings based on assessment of the lower-inflection point of the pressure–volume loop. A simple method of setting PEEP is based on tidal compliance. A set tidal volume is delivered and plateau pressure measured at increasing levels of PEEP. If plateau pressure remains the same, decreases or increases only slightly with increasing PEEP, this indicates improved lung compliance. If the plateau pressure increases by the same level (or greater) as the increase in PEEP, this suggests no improvement in compliance or potential overinflation. It should be noted that plateau pressures in the obese patient reflect stiffness of the respiratory system as a whole, including the pressure required to distended the chest wall mass, and may not accurately reflect an increase in alveolar pressure. Transpulmonary pressures, inferred from oesophageal manometry, may be a more accurate, if less practical.

There is little evidence to suggest a pressure- over a volume-controlled ventilatory strategy in this patient population. Whatever the mode of ventilation used, appropriate sedation and ensuring the patient is maintained in a head-up position of 30–45° is key to facilitate ventilation.

Acute Respiratory Distress Syndrome

Acute respiratory distress syndrome (ARDS) is an acute, diffuse inflammatory lung injury characterised by bilateral lung infiltrates and severe hypoxaemia. Diagnosis is based on the Berlin definition, relying on characteristic radiological findings and the presence of a reduced PaO_2/FiO_2 ratio (<300) despite adequate PEEP. In comparison to patients of a normal weight, obese patients are at increased risk of developing ARDS, with recurrent atelectrauma, decreased respiratory reserve and altered host response to inflammation (adipokines) being postulated as reasons for this.

Periodic prone positioning has been shown to provide a mortality benefit in severe forms of ARDS, with optimisation of V/Q matching and improved functional residual capacity leading to marked improvements in oxygenation. Although technically challenging, prone positioning has been shown to be particularly successful in the management of obese patients with ARDS, thought primarily due to recruitment of collapsed lung units, improving FRC. Particular attention should be paid to pressure areas and risk of unintentional tracheal extubation and vascular access lines displacement.

Veno-venous extracorporeal membrane oxygenation (VV-ECMO) has seen resurgence in recent years following its use during the influenza A (H1N1) pandemic in 2009. It is indicated in severe forms of hypoxaemic respiratory failure and carbon dioxide retention, despite optimisation of ventilatory settings, along with severe air leak syndromes and as a bridge to transplantation. Previously it was believed that obese patients would have poor outcomes on ECMO. A number of studies suggest the contrary, with trends to improved mortality in the obese population. Potential reasons include improved nutritional stores, immune modulation and earlier presentation due to pre-existing restrictive lung disease, with less severe parenchymal lung injury.

Cardiovascular Support

Pathophysiology

Increased baseline oxygen requirements along with the need to perfuse an increased tissue mass lead to blood volume and cardiac output increases. Chronically elevated pre-load and after-load lead to left ventricular dilation and hypertrophy with impaired diastolic function and eventually left ventricular systolic impairment. Chronically elevated filling pressure leads to left atrial enlargement and the development of atrial fibrillation. Pulmonary hypertension associated with sleep disordered breathing leads to right ventricular dysfunction along with chronically elevated right heart filling pressures resulting in dilation and hypertrophy.

Lines and Monitoring

Body habitus can impact on the accuracy of commonly used monitoring devices. Automated non-invasive blood pressure measurement can frequently underestimate systolic and overestimate diastolic pressures. The cuff bladder length should be at least 80% of the upper arm circumference, with a width of at least 50% of the upper arm length. The forearm may be a suitable alternative location. Invasive arterial monitoring provides accurate measurement of blood pressure in the obese population, with indexed

measurements of cardiac output by pulse contour analysis being as accurate as for the normal-weight population. ECG monitoring may demonstrate low-voltage complexes due to signal attenuation by the anterior chest wall.

Obesity can make the placement of intravenous lines challenging. Anatomy becomes distorted due to adipose deposition and skin surface landmarks are unreliable. Two-dimensional ultrasound is recommended for the placement of any central venous catheter to reduce the complications associated with multiple attempts. It may also be beneficial in the placement of peripheral venous lines and arterial catheters. Central venous pressure (CVP), although generally an unreliable measure of volume status, can be particularly misleading in the obese population owing to pulmonary hypertension and elevated right heart pressures.

Vasoactive Agents

The intricacies of pharmacology in the obese patient are discussed in Chapter 9, but it is worth mentioning that due to the rapidly titratable effect of vasopressors, body-weight adjustments are not required, with maximal concentrations based on adjusted body weight.

Obesity Supine Sudden Death Syndrome

Obesity supine sudden death syndrome (OSDS) describes oxygen desaturation and subsequent cardiac arrest associated with the supine position in patients with a BMI of greater than 50 kg/m^2. In morbidly obese individuals, with lying flat the large abdomen and extra thoracic soft tissue mass compress the thorax, causing an acute reduction in functional residual capacity with expiratory flow limitation. This results in acute hypercapnoea and hypoxaemia, with bradyarrhythmia and subsequent asystolic cardiac arrest. Clinicians need to be aware of this potential issue and ensure that a head-up position is maintained at all times.

Cardiopulmonary Resuscitation

Obesity can present considerable problems during cardiopulmonary resuscitation (CPR), with delays in positioning of defibrillator pads, securing the airway and difficulties in gaining intravenous access. Ventilation via supraglottic airway devices is unlikely to be adequate in a patient with higher BMI due to the inspiratory pressures required to overcome increased chest wall compliance. Tracheal intubation in an obese, poorly positioned patient is associated with difficulties previously discussed. Chest compressions are likely to be difficult to perform and increased thoracic impedance may attenuate defibrillation shocks. Despite this, a review of over 20 000 adult patients suffering a cardiac arrest in hospital, found no difference in survival amongst obese patients with a non-shockable presenting rhythm. In patients with a shockable rhythm, survival was equally poor in all patient groups, except those classed as overweight (BMI 25–29.9 kg/m^2). The American Heart Association suggests no changes to standard resuscitation algorithms in obese patients.

Renal

Obesity has been independently linked to the development of chronic kidney disease (CKD), due in part to associated co-morbidities such as diabetes, hypertension and hyperlipidaemia. Insulin resistance and the release of pro-inflammatory adipokines (leptin) and cytokines (TNF-α, IL-6) from adipose tissue, bring about a chronic pro-inflammatory state with associated renal damage. Obesity has also been linked to the development of acute kidney injury (AKI), with the incidence increasing with higher BMIs. It is worth noting, however, that commonly used systems for identifying AKI (such as the RIFLE, AKIN and KDIGO criteria) are defined on the basis of urine output measurements (indexed to body weight) and serum creatinine levels, and these can be inaccurate in the obese population. Increased muscle mass associated with increasing body weight can lead to higher baseline serum creatinine levels when compared to the ideal-weight population, which may be offset by an increased tubular filtration rate.

Elevated intra-abdominal pressures (IAPs) may also play a role in the development of AKI, with obese patients having elevated IAP at baseline when compared to normal-weight individuals. It is unclear at what pressure abdominal compartment syndrome should be diagnosed in the obese population and a high clinical index of suspicion should be maintained.

Obese patients are at increased risk of developing rhabdomyolysis and subsequent AKI, with excessive body weight leading to increased skeletal muscle compartment pressures and myonecrosis. Prolonged surgery (>4 hours), diabetes and intra-operative hypotension are associated factors. Treatment is as per the non-obese population with aggressive hydration, diuresis, urinary alkalinisation to increase myoglobin solubility and haemofiltration if necessary.

In general terms, the obese patient who develops AKI or a requirement for renal replacement therapy (RRT) has a higher mortality than their ideal-weight counterparts.

Nutritional Support

During critical illness, a catabolic state predominates. Increased basal insulin levels in the obese patient shift energy metabolism towards protein breakdown, as opposed to lipolysis of adipose tissue to drive gluconeogenesis, despite excess fat stores. This results in rapid lean muscle mass consumption, with detrimental effects on muscle strength, respiratory function, wound healing and immune function.

Controversy remains regarding the optimal nutritional regime in obese patients. Hypocaloric (80% daily requirement), high protein (1.5–2 g/kg/day) feeding regimes have been advocated, with the aim to reduce endogenous protein catabolism and promote steady weight loss, although supporting clinical trial data are lacking. As with all critically unwell patients, feeding should ideally be commenced within 24–48 hours of admission, with the enteral route being preferred where possible. Pro-kinetic agents can be used as per the non-obese population.

Logistics and Transfers

Caring for obese patients on the ICU poses a number of challenges for both medical and nursing staff. A number of these issues have already been touched on within the text of this chapter, including difficulties with intravenous access, monitoring modalities, airway management, skin care and pressure ulcer prevention. Specialist equipment should be available in any area with an expectation of managing the obese patient, with a thorough, but not exhaustive list suggested by the Association of Anaesthetists of Great Britain and Ireland (AAGBI) and the Society of Bariatric Anaesthesia (SOBA). Particular attention should be paid to the weight limitations and maximum size restrictions of commonly used imaging modalities (CT, MRI), which may be unable to accommodate patients with obesity.

Intra- and inter-hospital transfer of the obese patient can be problematic, with standard transfer trollies and ambulances being unable to accommodate patients of this size. This can be detrimental if time-critical interventions are required at tertiary centres (such as neurosurgical or cardiothoracic input), as appropriate transport equipment and personnel must be sourced prior to mobilisation.

The Obesity Paradox

The 'obesity paradox' describes the hypothesis that, against intuition, obesity is associated with a survival benefit. Being obese does not increase ICU mortality. It may, conversely be associated with a survival benefit, despite longer ICU stays and an increased number of ventilator days. Recent systematic reviews and meta-analyses seem to confirm this finding. Potential explanations may in part be due to selection bias, whereby multiply co-morbid critically unwell patients tend to have lower BMIs, with obese patients being admitted at an earlier point in their illness due to the risk of rapid deterioration and need for advanced nursing care. Obesity has previously been shown to be protective in chronic debilitating conditions such as end-stage renal disease and HIV/AIDS. Potential physiological factors conferring an improved survival in obese patients are various. An upregulation of anti-inflammatory and immunomodulatory adipokines act to positively modulate the immune response. Higher baseline pleural pressures may confer protection from ventilator-associated lung injury. Increased adiposity may act as a nutritional reservoir on recovery from critical illness (albeit unhelpful in the initial period). It should be noted that the heterogeneity of general ICU patients, both in terms of presenting illness, disease severity and pre-morbid state, make survival data difficult to interpret and the safest approach may be to say that obesity (up to a point) is not detrimental in critically unwell patients.

Summary

Obese patients necessitating critical care present multiple challenges, both physiologically and logistically. A thorough understanding of the underlying pathophysiology and appreciation of the increased risk of organ dysfunction and complications is essential in order to provide satisfactory care to this specialised patient group.

Further Reading

Cook TM, Woodall N, Harper J, Benger J; Fourth National Audit Project. Major complications of airway management in the UK: results of the Fourth National Audit Project of the Royal College of Anaesthetists and the Difficult Airway Society. Part 2: intensive care and emergency departments. *Br J Anaesth.* 2011;**106**:632–42.

Danziger J, Chen KP, Lee J, et al. Obesity, acute kidney injury, and mortality in critical illness. *Crit Care Med.* 2016;**44**(2):328–34.

De Jong A, Molinari N, Sebbane M, et al. Feasibility and effectiveness of prone position in morbidly obese patients with ARDS: A case-control clinical study. *Chest.* 2013; **143** (6):1554–61.

Druml W, Metnitz B, Schaden E, et al. Impact of body mass on incidence and prognosis of acute kidney injury requiring renal replacement therapy. *Intens Care Med.* 2010;**36**:1221–8.

Duarte AG, Justino E, Bigler T, et al. Outcomes of morbidly obese patients requiring mechanical ventilation for acute respiratory failure. *Crit Care Med.* 2007;**35**:732–7.

El Solh AA, Jaafar W. A comparative study of the complications of surgical tracheostomy in morbidly obese critically ill patients. *Crit Care.* 2007;**11**(1):R3.

Hibbert K, Rice M, Malhotra A. Obesity and ARDS. *Chest.* 2012;**142**(3):785–90.

Hogue CW,Jr, Stearns JD, Colantuoni E, et al. The impact of obesity on outcomes after critical illness: A meta-analysis. *Intensive Care Med.* 2009;**35**(7):1152–70.

Jain R, Nallamothu BK, Chan PS, American Heart Association National Registry of Cardiopulmonary Resuscitation (NRCPR) Investigators. Body mass index and survival after in-hospital cardiac arrest. *Circ Cardiovasc Qual Outcomes.* 2010;**3**(5):490–7.

Joffe A, Wood K. Obesity in critical care. *Curr Opin Anaesthesiol.* 2007;**20**(2):113–18.

McGrath BA, Wilkinson K. The NCEPOD study: On the right trach? lessons for the anaesthetist. *Br J Anaesth.* 2015;**115**(2):155–8.

Nightingale CE, Margarson MP, Shearer E, et al. Perioperative management of the obese surgical patient 2015: Association of Anaesthetists of Great Britain and Ireland Society for Obesity and Bariatric Anaesthesia. *Anaesthesia.* 2015;**70**(7):859–76.

Papazian L, Corley A, Hess D, et al. Use of high-flow nasal cannula oxygenation in ICU adults: a narrative review. *Intens Care Med.* 2016;**42**(9):1336–49.

Selim BJ, Ramar K, Surani S. Obesity in the intensive care unit: risks and complications. *Hosp Pract (1995).* 2016;**44** (3):146–56.

Shashaty MG, Stapleton RD. Physiological and management implications of obesity in critical illness. *Ann Am Thorac Soc.* 2014;**11**(8):1286–97.

Szeto C, Kost K, Hanley JA, Roy A, Christou N. A simple method to predict pretracheal tissue thickness to prevent accidental decannulation in the obese. *Otolaryngol Head Neck Surg.* 2010;**143**(2):223–9.

Chapter 35

Indications for Bariatric Surgery

Christos Tsironis

Introduction

Obesity is defined as a body mass index (BMI) over 30 kg/m^2. It is identified worldwide, in all age groups and according to the World Health Organization (WHO), more than 1.6 billion people are currently overweight and 400 million obese.

Obesity is related to many co-morbidities, including type 2 diabetes mellitus, hypertension, dyslipidaemias, ischaemic heart disease, sleep disordered breathing (SDB), non-alcoholic steatohepatitis, gastro-oesophageal reflux disease (GORD) and polycystic ovary syndrome (PCOS). Obesity also contributes to degenerative diseases of the joints, causing back, hip and knee pain. Depression is common among obese people and there is an increased cancer risk (colorectal, endometrial, breast and gall bladder cancer).

The term 'bariatric' is derived from the Greek words 'baros' meaning 'weight' and 'iatrikos' meaning 'medicine', and bariatric or metabolic surgery refers to the surgical procedures for management of obesity.

These operations involve volume restriction and/or nutrient malabsorption with mechanisms that limit the caloric intake, reduce caloric absorption and affect satiety and insulin sensitivity via hormonal pathways.

Revision bariatric surgery (further surgery after a primary procedure to facilitate further weight loss) should only be undertaken in specialist centres by surgeons, anaesthetists and other team members with extensive experience in these procedures because of the high rate of complications and increased mortality. These specialist procedures and indications will not be discussed in this chapter.

Bariatric Surgery

The contemporary operative procedures include the Roux-en-Y gastric bypass (RYGB), the sleeve gastrectomy (SG), the laparoscopic adjustable gastric band (LAGB) and the biliopancreatic diversion with duodenal switch (BPD-DS).

The RYGB is a combined malabsorptive and restrictive procedure, which consists of a small (approximately 30 ml) proximal gastric pouch, separated from the distal stomach and anastomosed to an alimentary Roux limb of the small bowel, 75 to 150 cm in length.

The SG, is essentially a partial gastrectomy where the greater curvature of the stomach including the fundus is excised, so that the remaining stomach is significantly smaller, with a 'sleeve' shape.

The LAGB is a restrictive procedure that consists of compartmentalisation of the proximal stomach by inserting a tight, adjustable band around the stomach just distal to the gastro-oesophageal junction (GOJ).

The mini gastric bypass (MGB) is relatively new. It is a safe and effective bariatric procedure. It consists of a long gastric pouch at the level of the incisura, separated from the gastric remnant, which is anastomosed to the jejunum approximately 200 cm distal to the ligament of Treitz.

Endoscopic bariatric procedures include intra-gastric balloon (IGB) insertion and newer procedures involving endoluminal suturing to restrict gastric volume.

Indications for Bariatric Surgery

In 1991 the National Institutes of Health (NIH) Consensus Development Panel was the first to define the indications for the surgical management of severe obesity that were subsequently reviewed by the American Bariatric Society in 2004.

Many bariatric surgery pathways require patients to participate in programmes for conservative management of obesity and lifestyle changes preoperatively to demonstrate their commitment.

There are currently several sources for guidelines/indications for bariatric surgery.

National Institute for Health and Care Excellence (NICE) Guidelines 2014

The current UK criteria for eligibility to undergo bariatric surgery in the UK are listed below. All criteria should be fulfilled.

1. The patient should have BMI of 40 kg/m^2 or more

or

   BMI between 35 kg/m^2 and 40 kg/m^2 with at least one obesity-related co-morbidity (such as type 2 diabetes mellitus or hypertension).

2. The patient should have attempted all the non-surgical pathways without achieving significant weight loss.

3. The patient has been receiving or will receive intensive management in a Tier 3 service.

4. The patient is generally fit for anaesthesia and surgery.

5. The patient is willing to engage with long-term follow-up.

Additional criteria were outlined in 2014 for people with type 2 diabetes mellitus:

1. Patients with a BMI of 35 kg/m^2 or greater who have recent-onset type 2 diabetes (within a 10-year time frame) should be offered an expedited assessment for bariatric surgery as long as they are also receiving or will receive assessment in a Tier 3 service (or equivalent).

2. People with a BMI of 30–34.9 kg/m^2 with recent-onset type 2 diabetes (within a 10-year time frame) can be considered for bariatric surgery as long as they are also receiving or will receive assessment in a Tier 3 service (or equivalent).

3. People of Asian origin who have recent-onset type 2 diabetes (within a 10-year time frame) can be considered for bariatric surgery at a lower BMI (reduced by 2.5 kg/m^2) than other populations as long as they are also receiving or will receive assessment in a Tier 3 service (or equivalent).

4. Surgery should be the option of choice (instead of lifestyle interventions or drug treatment) for adults with a BMI of more than 50 kg/m^2 when non-surgical interventions have not been effective.

NICE has also outlined recommendations regarding the pre-operative and post-operative management of the patient, as well as the decision-making for surgery in a Tier 4 service.

The candidate for bariatric surgery should be aware of the benefits of the operation, the long-term implications, and the related risks and potential complications, as well as the peri-operative mortality. These discussions should also include the patient's family.

The type of operation should be chosen jointly with the patient. This decision should take into consideration the patient's co-morbidities, the level of obesity and the available evidence on effectiveness and long-term effects of the chosen procedure. In addition, the facilities and equipment available and the experience of the surgeon who will perform the operation should also be part of this process.

Specialist peri-operative dietetic support is a vital part of the pathway. The provision of information on appropriate diet for the chosen bariatric procedure, monitoring of the patient's micronutrient status, individualised nutritional supplementation, support and guidance to achieve long-term weight loss and weight maintenance are key components.

The American Association of Clinical Endocrinologists, The Obesity Society, and the American Society for Metabolic and Bariatric Surgery

North American updated guidelines for obesity management, including indications for bariatric surgery were released in 2013.

These set the eligibility criteria for bariatric surgery to include:

1. Adults with a BMI ≥40 kg/m^2 without co-morbidity.

2. Adults with a BMI 35.0 to 39.9 kg/m^2 with at least one serious co-morbidity, including but not limited to type 2 diabetes mellitus, sleep disordered breathing (obstructive sleep apnoea, obesity hypoventilation syndrome), hypertension, hyperlipidemia, non-alcoholic fatty liver disease (NAFLD), non-alcoholic steatohepatitis (NASH), pseudotumour cerebri, gastro oesophageal reflux disease, asthma, venous stasis disease, severe urinary incontinence, debilitating arthritis, impaired quality of life, disqualification from other surgeries as a result of obesity (i.e. surgeries for osteoarthritic disease, ventral hernias or stress incontinence).

3. Adults with BMI between 30.0 and 34.9 kg/m^2 and uncontrollable type 2 diabetes mellitus or metabolic syndrome.

For Asian patients, the BMI criteria should be lowered by 2.5 kg/m^2 per class due to a higher prevalence of truncal obesity (i.e. visceral fat), which is associated with an increased adverse risk profile.

New guidelines on metabolic surgery for treatment of diabetes emerged from the Second Diabetes Surgery Summit (DSS-II), an international consensus conference held in London in 2015. This was jointly organised with the American Diabetes Association (ADA), International Diabetes Federation (IDF), Diabetes UK (DUK), Chinese Diabetes Society (CDS), and Diabetes India (DI).

According to these new guidelines, bariatric surgery is recommended to treat type 2 diabetes mellitus in patients with a BMI greater than or equal to 40 kg/m^2, as well as in those with BMI between 35 and 39.9 kg/m^2 when hyperglycemia is inadequately controlled by lifestyle and medical therapy. The consensus statement recognised that surgery should also be considered for patients with type 2 diabetes mellitus and BMI 30.0–34.9 kg/m^2 if hyperglycemia is inadequately controlled despite optimal treatment with either oral or injectable medications. These BMI levels should be reduced by 2.5 kg/m^2 for Asian patients.

Multidisciplinary Team Working

Every case should be discussed and 'approved' for surgery by a bariatric multidisciplinary team (MDT). This team consists of a surgeon, an anaesthetist, a dietitian, a psychologist and a specialist nurse as a minimum. Complete review of each case and input from all members allows a balanced decision to be made and this information to be provided to the patient. This will include a risk–benefit discussion, management of the complications of obesity, specialist assessment for eating disorder(s) and information on the different procedures, including potential weight loss and associated risks.

Bariatric Surgery in Children

NICE has provided guidelines for obesity surgery in children. Procedures are not generally recommended in children or young people. They may be considered for young people only in exceptional circumstances, and if they have achieved or nearly achieved physiological maturity.

Bariatric surgery in children should only be performed by a very specialist multidisciplinary team that can provide specialist pre-operative assessment, assessment for eating disorders, regular post-operative dietetic and surgical follow-up. Pre- and post-operative psychological support is very important. Genetic screening is recommended pre-operatively to exclude rare, treatable causes of obesity.

Conclusion

Obesity is an expanding disease worldwide, affecting all ages, and it is related to much co-morbidity such as type 2 diabetes, hypertension and ischaemic heart disease. Bariatric surgery refers to the surgical procedures that treat obesity and the related co-morbidities, currently including Roux-en-Y gastric bypass, sleeve gastrectomy, adjustable gastric banding, mini gastric bypass and biliopancreatic diversion/duodenal switch. Guidelines have been produced to define the indications for bariatric surgery, which include BMI over 40 kg/m^2, BMI 35–40 kg/m^2 with at least one obesity-related co-morbidity, BMI 30-35 kg/m^2 with uncontrolled hypoglycaemia. People of Asian origin should be considered for surgery with a BMI reduced by 2.5 kg/m^2 for the above categories. Indications also include previous failure of non-surgical methods for weight loss and attendance of Tier 3 or equivalent pathways. The patient needs to be generally fit for surgery and general anaesthesia. Patients need to agree to long-term follow-up. A multidisciplinary team should undertake surgery, including experienced bariatric surgeons and anaesthetists with specialised dietitians and psychologists. This should take place in appropriately equipped and experienced units.

Further Reading

Burguera B, Agusti A, Arner P, et al. Critical assessment of the current guidelines for the management and treatment of morbidly obese patients. *J Endocrinol Invest*. 2007;**30**(10): 844–52.

Deitel M, Gagner M, Erickson AL, et al. Third International Summit: Current status of sleeve gastrectomy. *Surg Obes Relat Dis*. 2011;**7**(6):749–59.

Elder KA, Wolfe BM. Bariatric surgery: a review of procedures and outcomes. *Gastroenterology*. 2007;**132** (6):2253.

Mahawar KK, Jennings N, Brown J, et al. 'Mini' gastric bypass: systematic review of a controversial procedure. *Obes Surg*. 2013;**23**(11):1890–8.

Majumder S, Birk J. A review of the current status of endoluminal therapy as a primary approach to obesity management. *Surg Endosc*. 2013;**27**(7):2305.

Mathus-Vliegen EM, Tytgat GN. Intragastric balloon for treatment-resistant obesity: safety, tolerance, and efficacy of 1-year balloon treatment followed by a 1-year balloon-free follow-up. *Gastrointest Endosc.* 2005;**61**(1):19.

Mechanick JI, Youdim A, Jones DB, et al. Clinical practice guidelines for the perioperative nutritional, metabolic, and nonsurgical support of the bariatric surgery patient–2013 update: cosponsored by American Association of Clinical Endocrinologists, The Obesity Society, and American Society for Metabolic & Bariatric Surgery. *Obesity (Silver Spring).* 2013;**21**(Suppl 1):S1–27.

NIH Conference Gastrointestinal surgery for severe obesity. Consensus Development Conference Panel. *Ann Intern Med.* 1991;**115**(12):956.

National Institutes of Health. Clinical guidelines on the identification, evaluation, and treatment of overweight and obesity in adults: the evidence report. *Obes Res.* 1998;**6** (Suppl 2):51S.

National Institute for Health and Care Excellence. National Clinical Guideline Centre (UK) *Obesity: Identification, Assessment and Management of Overweight and Obesity in Children, Young People and Adults: Partial Update of CG43.* London: National Institute for Health and Care Excellence (UK);2014.

Rubino F, Nathan DM, Eckel RH, et al.; Delegates of the 2nd Diabetes Surgery Summit. Metabolic surgery in the treatment algorithm for type 2 diabetes: a joint statement by international diabetes organizations. *Obes Surg.* 2017;**27** (1):2–21.

Chapter 36

Surgical Procedures for Weight Loss

Naim Fakih Gomez and Marco Adamo

Introduction

Bariatric procedures can be classified into restrictive and malabsorptive procedures. Malabsorptive operations reduce the absorption of calories, lipids, proteins and other nutrients. On the other hand, restrictive operations limit food intake and promote a feeling of fullness and satiety after meals. Some operations are a combination of both.

No operation is perfect. An ideal operation has been described as one that is safe, easy to perform, easy to revise and reversable. It should also have rare short- and long-term complications, be relatively inexpensive and highly satisfying for the patients. While the ideal bariatric operation might still be in evolution, different options are in place and others are still evolving to treat patients with obesity.

While surgery can offer a lasting control mechanism, it is not a cure and patients must always understand its limitations and that lifestyle change is important. It is only through an honest discussion with a bariatric surgeon that patients decide which procedure may be best suited for them and match their objectives. In our view, patient choice is a key factor in decision-making and plays a major role in enhancing the outcomes of the procedures. Bariatric units should offer their patients a wide variety of options and surgeons should seek training and continuously develop skills in different and new procedures, avoiding restricting patient's choice to certain operations. This is a task that every bariatric surgeon has to endeavour during their career.

This chapter will overview a historical perspective of these procedures, as well as describe the most common procedures being used and others that may play an important role in fighting obesity in the future.

Historical Perspective

Bariatric surgery began in the 1950s. The initial approach was deduced from the fact that extensive small bowel resections led to weight loss and thus the first intestinal bypass for obesity was performed. One of the first established operations was the jejunoileal bypass (JIB), which induced a state of malabsorption by bypassing most of the intestines, whilst keeping the stomach intact. Although weight loss with the JIB was good, too many side effects and complications resulted, such as diarrhoea, malnutrition, osteoporosis and liver failure.

Due to these complications, initial intestinal procedures were followed by gastric procedures, with development of the gastric bypass in the 1960s. This procedure was developed after observations that patients who had a partial gastrectomy for ulcers lost weight and struggled to regain weight afterwards. The initial approach was then modified into the Roux-en-Y configuration now standard for this procedure.

Biliopancreatic diversion (BPD) was developed in the 1970s and intended to have the benefits of JIB, but without its worst complications. This involved a distal subtotal gastrectomy (in contrast to the gastric bypass where the stomach was divided but left in situ) and a Roux-en-Y reconstruction with a lengthy biliopancreatic limb and a common channel of 50–100 cm. It showed excellent results, but required life-long follow-up, which decreased its popularity.

Different procedures have been developed since these original techniques. These are discussed in this chapter.

Surgical Procedures

Adjustable Gastric Band

The popularity of the adjustable gastric band (AGB) has reduced over the last few years. It is, however, an option for some patients. Widespread use of this technique in the first decade of twenty-first century has resulted in patients requiring revisional surgery as a result of complications due to their gastric band procedure.

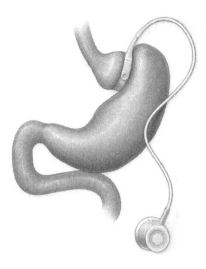

Figure 36.1 Adjustable gastric band.

Insertion of an AGB uses an adjustable silicone band around the stomach to provide restriction. It represented around 40% of the procedures worldwide in 2008, but its popularity fell to 10% in 2013, and this trend is continuing downwards at 5.5% during the 2013–2015 period.

The gastric band system (Figure 36.1) is designed to remain in situ for the patient's lifetime. As there is no malabsorption and the digestive tract is left intact, there is no risk of anaemia and dumping syndrome. It is also a reversible operation, and thus some patients may have preference for this procedure because of this.

A motivated, mobile, young patient is more likely to do well with an AGB. Regular follow-up is an important factor to achieve good results, as well as to identify complications at an early stage.

In addition to the general contraindications to bariatric surgery, the AGB should be avoided in patients with Crohn's disease or those with a diagnosis of an autoimmune connective tissue disease such as systemic lupus erythematosus or scleroderma.

The AGB is the procedure with the lowest early post-operative morbidity. However, even in the most experienced units between 6 and 60% of AGBs will require some form of re-operation over time. Although the majority of these re-operations for band complications are minor and rarely life threatening, some are high-risk, such as band erosion into the gastric lumen.

Complications of AGB insertion include:

1. *Band slip/prolapse*: This occurs when either the band migrates distally along the stomach or the stomach moves proximally through the band. This can occur acutely or chronically. Surgical placement of AGB by the 'peri-gastric' approach instead of the 'pars flaccida' approach decreased the rate of band slippage significantly (16% versus 4%). Symptoms can include dysphagia, vomiting, night reflux and food regurgitation. Diagnosis can be confirmed by plain abdominal X-rays with the band losing its 2 to 8 o´clock configuration and acquiring either a horizontal or a 4 to 10 o´clock position. Initial treatment after diagnosing a band slip is to deflate the band. Surgical intervention includes band removal or repositioning.

2. *Band erosions*: These occur in around 1–4% of patients and are generally thought to arise from ischaemia of the gastric wall due to an excessively tight band. They usually occur after 1 year of insertion. The symptoms are very variable, and can be totally asymptomatic to development of non-specific abdominal pain. Diagnosis can be made at gastroscopy.

Eroded bands must be removed, commonly via a laparoscopic approach. Revision surgery to other bariatric procedures can be performed at a later stage if appropriate.

3. *Port site problems*: These include infection, rotation or pain and usually require re-operation.

4. *Band/tubing leaks/disconnection*: These problems in addition to port site complications affect one in every five patients with AGBs. They clinically present as a sensation of lack of restriction and require re-operation.

Sleeve Gastrectomy

Sleeve gastrectomy (SG) (Figure 36.2) has become one of the most commonly undertaken bariatric procedures. It was popularized in the early 2000s as the first stage of a two-stage duodenal switch. Most patients lost significant amounts of weight and no second-stage operation was required. This established sleeve gastrectomy as a stand-alone operation. Evidence supports this as a safe and effective primary weight loss procedure.

During laparoscopic surgery, the patient is positioned supine in the reverse Trendelenburg position.

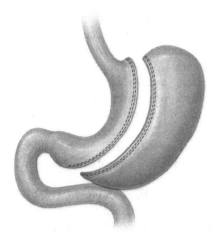

Figure 36.2 Sleeve gastrectomy.

The greater omentum is detached from the greater curvature of the stomach and the stomach fully mobilised from the short gastric vessels and posterior adhesions.

A 32–34 French gauge bougie is inserted via the mouth and oesophagus to lie along the lesser curvature of the stomach. Against this bougie the stomach is cut using a laparoscopic linear stapler. Careful attention should be taken so as not to create a narrow stomach, and thus before each firing, the size of the neo-gastric lumen should be checked moving the bougie alongside the lesser curvature. If any resistance alongside the movement of the bougie is felt, then the stapler should be repositioned to form a wider sleeve. The final volume of the gastric sleeve is around 70–100 ml.

SG presents various advantages over other procedures. It is technically simpler, with shorter operative times and continuity of the digestive tract is maintained. Data has demonstrated that SG achieves similar results to the gastric bypass in relation to diabetes remission and that long-term weight loss following SG is equivalent. This has contributed to the widespread acceptance of this as the main procedure offered in some bariatric units.

The only specific contraindication for SG is Barrett´s oesophagus. There is a variable effect of this procedure on acid reflux and the possibility of de novo reflux. Patients should be counselled about this possibility pre-operatively. If a hiatus hernia is observed during the procedure, it should be repaired.

Complications of SG include:

1. *Leaking*: Leaks from the staple line are a serious complication. They can be acute (presenting in the first week), early (<6 weeks), late (>6 weeks) or chronic (>12 weeks). The most common site (90% of leaks) is the proximal sleeve. Management is challenging and depends on the presentation. Options include drainage of collections, surgical exploration and endoscopic stenting across the leak.

2. *Bleeding*: The incidence of haemorrhage after SG is reported in up to 6% of patients. Haemorrhage can be extra-luminal or intra-luminal. Staple line bleeding is a common cause for extra-luminal bleeding. This risk can be reduced by avoiding intra-operative hypotension and high intra-abdominal pressure that could mask a bleeding vessel.

3. *Stricture*: This occurs in up to 2% of patients. Narrowing of the lumen in the first instance can be managed with endoscopic balloon dilatation. If this fails, then surgical intervention, most commonly requiring conversion to a gastric bypass.

Gastric Bypass

Mason developed this procedure in the 1960s after observing the weight loss obtained in patients undergoing gastrectomy for peptic ulcer disease. Initially the operation was performed as a loop bypass with a horizontal pouch. However, biliary reflux occurred with this loop configuration and a 'Roux-en-Y' reconstruction was undertaken. In 1997, the laparoscopic mini gastric bypass (MGB) was introduced by Rutledge, involving the initial loop configuration, but with a longer vertical pouch to avoid bile reflux.

The gastric bypass was the most common bariatric operation worldwide. It has now been surpassed by the sleeve gastrectomy.

Roux-en-Y Gastric Bypass

Roux-en-Y-gastric bypass (RYGB) (Figure 36.3) involves creation of a 15–30 ml proximal gastric pouch that is separated from the remnant stomach. The duodenum and proximal gastro-intestinal tract is bypassed by anastomosing a Roux limb of jejunum to the gastric pouch and the continuity of the GI tract is restored by a jejunojejunostomy. RYGB is both restrictive and malabsorptive.

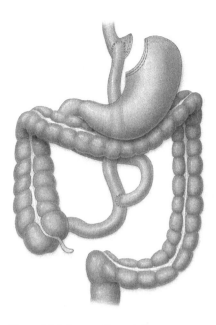

Figure 36.3 Roux-en-Y gastric bypass.

The RYGB involves different parts, including the formation of the gastric pouch, the gastrojejunal anastomosis, the jejunojejunal anastomosis and the closure of the mesenteric defects.

A gastric bypass is considered by many bariatric units as the 'gold standard' operation. It has more than 50 years of experience to rely on, offering sustainable, effective weight loss and co-morbidity resolution with acceptable morbidity and mortality.

Patients with previous intra-abdominal surgery (especially open surgery) or with large ventral hernias can present a challenge in performing an RYGB. In such cases, the risks of extensive laparoscopic adhesiolysis, conversion to open surgery or large abdominal hernia repair should be balanced with the benefits of the operation. Alternative procedures, such as a sleeve gastrectomy should be considered.

A history of Crohn's disease, anaemia, vitamin deficiency and risk of gastric cancer development are contraindications to RYGB surgery.

RYGB is associated with a low mortality rate; <1% at 30 days. The associated morbidity is approximately 21% (12–33%) with a re-operation rate of 3%.

Early complications include anastomotic leaks and bleeding. Other complications include internal herniation with small bowel ischaemia, marginal ulceration and nutritional/metabolic complications.

1. *Anastomotic leaks*: These occur in approximately 2–4% of cases and are associated with significant morbidity and mortality. They occur most commonly from the gastrojejunal anastomosis and less frequently from jejunojejunal anastomosis, staple lines or iatrogenic intestinal injury. Early detection and treatment is fundamental to reduce morbidity and mortality.

2. *Marginal ulceration*: The incidence is around 4%, and usually occurs at the gastrojejunal anastomosis, often on the jejunal side, between 1–6 months post-operatively. Ulceration presents with epigastric pain and/or as an upper GI bleed. Ulcers usually respond to treatment with proton pump inhibitors. Ulcer development is increased with the use of NSAIDS and cigarette smokers.

3. *Internal herniation*: Occurs in about 2.4%, commonly at around 1 year post-operatively.

Mini Gastric Bypass/One Anastomosis Gastric Bypass

MGB was first reported in 2001. The surgeon creates a long vertical gastric pouch with a Billroth type II loop gastrojejunostomy 200 cm or longer in length.

This operation is an attractive option as it has advantages over the RYGB. It is a simpler procedure

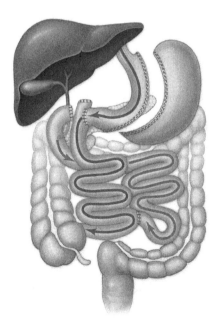

Figure 36.4 Bilopancreatic diversion procedure.

as it involves only one anastomosis, resulting in a shorter operative time and lower risk of anastomotic leak and internal hernias. In addition, results reveal better weight loss and co-morbidity resolution than the RYGB. This may be due to a larger portion of small intestine being bypassed.

However, the long biliopancreatic limb causes more malabsorption with associated anaemia and diarrhoea than with RYGB.

Duodenal Switch

The duodenal switch (DS) is a modification of the biliopancreatic diversion (BPD) (Figure 36.4). It was originally designed to prevent development of peptic ulcers, minimise the incidence of dumping syndrome and provide more restriction in comparison to the original BPD procedure. Acceptance worldwide is low, and it comprises about 1% of bariatric procedures worldwide. This is due to its technical difficulty, as well as related morbidity.

The procedure involves creating a sleeve gastrectomy with preservation of the pylorus, followed by transection of the first part of the duodenum. A Roux-en-Y reconstruction is fashioned with a duodenoileal anastomosis and an ileoileal anastomosis. The procedure combines malabsorption and restriction. Despite excellent results regarding weight loss and co-morbidity resolution, there is low acceptability among surgeons and patients due to its higher mortality and morbidity rates.

Single Anastomosis Duodenoileal Bypass with Sleeve Gastrectomy

This novel duodenal switch procedure (SADI-S) involves only one loop anastomosis of duodenum to ileum, 250 cm proximal to the terminal ileum. It has the advantage of a single anastomosis with respect to the DS, making the operation quicker, with a lower risk of anastomotic leak and internal hernias. Described as both a primary operation and revisional surgery after failed SG, the SADI-S can be performed in one stage. For higher risk individuals, a two-stage approach can be performed. Outcome data is limited for this procedure. It appears to be a promising technique and the preliminary short-term results are good, but larger series with a longer follow-up are necessary to draw definitive conclusions.

Further Reading

Angrisani L, Santonicola A, Iovino P, et al. Bariatric surgery worldwide 2013. *Obes Surg.* 2015;**25**(10):1822–32.

Buchwald H, Oien DM. Metabolic/bariatric surgery worldwide 2008. *Obes Surg.* 2009;**19**(12):1605–11.

Chang SH, Stoll CR, Song J, et al. The effectiveness and risks of bariatric surgery: an updated systematic review and meta-analysis, 2003–2012. *JAMA Surg.* 2014;**149**(3):275–87.

Himpens J, Cadiere GB, Bazi M, et al. Long-term outcomes of laparoscopic adjustable gastric banding. *Arch Surg.* 2011;**146**(7):802–7.

Kremen AJ, Linner JH, Nelson CH. An experimental evaluation of the nutritional importance of proximal and distal small intestine. *Ann Surg.* 1954;**140**(3):439–47.

Lee WJ, Ser KH, Lee YC, et al. Laparoscopic Roux-en-Y vs. minigastric bypass for the treatment of morbid obesity: a 10-year experience. *Obes Surg.* 2012;**22**(12):1827–34.

O'Brien PE, MacDonald L, Anderson M, et al. Long-term outcomes after bariatric surgery: fifteen-year follow-up of adjustable gastric banding and a systematic review of the bariatric surgical literature. *Ann Surg.* 2013;**257**(1):87–94.

Rutledge R. The mini-gastric bypass: experience with the first 1,274 cases. *Obes Surg.* 2001;**11**(3):276–80.

Chapter 37

Bariatric Surgery Complications

K. T. Yeung and Ahmed R. Ahmed

Introduction

The number of patients undergoing bariatric surgery worldwide is on the rise. There is increasingly convincing data demonstrating positive outcomes not only in weight loss, but in obesity-related diseases. In the United Kingdom, 16 928 bariatric operations were performed between 2012 and 2015. As this cohort of patients continue to grow, recognition and understanding of post-bariatric surgery complications becomes increasingly important. Early recognition in many cases will lead to action and subsequently, better outcomes.

This chapter will discuss complications relating to the three most common bariatric procedures performed in the United Kingdom: laparoscopic adjustable gastric band, sleeve gastrectomy and Roux-en-Y gastric bypass.

As a brief overview of current practice in the United Kingdom, approximately 95% of all bariatric procedures are performed laparoscopically. The average post-operative inpatient stay is 2.7 days. Nationally, the complication rate in primary procedures is 2.9%, with an overall 0.07% in hospital mortality. These figures compare well to current available international data.

General Post-operative Complications

Many obesity related co-morbidities such as diabetes mellitus, hypertension, cardiovascular disease, obstructive sleep apnoea, musculoskeletal disease and depression are present in bariatric patients. At any point, surgery may precipitate worsening of such diseases.

The principles of management are no different from non-bariatric patients and early recognition is essential. For example, presentation of sepsis in obese individuals may be atypical and may often present as a pyrexia, a rise in white cell count or may not even present as physiological derangement. Close monitoring and vigilance leads to early identification and improved outcomes. Contrast and cross-sectional imaging is often used to help identify any source of sepsis or pathology in the post-operative patient, but should not delay surgical intervention when needed.

Post-operative venous thromboembolic (VTE) events and pulmonary embolism (PE) risks are increased in older age groups, patients with a higher BMI, those undergoing open or revision procedures and in those with a history of VTE disease. Other contributing factors include a reduction in baseline mobility. A combination of mechanical and chemical prophylaxis intra- and post-operatively is used, with low molecular weight heparin the drug of choice. There are yet to be any randomised trials to determine the optimal VTE prophylaxis in bariatric patients in terms of appropriate dosage and length of usage post-operatively. In those clinically presenting with VTE/PE, subsequent investigations and treatment should be no different from ideal-weight individuals.

Sepsis in the post-operative bariatric patient needs to be taken very seriously. It is uncommon, but when it does occur, there is a high risk of morbidity and even mortality (30 times increased risk of death in laparoscopic gastric bypass patients).

One of the most common sources of sepsis is the chest. Obese patients are particularly susceptible to hospital-acquired pneumonia and almost always have a degree of basal actelectasis on a background of obesity-associated hypoventilation post-operatively. Preventive techniques include the use of incentive spirometery and early mobilisation is key in preventing respiratory complications.

Cardiac events can also occur particularly in patients with existing cardiac pathology, hypertension and diabetes.

Adjustable Gastric Band

The adjustable gastic band (AGB) is a restrictive procedure with no alteration to the patient's anatomy.

Weight loss is achieved by reducing the amount of food a patient can consume and promotes early satiety. It also requires significant alteration to a patient's eating habits in order to produce good results. The band can be adjusted through filling or removal of fluid from a port sited subcutaneously on the abdomen via a non-coring Huber needle.

The reported complication rate is approximately 8–36.9%, with a lifetime re-operation rate of 10–34%. A retro-gastric tunnel is created to allow the passage of a gastric band around the stomach. Possible early complications can include gastric or oesophageal perforation during dissection or days later from an unrecognised thermal (diathermy) injury, bleeding from the gastric vessels or injury to the spleen. The band also comes in a variety of sizes and is fitted according to intra-operative judgement.

Gastric or oesophageal perforation requires surgical repair. If discovered intra-operatively this should lead to abandoning of gastric band implantation. If bleeding from the spleen cannot be controlled with surgical clips or cautery, then a splenectomy may be required. Acute obstruction secondary to oedema from band placement may be managed conservatively, but if the symptoms fail to settle then re-laparoscopy and revision or removal of the AGB will be required.

Slipped or eroded gastric bands are the two most common long-term complications. Other long-term complications include dilatation of the gastric pouch or oesophagus and port complications such as malposition or tube fracture.

Gastric band slippage occurs in approximately 2–4% of patients. The stomach herniates through the band at the proximal end causing a range of symptoms, including vomiting, dysphagia, reflux and inadequate weight loss. This can be acute and/or chronic. Pain is uncommon in band slippage, but should prompt the clinician into thinking about gastric ischaemia that requires emergency surgical treatment with immediate band emptying followed by laparoscopic band removal.

In order to assess the cause of pathology, a logical sequence of investigations must be performed. An assessment of the patient's physiology and biochemistry, including lactate levels is helpful. The American Society for Metabolic and Bariatric Surgery (ASMBS) suggests a routine as follows:

1. Plan abdominal X-ray to assess the band position and an upper GI contrast swallow to assess for stenosis or obstruction.

2. If slippage is seen then the band must be deflated and will need subsequent surgery – re-positioning or removal.

3. Removing fluid from the band in this scenario will alleviate or improve symptoms. More importantly it improves any ischaemia.

Gastric band erosion occurs in approximately 1–3% of patients and is one of the most serious complications associated with AGB. A common presentation of erosion may be port site infection. Thus, all patients with port site infections must be investigated with an upper GI endoscopy to rule out AGB erosion. Other features can include unexplained weight re-gain, abdominal pain and even obstruction. If a significant portion of the band is eroded, retrieval of the band can be performed endoscopically, otherwise laparoscopic removal with suture repair of the erosion site is required.

Complications relating to the port and tubing can also occur. This includes leakage, infection or displacement and rotation of the port within the subcutaneous space. Leakage may be related to damage to the system through improper filling, leading to needle stick injury to the band tubing as it joins the port, and commonly requires surgical replacement of the port. It is important to adhere to strict aseptic techniques while filling or deflating gastric bands to prevent infection. The port is normally fixed to the abdominal fascia to prevent displacement, rotation and flipping. If this occurs, surgical re-positioning/replacement is required.

Overall there is a 1–8% and up to 50% rate of overall lifetime band removals reported in current literature.

Sleeve Gastrectomy

Sleeve gastrectomy (SG) is a restrictive procedure. The stomach is 'trimmed' using a series of surgical staples to create a gastric tube. The reported major complication rate is 1–2%. Patients commonly suffer nausea in the first 48 hours post-operatively. A theory is that SG increases intra-luminal pressures within the newly created gastric tube, leading to nausea.

Complications in the early post-operative period are rare, but more serious complications include leaks and bleeding from the gastric staple line. Presentation of a leak may be variable, with sepsis being the most common. This occurs in approximately 1.1–4% of all cases and can occur at any stage from a day after surgery (typically from a technical staple line failure) to days or weeks later (more in keeping with ischemic or thermal injury). Leaks, particularly from the proximal staple line can be difficult to treat. A variety of strategies exist, including the use of endoscopic stents or even surgical revision to Roux-en Y fistulojejunostomy or RYGB as a salvage procedure. Bleeding may require surgical intervention and patients should be resuscitated and managed as per any post-operative bleed prior to and during re-operation. There is increasing evidence that using staple line reinforcement can reduce both bleed and leak incidence rates.

Late complications may include gastro-oesophageal reflux, gastric tube stricture/stenosis, leaks and weight re-gain.

Symptoms of reflux or dysphagia should be investigated initially with radiological contrast swallow and endoscopy. This will help identify any anatomical pathology for the symptoms. If these two investigations suggest a problem, further imaging by CT may assist further evaluation. Strictures can be dilated with the aim of improving symptoms. Medical treatment with proton pump inhibitors and pro-kinetic agents may also help improve reflux symptoms. The presence or absence of a hiatus hernia is also important to establish.

With regards to weight regain after SG, the exact mechanism is unknown. There may be patient-related factors (poor dietary choices, chronic over-eating) and hence all patients with weight re-gain need follow-up with a dietitian and psychiatrist. That being said, surgeons should investigate for anatomical causes such as a misshapen sleeve with excess fundus or, in rare cases, dilatation of the gastric tube. Subsequently the patient may be able to ingest larger volumes of food with less restriction. This can also be identified on contrast imaging. Despite initial concerns regarding the suitability of sleeve gastrectomy as a primary weight loss procedure, there is now widespread published data demonstrating positive outcomes at 5 years regarding weight loss and related co-morbidities.

Nutritional deficiencies in this procedure are less common, but can occur. This includes deficiencies in iron, vitamin D, folic acid, and vitamins B1 and B12. Lifelong monitoring and replacement is essential.

Roux-en-Y Gastric Bypass

Roux-en Y gastric bypass (RYGB) is one of the most common bariatric procedures worldwide. Its precise mechanism leading to weight loss is unknown. In the United Kingdom, at least 52% of all bariatric procedures performed are a RYGB. Serious early complications are rare. Again, leaks, bleeding, ileus and GI tract obstruction can occur.

The most serious complication in RYGB is an anastomotic leak. Current literature reveals an anastomotic leak rate of between 0.4 and 1.9%. Patients can present with abdominal pain and signs of peritonitis. Some cases may present with fever and shoulder tip pain and should prompt consideration of an intra-abdominal abscess. Other subtle signs include persistent ileus, failure to progress or even respiratory symptoms. The most common site of leaks is the gastrojejunal anastomosis. A blow out from back pressure secondary to bowel obstruction should be excluded, particularly in cases of jejunojejunal anastomosis leaks. Leaks can also occur at the staple lines of the gastric remnant and divided jejunum. Risk factors for an anastomotic leak include open or revisional surgery, advancing age, male gender and chronic heart, lung and renal disease.

Bleeding can present both as an early or a late complication. Approximately 1% of patients develop bleeding as a post-operative complication. Sources can be intra- or extra-luminal or both. Presentation may include physiological derangement, haemodynamic instability and haematemesis or fresh per rectal (PR) bleeding. Not all cases require surgical re-exploration, but the timing and physiological picture will help determine the urgency of treatment.

Late presentation of complications often relates to ulcers and should be investigated with oesophagogastric endoscopy. There is a 4% incidence of marginal ulcers post-operatively. Presentation can range from post-prandial epigastric pain, haematemesis, malaena and or fresh PR bleeding. A major risk factor is the continuation of smoking post bariatric surgery. Treatment is primarily supportive with medical therapy using proton pump inhibitors and in some cases endoscopic intervention for bleeds.

Bowel obstruction presents with abdominal pain and or distension, nausea and vomiting, and commonly reduced bowel function. Internal hernia and anastomosis stenosis/stricture are the most common causes of obstruction in patients who have had RYGB. Bezoars and intussception are rare causes of obstruction.

Internal hernias are unusual, but a potentially serious complication. The reported incidence ranges from 3 to 16%. Due to the nature of the procedure, defects are created in the mesentery as a result of the re-organised anatomy. Common sites include the opening where the Roux limb, or its mesentery (Petersons defect), overlies the transverse mesocolon and small bowel mesentery defect at the JJ anastamosis. Herniation through these defects can cause obstructive symptoms, but more worryingly bowel ischaemia.

Routine cross-sectional imaging does not always reveal the presence of internal hernias. There is a low threshold for re-laparoscopy in patients who suffer from symptoms of unexplained abdominal pain or bowel obstruction. A bariatric specialist should always review bariatric patients who present with such symptoms.

Recent evidence suggests these defects should routinely be closed during the primary surgical procedure. However, closure at this time does not guarantee that the defects remain closed. Closure is associated with a risk of early bowel obstruction caused by bowel kinking.

Port site and incisional hernias present similarly and will be evident on clinical examination and by radiological imaging. Surgical intervention is often required.

Strictures can develop at any anastomotic site, most commonly at the gastrojejunal anastomosis. Presentation is chronic in nature; patients present with progressive reduction in oral intake with associated abdominal pain and vomiting. Assessment involves contrast studies and endoscopic inspection. Treatment comprises endoscopic or radiological dilatation and finally surgical revision if all other methods fail.

Dumping syndrome involves a neural and hormonal response as a result of rapid hyperosmolar fluid entry from the stomach pouch to the small bowel related to the bypass anatomy. Patients suffer symptoms such as dizziness, abdominal pain and diarrhoea shortly after eating. Treatment is by modification of food intake content. Revisional surgery is reserved for extreme cases.

Reduced oral intake after RYGB leading to nutritional deficiencies is a common problem. Patients can develop deficiencies in vitamins B1, B12 and D, iron, calcium, copper, zinc and selenium. Lifelong monitoring and replacement is important. Diet-related problems account of 33% of bariatric surgery re-admissions.

Biliary Pathology

Rapid weight loss with any bariatric procedure is a significant risk factor for gallstone formation. Ursodeoxycholic acid has been shown to be an effective prophylactic agent and is used routinely in some units post-operatively. Biliary symptoms can still develop after surgery and treatment post-RYGB can be challenging due to the altered anatomy. A variety of techniques is available to clear gallstones from the common bile duct. This includes transgastric endoscopic retrograde cholangiopancreatography (ERCP) or laparoscopic bile duct exploration. Prophylactic cholecystectomy performed during bariatric procedures in asymptomatic patients has not been shown to be justified and is not performed.

Revisional Procedures

A revisional procedure refers to surgical procedures for correction, conversion or reversal of prior bariatric surgery. For example, revision of gastric band position or conversion of gastric band to sleeve gastrectomy or Roux-en-Y gastric bypass. Up to 11% of patients will at some point undergo revisional surgery.

The main indication for such procedures is treatment of side effects. A common scenario is: worsening reflux after sleeve gastrectomy in the absence of a hiatus hernia and thus conversion to a Roux-en-Y gastric bypass. Other side effects requiring further treatment include, but are not limited to, nausea and vomiting, and dumping syndrome. The other slightly more controversial indication for revisions is inadequate weight loss.

Revision procedures have a significantly higher surgical risk with all complications. Surgical time is often longer with more blood loss. Post-operatively, the complication rates of leaks, bleeding, cardiac events and VTE are higher. Despite this, it has been shown to further improve weight loss and further reduce co-morbidities. Mortality, however, is thought to be no different from primary procedures.

Psychology

It is worth mentioning that weight re-gain is not solely a surgical and medical issue. There is a large cohort of patients where psychological and behavioural factors contribute to their poor outcomes. Input from the psychological team with the aim of identifying and modifying such factors may be useful in achieving desired outcomes and patient satisfaction.

Further Reading

Berg P, McCallum R. Dumping syndrome: a review of the current concepts of pathophysiology, diagnosis and treatment. *Dig Dis Sci.* 2016;**61**(1):11–8.

Blair LJ, Huntington CR, Cox TC, et al. Risk factors for postoperative sepsis in laproscopic gastric bypass. *Surg Endosc.* 2016;**30**(4):1287–93.

Brethauser SA, Kothari, S, Sudan R, et al. Systematic review on reoperative bariatric surgery: American Society for Metabolic and Bariatric Surgery Revision Task Force. *Surg Obes Relat Dis.* 2014;**10**(5):952–72.

Chang SH, Stoll CRT, Song J, et al. The effectiveness and risks of bariatric surgery: an updated systematic review and meta-analysis 2003–2012. *JAMA Surg.* 2014;**149**(3):275–87.

Elie C, Younan A, Alkandari M, et al. Roux-en-Y fistula-jejunostomy as a salvage procedure in patients with post-sleeve gastrectomy fistula: mid-term results. *Surg Endosc.* 2015;**30**(10):4200–4.

Hamdan K, Somers S, Chand M. Management of late postoperative complications of bariatric surgery. *Br J Surgery.* 2011;**98**(10):1345–55.

Ma IT, Madura JA. Gastriointestinal complication after bariatric surgery. *Gastroenterol Hepatol(NY).* 2015;**11**(8): 526–35.

Masoomi H, Kim H, Reavis KM, et al. Analysis of factors predictive of gastrointestinal tract leak in laparscopic and open gastric bypass. *Arch Surg.* 2011;**146**(9):1048–51.

Nguyen NT, Rivers R, Wolfe BM. Early gastrointestinal haemorrhage after laparoscopic gastric bypass. *Obes Surg.* 2003;**13**(1):62–5.

O'Brien PE, MacDonald L, Anderson M, et al. Long-term outcomes after bariatric surgery: fifteen-year follow-up of adjustable gastric banding and a systematic review of the bariatric surgical literature. *Ann Surg.* 2013;**257**(1):87–94.

Snyder B, Wilson T, Mehta S, et al. Past, present, and future: critical analysis of use of gastric bands in obese patients. *Diabetes Metab Syndr Obes.* 2010;**3**:55–65.

Varban OA, Cassidy RB, Sheetz KH, et al. Technique or technology? Evaluating leaks after gastric bypass. *Surg Obes Relat Dis.* 2016;**12**(2):264–72.

Welbourn, R, Small P, Finlay I, et al.; NBSR Data Committee. *The National Bariatric Surgery Registry of the British Obesity and Metabolic Surgery Society – Second Registry Report.* London: British Obesity and Metabolic Surgery Society; 2014.

Anaesthesia for Bariatric Surgery

Jonathan Cousins and Christopher Bouch

Introduction

Obesity is an increasing global issue with approximately 600 million individuals affected in 2014. To date the only intervention that has consistently delivered sustained weight loss with reversal of co-morbidities is weight loss surgery.

This chapter reviews anaesthetic management of patients for weight loss surgery. Many chapters of this book relate to management of this unique patient group and the reader is referred to these as required.

Without question bariatric surgery should only be performed in appropriately staffed and equipped centres frequently performing these procedures. Attention to detail and a simple anaesthetic management approach beneficially influence the surgical outcomes seen.

Bariatric Data

The National Bariatric Surgery Register (NBSR) collates data for weight loss surgery in the UK. The most recent report for 2014 demonstrated that 16 956 operations were performed of which 95% were laparoscopic with an associated complication rate of 2.9% and in-hospital mortality of 0.07%.

Patient data 1 year post-surgery demonstrated loss of 58.4% of excess weight and 61% had complete resolution of sleep disordered breathing. After 2 years nearly 65% of type 2 diabetics progressed to a non-diabetic state.

Currently, little anaesthetic data is collected by the NBSR. It is likely in the future that anaesthetic data will be collected recognising the important component that anaesthesia plays in the team approach to peri-operative bariatric care.

Anaesthetic Management

Weight loss surgery is a low-risk procedure. This is achieved by an experienced, multidisciplinary team (MDT) approach to patient assessment and

optimisation as well as peri-operative care delivery. Care must be tailored to each patient and combined with early post-operative mobilisation with adherence to an enhanced recovery approach to facilitate good outcomes.

Currently in the UK there is no guidance on the minimum number of cases that should be undertaken annually by an anaesthetist to be deemed competent in the field of bariatric anaesthesia. Ideally anaesthetists who undertake weight loss procedures should have a special interest in this area and a regular commitment to these cases.

Pre-operative Management

Prior to any patient undergoing weight loss surgery there is a lengthy process of assessment and management to ensure patient optimisation and consent. This can take many months. The MDT includes dietitians, psychologists, metabolic physicians, surgeons and specialist weight loss nurses. Bariatric anaesthetists play an important role in this process, not only with assessment and management of co-morbidities, but planning the peri-operative period. In line with NECPOD and other reports, anaesthetists should always be a part of this process.

Questions that need to be addressed by the bariatric MDT include:

- Is the patient suitable for surgery?
- Is the patient motivated and well informed?
- What drug therapy is the patient receiving?
- What co-morbidities exist?
- Which co-morbidity can be further optimised?
- Is a higher level of post-operative care required?

These discussions may direct that more in-depth specialist review and investigations are appropriate, e.g. to cardiology, respiratory, endocrine, psychiatry/psychology. It is important that investigations are individualised to each patient, their co-morbidities and the type of procedure planned. Blanket or standard investigation requests are rarely useful and can result in patient harm/delay to surgery.

In addition to management of medical conditions, engagement of the patient and balancing their views and expectations with reality of the procedure planned is very important.

Airway Assessment

All obese patients need an airway assessment using standard clinical examination tools. It is a common misconception that obesity results in problematic airway management. Numerous studies have demonstrated no association between weight or BMI and difficult intubation. However, when managing the obese patient, airway caution is indicated as certain conditions can increase the risk of difficult bag-mask ventilation, including short obese neck, history of snoring, large tongue and presence of a beard. This is classically seen more frequently in males and the 'apple' distribution of fat in bariatric cases.

Respiratory Assessment

Obesity is associated with numerous pulmonary changes, including decreased lung and chest wall compliance, increased oxygen consumption and reduced FRC with encroachment upon closing capacity. As a result, dyspnoea from obesity is a common symptom. Assessment must aim to define the reason for shortness of breath; simple obesity with pulmonary changes or heart failure with potential pulmonary hypertension.

Sleep disordered breathing is present in approximately 70% of obese individuals presenting for weight loss surgery. This is commonly undiagnosed at presentation. General history and examination are poor tools, thus many screening and scoring systems exist. The STOP-BANG questionnaire is the most specific and easy to use screen. The addition of a venous bicarbonate level >28 mmol/l increases the sensitivity to a point where STOP-BANG (bicarbonate) may be used in local referral to sleep services to identify high risk cases.

Cigarette smoking is associated with adverse peri-operative events, including oxygen desaturation, poor wound healing, unplanned ITU admission, cardiac events and laryngospasm. All patients should therefore stop smoking pre-operatively. This forms part of the 'patient contract' between the treating team and the weight loss surgery patient. Studies suggest a minimum of 12 to 24 hours to improve oxyhaemoglobin levels, but an association with increased pulmonary complications implies cessation for greater than 4 weeks to deliver the best risk reduction overall.

Cardiovascular Assessment

The majority of obese patients are physically deconditioned, yet most can move their body frame through the activities of daily living. Their ability to exercise is limited by being obese and having co-existing cardiorespiratory changes or disease. In addition, social isolation due to societal views lead these individuals to withdraw behind closed doors and can result in loss of functional capacity.

Assessment of cardiovascular function should be based on functional capacity and ability to undertake activity. The ability to undertake at least 4 metabolic equivalents (METs) is considered to predict a reasonably low risk of a cardiovascular complication. This is the ability to walk up a hill or flight of stairs. The exact MET in obese individuals is undefined. A flight of stairs for a 200 kg man requires more METs than for an 80 kg man. A confounding factor is that some obese (high BMI) individuals may have a relatively low muscle mass – called sarcopenic obesity – these individuals may be a high risk sub-group and warrant special clinical evaluations.

There is potential for the use of cardiopulmonary exercise testing in those presenting for weight loss surgery. However, difficulties commonly related to obesity and equipment has proven problematic for a consistent approach. Data suggests the ability to achieve an anaerobic threshold of at least 11 ml/kg/min is associated with increased complications.

The patient who presents for surgery without any relevant history, but with functional limitation is a difficult scenario. Specialist cardiology assessment and investigation may be required to ensure true optimisation. Shortness of breath is a common symptom of obesity and is not always due to pathology. Pre-assessment should aim to identify those with heart failure and elucidating the primary cause to direct relevant therapy.

Emerging data suggests that the use of exercise training pre-operatively can reverse some deconditioning/sarcopenia and thus may improve perioperative outcomes. For the obese patient, when combined with continuing weight loss pre-operatively, this could be anticipated to facilitate improvements in cardiorespiratory function.

A high BMI patient with good exercise tolerance/ METs (high muscle mass) is different to the sarcopenic low muscle mass, more immobile, high BMI patient. Assessment to exclude occult cardiopulmonary disease is advised in the latter group, e.g. exercise testing and stress echocardiography

Hypertension is a common condition in obesity. Management should follow the national guidance for normal-weight individuals. Obesity-related hypertension is frequently resistant to mono-therapies and early escalation is appropriate.

All patients regardless of age should have a baseline ECG. Arrythmias and conduction defects are commonly identified at pre-assessment as common symptoms of these may be masked by obesity.

Obese individuals are at an increased risk of thomboembolic disease. It is important as part of assessment to identify those with a higher than normal risk, including a past history of thromboembolic disease, to facilitate investigation of any underlying prothrombotic disease. With simple protocolled therapies for VTE prophylaxis, low rates can be achieved. The UK NBSR database demonstrates VTE rates of less than 1%. The use of multiple prophylactic therapies: body-weight corrected doses of LMWH, use of pneumatic compression devices (and with less evidence, the use of graduated compressions stockings) combined with very early mobilisation all aid in delivering this low VTE rate.

Examination of peripheral venous anatomy can reveal potential issues with gaining venous access and can identify the rare occurrence that elective central venous access may need to be planned.

Metabolic Management

Diabetes mellitus is common in obesity. The pre-operative aim should be to achieve good glycaemic control as evidenced by blood glucose readings and HbA_1c. Exact targets vary between surgical units. However, there is no relation between pre-operative glucose control and long-term outcomes with bariatric surgery. An HbA_{1c} of less than 8.5% reflects good control. For some patients though, such idealistic control may be hard to achieve. In these cases, specialist diabetic physician management can prove useful. Ultimately, improved control can sometimes only be achieved with bariatric surgery and a balance of risk versus a delay for optimal therapy is required.

The metabolic syndrome is also common in obesity; for diagnosis it requires three of the following conditions:

- central obesity;
- systemic hypertension;
- raised triglycerides;
- impaired glucose tolerance/diabetes mellitus;
- low HDL-cholesterol.

The presence of this syndrome is associated with a significant increase in peri-operative morbidity and mortality for non-bariatric patients. In the bariatric population, risks are not increased with its presence. This likely reflects the pre-operative assessment and optimisation that occurs, requiring a coordinated, multidisciplinary approach to patient and pathology optimisation.

Intra-operative Management

The peri-operative period requires a good team approach to ensure a smooth course. It is vital to ensure that there are adequate, experienced team members present for the duration of the procedure and through the recovery period. All involved need to be aware of any potential issues, patient or otherwise, that relate to the proposed procedure and the obesity co-morbidities.

Equipment

Prior to commencing any weight loss surgery, it is essential to ensure that appropriate equipment is available for all aspects of care. An appropriate anaesthetic ventilator that can generate high inspiratory pressures and deliver appropriate levels of PEEP is required and advanced airway equipment that is immediately available to deal with difficult or failed intubations. Appropriate beds and operating tables, and devices to facilitate patient movement are also required.

Patient Positioning and Monitoring

All aspects of patient care should be undertaken in the operating room. There is no role for induction in the anaesthetic room and the transfer of an obese, anaesthetised patient into the operating room is ill advised. The risks of injury to patient and/or staff, oxygen desaturation with gas disconnection are obvious, with a risk of anaesthetic awareness included. These risks may be mitigated if the patient walks from ward to operating room and positions themselves on the operating table in a ramped, head-up position from the outset. This ideal position ensures the external auditory meatus is level with the manubrium sterni and delivers a comfortable patient position, whilst maintaining good lung volumes with increased apnoea to desaturation time. Additionally, this allows easier airway management with both bag-mask ventilation and tracheal intubation. Various commercial devices are available to assist in achieving this 'ramped' position. In the experience of the authors, appropriate positioning can easily be achieved by moving the operating table and use of pillows/towels.

Monitoring should conform to AAGBI standards. Difficulty can arise with blood-pressure cuff placement due to upper arm size. An easy and reliable solution to this, which avoids the use of intra-arterial pressure monitoring, is to place a normal size adult cuff on the forearm, which can be used throughout the hospital stay.

Bariatric procedures are performed in a steep head-up position to facilitate the surgical view. This presents the following anaesthetic challenges: safe ongoing management of the airway, venous pooling with a pneumoperitoneum affecting venous return and cardiac output, access to limb and central veins and pressure points and limb joint pressure in the near-standing position.

The operating table needs to be 'rated' for the weight of the patient in all positions, as this varies from a supine to a head-up position. Consideration must be given to the period of time that a patient will be motionless during surgery, as during this time perfusion to the lowermost skin, adipose and muscles may be compromised. In high weight cases, rhabdomyolysis may be noted after long surgery due to buttock area crush and reduced muscle perfusion. Appropriate mattress use whilst maintaining a high/normal perfusion pressure and limiting operating time is essential for prevention.

Vascular Access

Peripheral venous access can be difficult. Fat, particularly on the dorsum of the hand, is compressible and pressure applied here assists in unmasking venous structures. On occasion, unique sites can be used, e.g. anterior chest wall. With care, experience and patience, vascular access can be achieved in the majority of patients. It is always sensible to site two

intravenous cannulae prior to induction of anaesthesia. This provides security in the event of cannula 'tissuing'.

Ultimately, should peripheral venous access not be achievable, then central venous access is required. Thankfully this is a rare occurrence. If a possibility exists of ongoing access requirements then an elective peripherally inserted central catheter (PICC) line should be considered before surgery.

Induction and Maintenance of General Anaesthesia

There is no specific recipe for induction of general anaesthesia for weight loss surgery. After careful and considered pre-oxygenation, administration of an induction agent with a short-acting opiate and muscle relaxant would be routine. Drug doses should be based for the majority of agents on either IBW or LBW. Given the difficulty with drug dosing and the increased risk of awareness of obese patients at induction, a low threshold for using EEG/collated EEG systems like BIS or Entropy is advised.

Pre-oxygenation prior to induction of anaesthesia combined with ramped positioning should assist time to desaturation. The emerging technique of apnoeic oxygenation – THRIVE (transnasal humidified rapid insufflation ventilatory exchange) is increasingly adopted to assist in this aim.

The majority of anaesthetists in the UK maintain anaesthesia for weight loss surgery with a volatile agent, commonly desflurane or sevoflurane. Desflurane has a rapid excretion when administration ceases, with earlier recovery time of airway reflexes. Studies demonstrate that at discharge from the recovery room there is no difference between desflurane, sevoflurane and isoflurane. Of note, nitrous oxide is not routinely used due to risk of stomach and small bowel distension causing poor surgical views in an already apdipose-filled pneumoperitoneum and increased risk of post-operative nausea and vomiting.

Total intravenous anaesthesia is not commonly employed in bariatric surgery partly due to algorithms being unreliable in the obese patient.

Routine rapid sequence induction (RSI), whilst theoretically attractive in this patient group for a number of reasons, is not routinely employed unless a risk of regurgitation is pre-demonstrated.

Airway Management and Ventilation

For all bariatric surgical procedures, tracheal intubation is the only method. Alternative airway management may need to be utilised in the case of a failed intubation. Difficult Airway Society guidelines should be adhered to for optimum management in these thankfully rare cases. Airway management is straightforward in the majority of patients when facilitated by appropriate positioning and pre-oxygenation.

There is no role for a spontaneous breathing technique under general anaesthesia. Functional residual capacity (already reduced by the obese state) reduces by a further 50% with supine position and induction of general anaesthesia. This leads to development of atelectasis and shunting. These issues, combined with the pneumoperitoneum and the detrimental effects of any hypoxaemia, hypercapnia, pulmonary hypertension and right heart failure can lead to cardiorespiratory instability.

There is no best mode of ventilation. Attention to avoid large tidal volumes and the associated barotrauma with cyclical alveolar shearing force is paramount for lung protection. Tidal volumes of 6 ml/kg of ideal body weight and application of PEEP, after simple recruitment manoeuvres, seem to offer the best simple approach to minimising potential damage, whilst maintaining oxygen delivery, carbon dioxide removal and prevention of airspace collapse. The ideal level of PEEP is unknown. The international PROBESE trial (NCT02148692) is ongoing, comparing high versus low PEEP and recruitment manoeuvres in obese patients. The results of this study are awaited, but may shed more light on best management of PEEP in the obese patient. Current practice by most anaesthetists would be the use of between 5 and 10 cmH$_2$O PEEP for the duration of the surgical procedure.

Analgesia

The aim is to ensure patient comfort and promote early mobilisation. Most bariatric procedures are laparoscopic and as such do not result in significant post-operative discomfort. Peritoneal discomfort may present as: nausea, indigestion, shoulder pain, hypertension and irritability.

Sleep disordered breathing is of course common in the obese. This results in increased sensitivity to opioids, specifically the depressant effects on consciousness and respiratory function rather than the analgesic effects. Avoidance of these drugs or administration of short-acting agents is therefore preferred.

Optimal analgesic management should be multimodal and opioid sparing. This approach utilises paracetamol, NSAIDs and atypical agents, e.g. clonidine or ketamine, and should also continue in the post-operative period.

There is some evidence that pre-emptive analgesia can reduce post-operative pain scores. Gabapentin has received attention in this regard, but may precipitate undiagnosed sleep disorders or potentiate opioid side effects.

Local anaesthetic administration is a useful adjunct to the multimodal recipe. Skin infiltration is not generally useful. Local anaesthetic instilled into the peritoneal cavity may provide high-quality analgesia and reduce rescue opioid requirements. Intravenous administration of lidocaine as a bolus dose and continued as an infusion facilitates a true non-or low-opioid anaesthetic and its popularity is increasing for this group of patients, as it provides very good analgesia.

Simple, regular post-operative analgesia should be prescribed, e.g. paracetamol and NSAIDs. For breakthrough analgesia, sublingual sufentanil may have helpful drug qualities and is available as a simple PCA system. Opioid IV PCA systems are rarely seen outside of open surgery and often predict level 2 care post surgery.

Regional analgesia is essentially obsolete in bariatric practice, but intrathecal delivery is effective. Low post-operative pain levels are commonly obtained and the technical difficulties of neuraxial block, insertion and maintenance, frequently render this technique unattractive to the operator. The associated reduced need for urinary catheterisation and limitation of mobility are additional detractors to these blocks.

Transversus abdominus plane (TAP) blocks are described in some centres, but their true impact and difficulty in reliable insertion have seen a decline from widespread use.

Ultimately, the best way to reduce post-operative pain is to encourage the patient to mobilise and accept the post-surgery reality of peritoneal discomfort. This forms part of patient education at pre-assessment. At very high BMI levels, the abdominal wall and peritoneum do not move in awake spontaneous respiration, thus analgesic requirements can be far lower than otherwise anticipated.

Post-operative Care

At the end of the surgical procedure, tracheal extubation should occur after full reversal from neuromuscular paralysis. Blockade of the neuromuscular junction (NMJ) should be monitored in every case and consideration given to drugs of reversal. Many units consider a high BMI an indication for the use of sugammadex over neostigmine, but this is a local decision. The patient should be sitting up, fully awake and cooperative, with return of airway reflexes, prior to discharge from the operating room.

The location of post-operative care is determined by patient co-morbidities and procedure performed. Routine admission of patients to critical care post-weight-loss surgery based on their size has been demonstrated to be detrimental to their recovery and care by limitation of mobilisation and lack of high BMI facilities.

In the case of surgical units that undertake elective bariatric surgery in hospitals without critical care on site, there is no large increase in complications, however a clear escalation pathway to critical care is essential.

For the majority of bariatric surgical procedures with pre-operative identification and optimisation of co-morbidities, routine admission to a post-anaesthesia care unit area (PACU) is entirely appropriate. Factors that have been demonstrated to prolong recovery time include known hypertension, minimal prophylactic anti-emetics administered, and long surgical duration and open surgery.

Patients with more severe co-morbidities or complicated surgery will require a higher level of post-operative care and admission to a critical care unit is then appropriate.

Early identification of physiological changes and targeted management plans are required to facilitate a smooth post-operative course. The use of track and trigger systems should be routine. Any patient with persistent tachycardia or inability to maintain oxygen saturations should have immediate review and management. Early surgical intervention should be the standard approach and not a 'watch and wait' process. Re-laparoscopy is recommended at an early stage of clinical suspicion to exclude bleeding or anastomotic leak often masked by the physiological changes of morbid obesity.

Enhanced recovery protocols have major beneficial effects for the bariatric surgical population. The essence of these is to reduce pre-operative fasting times and in the post-operative period promote early mobilisation and feeding, avoiding excessive fluid administration and respiratory depressant drug administration. This is ideal for the bariatric patient, where an earlier return to independence is associated with reduced morbidity, safe/early discharge and reduced readmission rates.

Special Considerations Specific to Bariatric Surgery

Nasogastric Tubes/Drains

Some centres insert these after induction to drain gastric contents. Given their calibre, they may be inadvertently stapled by a surgical device, so a clear, careful agreed policy for insertion and removal are crucial to avoid this error. Many centres simply use an orogastric bougie to prevent this rare but serious complication.

Orogastric Bougie

Bariatric surgery involves the use of a bougie that allows the surgeon to visualise the size and calibre of the gastric pouch, allowing patency checks after construction and toileting/venting of the lumen undergoing stapling. This is a specific procedure in itself, often completed by the anaesthetist. It requires consideration and in some areas a specific consent due to the inherent risks. Bougie size is a local choice, but ranges from 28–34Ch commonly with some units even using 40Ch. These large devices are inserted under anaesthesia (blindly) and carry the risk of damage to any structure passed. Specific considerations include avoiding damage to the oesophagus, hiatus hernia and stomach itself, e.g. rupture of the thoracic oesophagus in a large hiatus hernia can be a fatal complication.

Leak Testing

Once surgical anastomoses are complete, usual practice is to 'leak test' them before concluding surgery. There are two techniques favoured by proponents, neither having evidence of greater effectiveness at detection of an occult leak over the other. In both, the distal segment of gut should be soft clamped. A saline leak test involves gravity pressured 50–100 ml of blue dyed saline passed down the oral or nasogastric tube and the surgeon checks for blue dye extrusion in the surgical field. A gas (oxygen) leak test involves the head-down/Trendelenburg position, instillation of saline over the surgical zone of interest and then pressurised oxygen being passed down the oral or nasogastric tube to reveal any gas leakage by bubbles. Following a leak test the anaesthetist must ensure gas or saline is adequately drained from the gut and the oropharynx is carefully suctioned to prevent aspiration at the end of anaesthesia.

Endoscopic Bariatric Procedures

Endoscopic weight loss procedures can be undertaken reasonably quickly, but without the physiological disturbance of laparoscopic intervention. The commonest procedure is insertion and removal of an intra-gastric balloon.

Intra-gastric balloon operations are day-case procedures. Most are performed under general anaesthesia or anaesthetic sedation for patient tolerance. There is little pain associated with insertion, but nausea due to the 600 ml balloon can be an issue. Administration of multiple anti-emetics and continuation of these in the post-operative period is required.

Further development of endoscope technology has facilitated the ability to suture and resulted in procedures such as endoscopic sleeve gastroplasty (ESG) that restrict stomach size.

ESG procedures cause some discomfort in the post-operative period. This does not usually require high-dose opiate administration. Similar to gastric balloon procedures, post-procedure nausea is a concern and appropriate multiple therapies must be given.

Revision Procedures

There has been an increase in patients presenting for revision of previous bariatric surgery. This is high-risk surgery due to patient expectations, complication rates – bleeding, bowel injury, stricture formation, to name a few. Surgery can be prolonged, so positioning and drug dosage need clear planning. It is very important to ensure optimisation and plan for predicted surgery. Post-operative care must be delivered by an experienced team with understanding of the potential surgical complications in an appropriate institution or area.

Surgery Post Weight Loss Surgery

It is increasingly common for patients who are post weight loss surgery to present for non-weight loss procedures. In very general terms insertion of naso-gastric tubes (NGTs) or probes should be avoided due to the risk of perforating the smaller stomach or displacing a gastric band. The exception to this would be the patient with acute abdomen or bowel obstruction, where the small stomach and anastomoses are at risk of rupture. In these instances, early NGT insertion can be life-saving.

Patients with a gastric band should not have this deflated when presenting for surgery. The risk of introducing infection is too high, unless there is a risk of vomiting or peri-operative aspiration.

Standard airway management for all post-weight-loss surgery patients should be tracheal intubation. There is a risk of reflux of gastric contents after gastric band and sleeve surgery, and development of a silent mega-oesophagus with the presence of a gastric band. Reflux or oesophageal dysmotility may require induction of anaesthesia with RSI to prevent risk of aspiration.

In general, non-weight-loss surgery in patients with a gastric bypass should not result in increased risk of reflux. However, assessment of nutritional status is important pre-operatively.

Key Points

1. A multidisciplinary team approach is required for weight loss surgery.
2. Pre-operative assessment and optimisation is paramount.
3. A multimodal analgesic technique is best to minimise opioid use.
4. Routine critical care admission is not required.
5. Application of enhanced recovery protocol is advantageous.

Further Reading

Abdullah HR, Chung F. Perioperative management for the obese patient. *Curr Opin Anesthesiol.* 2014;**27**(6): 576–82.

Alvarez A, Singh P, Sinha A. Postoperative analgesia in morbid obesity. *Obes Surg.* 2014;**24**: 652–9.

Awad S, Carter S, Purkayastha S, et al. Enhanced recovery after bariatric surgery (ERABS): clinical outcomes from a tertiary referral bariatric centre. *Obes Surg.* 2014;**24**: 753–8.

Carron M, Veronese S, Foletto M, et al. Sugammadex allows fast-track bariatric surgery. *Obes Surg.* 2013;**23**: 1558–63.

De Baerdemaeker L, Margarson M. Best Anaesthetic drug strategy for morbidly obese patients. *Curr Opinion Anaesthesiol.* 2016;**29**:119–28.

Fernandez-Bustamante A, Hashimoto S, Neto A, et al. Perioperative lung protective ventilation in obese patients. *Anaesthesiology.* 2015;**15**: 56.

Gildasio S, Kenyon D, Fitzgerald P, et al. Systemic lidocaine to improve quality of recovery after laparoscopic bariatric surgery: a randomised double-blind placebo controlled trial. *Obes Surg.* 2014;**24**:212–18.

Hodgson LE, Murphy BM, Hart N. Respiratory management of the obese patient undergoing surgery. *J Thorac Dis.* 2015;**7**(5):943–52.

Lemanu D, Srinivasa S, Singh P, et al. Optimizing perioperative care in bariatric surgery patients. *Obes Surg.* 2012;**22**:979–90.

Morgan DJR, Kwok MH. A comparison of bariatric surgery in hospitals with and without ICU: a linked data cohort study. *Obes Surg.* 2016;**26**:313–20.

Schulmeyer M, De la Maza J, Ovalle C, et al. Analgesic effect of a single dose of pregablin after laparoscopic sleeve gastrectomy. *Obes Surg.* 2010;**20**:1678–81.

Ushma S, Wong J, Wong T, et al. Preoxygenation and intraoperative ventilation strategies in obese patients: a comprehensive review. *Curr Opin Anaesthetsiol.* 2016;**29**: 109–18.

Weingarten TN, Hawkins NM, Beam WB, et al. Factors associated with prolonged anesthesia recovery following laparoscopic bariatric surgery: a retrospective analysis. *Obes Surg.* 2015;**25**:1024–30.

Chapter

39

Management of Patients Post Bariatric Surgery

David Bowrey, Tom Palser and Melanie Paul

As with other facets of surgery, the peri-operative management of the patient undergoing bariatric surgery requires dedicated attention from staff familiar with this patient group. A specialist nurse-led service is imperative, both as a point of contact for the patient throughout their pre-hospital journey and to ensure delivery of any enhanced recovery protocols while in hospital. Knowledge of the practical aids to assist the recuperation of this patient group are key.

Most patients can be safely admitted on the day of surgery. A clear explanation of what the inpatient journey will look like helps patients prepare for their stay. This information should be provided to patients in advance of their surgery.

This chapter considers, for the most part, the normal or usual care pathway followed by patients after surgery and what to look out for, to indicate that something is amiss. The recommendations are based largely on the authors' personal practice, accepting that there is no strong evidence base for the majority of clinical management, and that practice evolves continuously. Most patients currently have a 23-hour stay after sleeve gastrectomy or gastric banding, and a 48-hour stay after gastric bypass.

The patient care plan (Figure 39.1) should address each of observations, diet, medications, patient care, investigations and ancillary reviews.

Antibiotics

There is limited evidence of the utility of antibiotic prophylaxis for surgical site infection. It is common practice to administer a single dose of a broad spectrum antibacterial at the time of surgery, to patients undergoing gastric bypass, on the basis of greater potential contamination compared to other types of weight loss surgery. No antibiotic therapy is given to patients undergoing gastric banding or sleeve gastrectomy.

Thromboprophylaxis

All patients should wear anti-embolism stockings from the time of admission until fully ambulant at home. Intermittent pneumatic compression devices are employed during surgery. Low molecular weight heparin is administered at a dose of 5000 IU or 7500 IU, depending on patient weight. This is continued for 14 days after discharge. Selected patients triaged to be at higher risk, e.g. a previous history of venous thromboembolism continue pharmacological thromboprophylaxis for 30 days.

Urinary Catheter

It is not routine practice to place a urinary catheter in patients undergoing weight loss surgery. However, in selected patients, it may be necessary due to the length of the procedure, especially revisional surgery. The catheter is removed at the end of the procedure. In general, placement of a catheter discourages early mobilisation and prolongs hospital stay.

Nasogastric Tube

It is usual to place a nasogastric or orogastric tube at the time of surgery to decompress the stomach of air and fluid. The tube is either removed completely to ensure its absence from the stomach during stapling, or if an air or methylene blue leak test is planned at the end of the procedure, the tube is withdrawn into the oesophagus. Unless there have been intra-operative problems with the anastomosis, the nasogastric or orogastric tube is removed before the patient is extubated.

Post-operative Analgesia

At the end of the procedure a local anaesthetic admixture comprising lidocaine 1% and levobupivacaine 0.5% is instilled into the peritoneal cavity over the site of the surgery and beneath each hemidiaphragm. Intravenous analgesics, avoiding opiates, are administered

OBSERVATIONS
- Record observations every hour for 8 hours **THEN** every 2 hours as a minimum

ACTIVITY
- Get out of bed within 2 hours of returning to ward
- Walk around the ward every hour during the day
- Ensure head of bed is greater than 30°
- Flexion/ extension exercises every hour while awake for prevention of DVT

DIET
- Operation day – 60 ml water or coloured fluid/hour
- Day 1 – Commence Complan regime.
- If patient unable to tolerate Complan on day 1, offer milk or Fortijuce instead.

MEDICATION
- Ensure patient is prescribed liquid/crushable/soluble or sublingual medication
- Refer to surgical medication review (attached to drug chart)
- Dalteparin 5000 units daily while in hospital, to continue for 2 weeks after discharge
- Regular ondansetron sublingually
- Lansoprazole oro-dispersible 30 mg daily. To continue for 2 months after discharge
- Forceval Soluble daily (for gastric bypass patients only), to be taken lifelong
- Appropriate analgesia – avoid opiates

PATIENT CARE
- Strict intake and output chart every 4 hours
- Wound drain to stay until day of discharge
- NGT removed at end of procedure unless having CPAP
- Administer oxygen if required
- Maintain SPO_2 above 92%
- Cough and deep breath every hour while awake
- If diabetic, monitor blood glucose every 2 hours
- Ensure VTE stockings are worn daily
- AVOID CPAP IN FIRST 48 HOURS POST-OPERATIVELY. IF CPAP NECESSARY, RETAIN NGT FOR 48 HOURS
- Ensure early warning score (EWS) is recorded within 2 hours prior to discharge and is <2

INVESTIGATIONS
- Post-op bloods on day 1

REFERRALS
- Refer to physiotherapist first day post-op
- If diabetic review by diabetic team prior to discharge

If patient is well discharge home on Day 2 post-op.

Figure 39.1 Gastric bypass/sleeve gastrectomy post-operative pathway

intra-operatively and are continued in oral format for the first 5 days. Non-steroidal anti-inflammatory agents are given for the first three days. The use of opiate patient-controlled analgesia is avoided as it is associated with reduced mobility and a longer hospital stay.

Observations

Hourly observations, with calculation of the early warning score (EWS), are undertaken for the first 8 hours, reducing to 2 hourly after that for hours 8–24, then 4 hourly. Use of the early warning scoring systems facilitates prompt recognition of change from baseline. Minor aberrations in the early warning score (scores of between 1 and 3) are common in the first 24 hours after surgery. Most patients experience an uneventful post-operative recovery.

Causes for Concern

These include aberrations in the early warning score, in excess of 3. These should prompt clinical review by a senior member of the surgical team (registrar grade or above). Early cross-sectional imaging is advised with a low threshold for repeat laparoscopy if any abnormality is demonstrated on imaging. The principal hazard in the first 24 hours is intra-abdominal bleeding from the short gastric vessels (gastric bypass or sleeve gastrectomy) or the staple line (sleeve gastrectomy). Anastomotic leak is rare and typically manifests after 48 hours or later (gastric bypass). Staple line leak after sleeve gastrectomy typically manifests 2–3 weeks after hospital discharge. Clinical examination is less reliable in morbidly obese patients, so the conventional signs of tenderness associated with peritonitis may be absent or diminished, due to the distance of the peritoneum from the anterior abdominal wall. The threshold for obtaining an oral contrast study is lower than in the non-bariatric patient cohort, and would be indicated with what might be considered subtle signs such as deterioration in pain scores, left upper quadrant or shoulder tip pain or reduced oxygen saturations.

Mobilisation

Pre-operative patient counselling about what is expected in relation to mobilisation is vital. Patients are mobilised on the day of their surgery, within 2 hours of returning to the ward. During the daytime, patients are expected to walk around their bed space and ward at least every hour.

Drain Placement

A suction drain is typically left at the level of the anastomosis or staple line. This is kept in place and removed just before the patient is discharged home. Its main purpose is to evacuate any wash fluid and as an indicator of a problem such as a leak or bleed.

Causes for concern

The presence of clotted blood in the drain should prompt imaging to exclude a haematoma. Signs of a leak include the presence of turbid fluid or frank gastro-intestinal contents in the drain or a greater volume of fluid than usual (>100 ml daily).

Oral Intake and Diet

Oral intake should be recommended as soon as the patient has recovered from the anaesthetic. A common approach is to start patients on 60 ml fluid hourly on the day of surgery, and then commence an unrestricted oral fluid regimen on the first post-operative day. As with early mobilisation, pre-operative counselling about what is expected from an oral intake point of view is vital. Patients are reviewed on the ward by the dietitian or nurse specialist and discharged home on a liquid/pureed diet for the first 4 weeks, with the goal of providing 2000 ml of fluid and 60 g of protein daily. A soft diet is started during week five and then, more textured foods are re-commenced in week seven after the surgery. At this point, the intention is for patients to consume 60 g protein daily and between 800 and 1200 kcal/day.

Antacid Medications

Because of the theoretical risk of stomal or staple line ulceration, patients are routinely discharged home on a once-daily proton pump inhibitor for the first two months after surgery.

Review of Existing Medications

Where feasible all medications are switched to a dispersible or suspension format for the first month after surgery. No dose modifications are required for patients undergoing gastric banding or sleeve gastrectomy. Patients undergoing gastric bypass may require dosage modifications to those medications absorbed preferentially in the upper small intestine.

Special Considerations

Diabetes Mellitus

Patients receiving oral hypoglycaemic agents should stop their medication on the evening before surgery. Typically, these patients will not require any therapy during their hospital stay. Patients requiring insulin as part of their usual treatment should take 50% of their usual dose the evening before surgery and have a sliding scale insulin-glucose infusion established on the day of surgery. Conversion to subcutaneous insulin the day after surgery is in accordance with blood glucose levels, but will often be 50% of pre-surgery requirements. Review by the diabetic team is mandatory prior to hospital discharge.

Sleep Disordered Breathing

Patients who require continuous positive airways pressure (CPAP) support have their CPAP face mask applied in the theatre recovery. In these patients, consideration should be taken of leaving a nasogastric tube in place to prevent air distention of the gastric pouch (sleeve gastrectomy, gastric bypass). This is removed on the second day after surgery.

Anti-coagulation

Patients who receive oral anti-coagulation should have a bridging plan agreed with the anti-coagulation service in advance of their admission. It is usual to switch to therapeutic low molecular weight heparin for the first month after surgery, and re-commence oral anti-coagulants after that time. Warfarin dosage is typically one-third lower than pre-operative requirements in the initial months.

Vitamin and Trace Element Supplementation

It is advisable to routinely screen for micronutrient deficiencies in advance of surgery and correct any aberrations. There is emerging evidence that bone mineral density is better preserved if vitamin D levels are normalised prior to surgery. No specific supplementation is required after gastric banding. Patients undergoing sleeve gastrectomy or gastric bypass should take a combined multivitamin, calcium, iron and vitamin D supplement indefinitely after surgery. Patients who have undergone gastric bypass should also have 3-monthly vitamin B12 injections. Patients who have undergone sleeve gastrectomy should either be screened for vitamin B12 deficiency or have scheduled replacement, as up to a third will demonstrate deficiency during follow-up. All patients after weight loss surgery should have annual screening blood tests, including full blood count and haematinics, bone profile, including vitamin D, parathyroid hormone, vitamin and trace elements, and any deficiencies treated on an ad hoc basis. Patients who have undergone limb gastric bypass or duodenal switch will also require supplementation with fat-soluble vitamins.

Activity and Return to Work

The general advice given to patients after surgery is in line with that given to patients having other laparoscopic procedures. Typically, patients are able to perform administrative tasks the day of discharge from hospital, but they are not able to perform heavy manual work for several weeks. Patients are advised to refrain from driving for 1 week after surgery and to plan on taking at least 3 weeks off work. In practice, many patients require 1–3 weeks longer off work, depending on the flexibility of their work and their employer.

Post-discharge Follow-up

Patients are contacted by telephone within the first 2 weeks by either the nurse specialist or dietitian and any queries addressed. Adjusting to the reduced gastric pouch size is often a struggle for patients in the first few weeks after surgery. Reassurance is required that this is a normal part of the recovery process. Surgical review is typically 6 weeks after surgery to assess the surgical wounds and give advice on building up exercise. Gastric bands are filled for the first time 6 weeks after placement. It is common to experience discomfort in the operating port used for specimen extraction (sleeve gastrectomy) or for anastomosis (gastric bypass) if a circular stapler has been used. This port will require a larger fascial defect than the other operating ports, that will require closure to prevent incisional herniation. The transfascial sutures typically used to close these ports tend to cause a pulling sensation, as is common with laparoscopic incisional hernia repairs. Avoiding overtightening of the suture material may reduce the associated discomfort. Patients should have a surgical review on the first and second anniversaries of their surgery to assess co-morbidities resolution and to address any queries. Dietetic follow-up is timed to fall in the intervals between surgical reviews with additional open-access clinic appointments provided on an ad hoc basis.

Causes for Concern

Gastric Banding

Patients who report new onset reflux symptoms, dysphagia or vomiting require urgent evaluation to ensure that they have not experienced band slippage or to determine whether band deflation is required. A drop-in body mass index below 25 kg/m^2 likewise merits further investigation.

Sleeve Gastrectomy

Reflux symptoms may be exacerbated after this procedure and for this reason, a gastric bypass is the preferred procedure for an obese patient with significant reflux. Up to 10% of patients develop de novo reflux symptoms after sleeve gastrectomy. If not controlled with antacid medications, conversion to gastric bypass may be required.

Gastric Bypass

The development of abdominal pain after eating should be investigated to exclude stomal ulceration or internal herniation. The former can be confirmed endoscopically, the latter by cross-sectional imaging.

Physical Exercise

Patients are encouraged to incorporate physical activity into their weekly routine. This is especially relevant for patients beyond the first year when late weight regain can occur. Use of a structured activity programme at this time point, comprising moderate intensity exercise for three times weekly is associated with improved metabolic parameters and better weight control.

Summary

The majority of patients experience a predictable uneventful journey through their bariatric surgery. An important component of planning surgery includes careful information-giving to the patients about what is expected of them when in hospital. The use of standardised care pathways facilitates earlier discharge from hospital and potentially an earlier return to normal activities.

Further Reading

Aminian A, Andalib A, Khorgami Z, et al. Who should get extended thromboprophylaxis after bariatric surgery. *Ann Surg.* 2017;**265**:143–50.

Badaoui R, Alami Chentoufi Y, Hchikat A, et al. Outpatient laparoscopic sleeve gastrectomy: first 100 cases. *J Clin Anesth.* 2016;**34**:85–90.

British Obesity and Metabolic Surgery Society. *GP Guidance: Management of Nutrition Following Bariatric Surgery*; 2014. www.bomss.org.uk/nutritional-guidelines/ (accessed May 2018).

El Chaar M, Stoltzfus J, Claros L, Wasylik T. IV acetaminophen results in lower hospital costs and emergency room visits following bariatric surgery: a double-blind, prospective, randomized trial in a single accredited bariatric center. *J Gastrointest Surg.* 2016;**20**: 715–24.

Eltweri AM, Bowrey DJ, Sutton CD, Graham L, Williams RN. An audit to determine if vitamin B12 is necessary after sleeve gastrectomy. *SpringerPlus* 2013;**2**:218.

Herring LY, Stevinson C, Carter P, et al. The effects of supervised exercise training 12–24 months after bariatric surgery on physical function and body composition: a randomised controlled trial. *Int J Obes.* 2017;**41**:909–16.

Herring LY, Stevinson C, Davies MJ, et al. Changes in physical activity behaviour and physical function after bariatric surgery: a systematic review and meta-analysis. *Obes Rev.* 2016;**17**:250–61.

Kalarchian MA, Marcus MD, Courcoulas AP, Cheng Y, Levine MD. Self-report of gastrointestinal side effects after bariatric surgery. *Surg Obes Relat Dis.* 2014;**10**:1202–7.

Lemanu DP, Singh PP, Berridge K, et al. Randomized clinical trial of enhanced recovery versus standard care after laparoscopic sleeve gastrectomy. *Br J Surg* 2013;**100**:482–9.

O'Kane M, Barth JH. Nutritional follow-up of patients after obesity surgery: best practice. *Clin Endocrinol.* 2016;**84**: 658–61.

Parretti HM, Hughes CA, O'Kane M, Woodcock S, Pryke RG. Ten top tips for the management of patients post-bariatric surgery in primary care. *J Obes* 2015;**1**:68–73.

Paediatric Bariatric Surgery and Anaesthesia

N. Durkin, S. Noor, Ashish Desai and Meera Kurup

Childhood Obesity: Defining the Problem

Childhood obesity is increasingly a global issue with the prevalence in the UK one of the highest in Europe. The Health Survey for England began collecting annual data on childhood obesity from the 1990s, which demonstrated a constant increase in the prevalence of obesity by 1% every 2 years. The National Child Measurement Programme (NCMP) was established in 2006 to formally measure the weight of all children in state school at two time points. In 2014–2015, over one million measurements were taken, which represented 95% of the eligible population with staggering results; 21.9% of children aged 4–5 were classified as overweight or obese, a figure which rose to one-third (33.2%) of 10–11 year olds. Over recent years this appears to be a trend, which is plateauing, although there is no convincing evidence that it is declining. Unsurprisingly, there is also a considerable health inequality with regards to social deficit, with prevalence for children living in the most deprived areas double that of those living in the least deprived areas. Sadly, this is a disparity that is continually increasing. A recent government White Paper highlighted that if the trends continued, 60% of men, 50% of women and 25% of all children would be obese by 2050.

Terminology

Defining obesity in children presents slightly different challenges to that in adults. The body mass index (BMI) provides a relatively good gauge of body fat, whilst being easy to measure and calculate. Standardised levels of BMI classify obesity in adults; if the BMI >30 kg/m^2 this is considered obese. Children have varying proportions of body fat at varying ages, which also differs depending on gender. As such, fixed levels of BMI provide inaccurate comparisons.

In children, BMI growth charts of large referenced populations are used. These are gender and age specific and also consider the pattern of growth over time. In the UK, the UK90 is the growth chart used for clinical assessment and monitoring using BMI Z-scores, a measure of how many standard deviations a child's BMI is above (or below) the mean. The UK90 provides centile curves for British children from birth to 23 years based on measurements of over 30 000 children between 1978 to 1994. Using NICE guidance, a child on the 91st–98th centile is considered overweight, and obese if on or above the 98th centile. Since the initial UK90, the curve has shifted to the right, indicating that as a whole the population is heavier than it was 20 years ago. Other growth references available include the International Obesity Task Force (IOTF), Centres for Disease Control and WHO growth references. These are infrequently used in the UK, however they can be used to make international comparison of obesity prevalence.

Rationale for Surgery in Adolescents

The increased prevalence of adolescent obesity has been paralleled by an increased incidence of associated co-morbidities. Specifically, obese children are at risk of metabolic syndrome. This constellation of glucose resistance, hypertension and high cholesterol predisposes to long-term sequelae of cardiovascular disease, which has now been observed in practice. A recent retrospective review with over 6000 children found a strong association between obesity and further co-morbidities, including hypertension, diabetes and asthma. The link between childhood obesity and diabetes mellitus is exacerbated by physiology: growth itself creates a relative insulin resistance that makes adolescents more vulnerable to developing diabetes. Non-alcoholic fatty liver disease (NAFLD), gallstones and orthopaedic complications such as slipped upper femoral epiphysis (SUFE) in childhood have also been attributed to obesity.

It has become clear that adolescent obesity is strongly associated with severe obesity in adulthood. As such, these children are experiencing obesity-associated co-morbidities at even earlier ages. A follow-up study over 53 years, from Harvard, demonstrated an increased relative risk of all-cause mortality from coronary heart disease. The consequences for psychosocial wellbeing are also not to be underestimated. Multiple studies have demonstrated significant reductions in global self-esteem and quality of life in obese youths that fluctuates relative to weight. These children have also been found to have lower attainment in education and training.

The rising incidence of obesity-associated co-morbidities at a younger age also has a financial implication. Currently, obesity has been estimated to cost the NHS £5.1 billion each year. In an increasingly stretched NHS, this is 5–6% of the total budget. The current cost to society has been estimated at £16 billion, 1% of our GDP, which is forecast to rise to £50 billion by 2050. Why not, then, make a sustained intervention prior to the development of these co-morbidities and their complications? Whilst primary prevention is clearly the best solution, community-based interventions have yet to demonstrate significant and definitive positive results. Childhood obesity is, therefore, a growing problem worth treating at an early stage and as such has evolved into an increasingly surgical issue.

Eligibility Criteria: NICE Guidelines, Assessment and the Role of the MDT

Patient selection is key and surgery is only considered in exceptional circumstances. Children identified at risk in the community are referred from their general practitioner to a lifestyle weight management programme. The main aim of these programmes involves maintaining the child's existing weight as they grow taller, which can lead to a significant reduction in BMI. Should community-based measures not make a sustained improvement, adolescents are referred to a Tier 3 centre comprising professionals who specialise in adolescent weight management. BMI Z-scores >3.0 standard deviations from the mean for pre-pubertal children or a BMI >35 kg/m^2 in post-pubertal children are generally considered at highest risk. All potential surgical patients undergo medical evaluation by a paediatric endocrinologist. Initial assessment involves an understanding of:

1. history of weight excess;
2. risk factors;
3. activity;
4. diet;
5. history of weight loss surgery in family;
6. complication and co-morbidity screening including menstrual history;
7. past medical history;
8. birth history;
9. family and social history;
10. examination, including anthropometric measurements and behaviour.

Further essential components include a comprehensive psychological, educational, family and social assessment performed by a specialist psychologist or psychiatrist with exclusion of eating disorders; a contraindication to surgery. A trained paediatric bariatric dietitian establishes eating patterns and behaviours using a food diary. They advise the patient and their family on healthy eating and post-operative requirements. The entire assessment process does not have a defined time scale; however, it may take 6–12 months.

If medical management in a Tier 3 centre fails to make a sustained improvement, the patient is offered surgical intervention. The decision to refer for surgery is one taken by the whole MDT and is only done once co-morbidities have also been established. This involves a combination of the following investigations:

1. cardiovascular examination including blood pressure;
2. oral glucose tolerance testing, insulin levels and HbA1c;
3. Fasting bloods including:
   a. cholesterol and triglycerides;
   b. ferritin, folate, vitamin D and B1, with appropriate supplementation if deficiency found;
   c. thyroid stimulating hormone and T4;
   d. follicle-stimulating hormone (FSH), luteinising hormone (LH), testosterone, free androgen index;
   e. liver function;
4. ultrasound liver to assess for evidence of NAFLD and gallstones.
5. psychological assessment: Child Anxiety and Depression Scale, Rosenburg Self Esteem Scale;
6. sleep study.

NICE guidance states that adolescent bariatric surgery should only be offered if the BMI is >40 kg/m^2 or >35 kg/m^2 with significant co-morbidities that would improve with weight loss. Age of surgery is an important consideration. In adults, calorie restriction and subsequent metabolic changes following bariatric surgery result in a reduced metabolic rate, muscle wasting and nutritional deficiencies. Children undergoing bariatric surgery undergo all these changes with the superimposed effect of increased growth hormone resistance and subsequent growth failure. Additionally, vitamin D depletion results in bone demineralisation. As such, UK bariatric surgery is predominantly offered to those who have achieved or nearly achieved physiological maturity to ensure they have finished bone growth. The additional ethical consideration of whether bariatric surgery at a pre- or peri-pubertal age respects the child's autonomy is yet to be established.

The bariatric surgeon can be either adult or paediatric trained in specifically performing adolescent bariatric surgery. Plastic surgical procedures such as apronectomy may be necessary in due course and it is advantageous if this is an established service in the tertiary hospital. Other than the correct team members, the centre must also have the appropriate equipment to care for paediatric bariatric patients, including scales, theatre table, hoists, pressure-relieving mattresses and staff skilled in using this equipment.

Practical Considerations

Procedure and Consent

Of all bariatric procedures, only two are predominantly performed in adolescents; sleeve gastrectomy and gastric bypass. The operative procedures are discussed in other chapters and are the same as in adults. The procedure is decided in conjunction with the patient and their family, taking into consideration the degree of obesity, co-morbidity, effectiveness and risks of the procedure, including surgeon experience. There is a predilection for sleeve gastrectomy as there is potential to convert this to a gastric bypass in the future if the primary operation is not successful. Potential excess weight loss is the same as that in adults and quoted to be 50–60% with gastric sleeve and 60–70% with bypass surgery.

If aged 16 to 17, the patient is presumed to have sufficient capacity to consent. Those under 16 can also consent if considered to have enough intelligence, competence and understanding to fully appreciate the procedure and its risks (Gillick competence). An assessment of the understanding and expectations of the operation itself and post-operative course are usually assessed in depth prior to surgery by a clinical psychologist, which can further be used to guide the clinician.

Operative Set-up

If mobile, patients should be encouraged to walk to the operating theatre and transfer themselves onto the operating table. Due to the risk of pressure damage to tissues, self-positioning should be encouraged. Areas where binders, supports or equipment are in contact with the patient should be assessed throughout surgery, as in adult patients. Children with associated bone disease (achondroplasia/osteogenesis imperfecta) need special care during positioning to avoid inadvertent fracture.

Once anaesthetised, a urethral catheter is inserted for close monitoring of urine output post-operatively. Single dose, standard, broad-spectrum antibiotics are given at induction and continued for approximately 5 days. An intermittent pneumatic device and thromboembolic disease (TED) stockings are positioned to reduce the risk of venous thromboembolism.

Intra-operative Anaesthetic Considerations

Airway Optimisation

Obstructive sleep apnoea (OSA) is a common condition in children, but particularly in those who are obese. Obese children are at increased risk of airway complications in the peri-operative period, including difficult mask ventilation, desaturation and hypoventilation. Literature reveals an increased incidence of respiratory adverse events in obese children and that bronchospasm, although not raised in obesity alone, is associated with OSA. Use of positioning pillows and head supports can aid induction and allow for improved ventilation and tracheal intubation conditions intra-operatively. Pre-oxygenation in a head-up/sitting-up position is followed routinely. Once full neuromuscular paralysis is obtained tracheal intubation occurs.

Monitoring and Access

As there may be difficulties in monitoring non-invasive blood pressure (NIBP), consideration of invasive monitoring is needed. For the majority of patients NIBP monitoring is achievable, especially when placed in the distal portion of the limb. Peripheral intravenous access using a mid-length cannula can be helpful, since short-length cannulas can be easily displaced.

Pain Management

Pain management is a challenge in obese children; those with OSA have reduced sensitivity to carbon dioxide and increased sensitivity to the respiratory depressant effects of opiates. These children require post-operative oxygen supplementation and monitoring of oxygen saturations. Judicious opioid therapy should therefore be provided. Our institution follows the regime of intravenous patient-controlled analgesia for a minimum of the initial 24 hours post-operatively. Regular paracetamol and ibuprofen is prescribed unless contraindications exist.

Drug Dosing

Drug dosing is critical in paediatric care and knowledge of pharmacokinetics essential. Most commonly used anaesthetic drugs are dosed on lean body weight (LBW) including muscle relaxants, although suxamethonium is based on total body weight (TBW), see Table 40.1.

Table 40.1 Drug dosing for paediatric anaesthesia

Drug	Dosing weight
Fentanyl	Corrected weight = LBW + (0.4 × excess body weight)
Alfentanil	LBW
Morphine	LBW
Remifentanil	LBW
Propofol	Induction: LBW Maintenance: TBW or LBW + (0.4 × excess weight)
Thiopentone	LBW
Midazolam	TBW for initial dose Infusion: LBW
Atracurium	TBW
Cisatracurium	TBW
Suxamethonium	TBW
Rocuronium	LBW
Paracetamol	LBW
Neostigmine	TBW

Immediate Post-operative Care

The majority of patients have a planned admission to the paediatric high-dependency unit for the initial 24 hours post-operatively for monitoring of respiratory, cardiovascular and renal function. Children who are already on CPAP as a treatment for OSA can be prescribed CPAP up to 10 cmH$_2$O. Post-operative physiotherapy and incentive spirometry is essential to reduce the risk of lower respiratory tract infections.

A pressure-relieving mattress is used with intermittent pneumatic devices and graduated compression stockings in situ. The use of low molecular weight heparin (LMWH) with weight-dependent dosing further reduces the risk of post-operative thrombosis.

Nasogastric tubes are not routinely required and are actively discouraged due to undue pressure on the anastomosis. However, post-operative nausea and vomiting must be treated vigorously, as this can place undue stress on the suture line. Management of intake is protocolled over the following 8 weeks and managed by adolescent bariatric dietitians.

Long-term Follow-up

Long-term follow-up is essential to the success of the procedure. Surgical follow-up is at 6 weeks with additional regular dietitian review. On discharge, multivitamins are prescribed along with urosdeoxycholic acid (UDCA) for 6 months. LMWH is administered for a further 4 weeks with TED stockings. Vitamin B12 is not routinely given unless it is low. Full blood count, urea and electrolytes, liver function and blood coagulation tests, lipid profile, zinc, calcium, glucose, ferritin, folate and B12 are monitored annually and replaced as appropriate.

Results

Paediatric bariatric surgery is a relatively new subspeciality and results are only now becoming available. The UK National Bariatric Surgery Registry was established in 2010 and provides nationwide analysis of patients undergoing bariatric surgery in the UK, including the first record of adolescent bariatric cases. Over 3 years (2011–2013), 62 patients aged 18 and under were reported to have undergone bariatric surgery, including a child as young as 12. The gender disparity frequently seen in the adult population is reflected in paediatrics; 77% were in girls. This data also demonstrates that for those in the <25 age group, BMI at initial operation was fairly comparable to that of older patients with 39.5% already in the super-obese category, with a BMI >50 kg/m². This highlights a very real concern that even at such a young age, these patients already had a comparable BMI to their adult peers, indicating that preventative measures are currently not working to tackle obesity.

Currently this database does not provide specific outcome data for the adolescent population or information on which operations are being performed in the UK. The largest UK series published included six patients whose Z-score fell from +4.4 to +3.1 at 2 years with no procedural complications and associated resolution of hypertension, no progression to diabetes and improved school attendance found.

The majority of long-term results of adolescent bariatric surgery have therefore come from the USA; from the teen-LABS consortium. Prospectively collected data on 242 adolescent patients with a mean age of 17.6 and BMI of 53 was analysed. In this cohort, the mean weight of patients decreased by 28% with gastric bypass and 26% with sleeve gastrectomy. This was a result that was sustained after 3 years. Convincing improvements were made in obesity-related co-morbidities; remission of diabetes was seen in 95% of patients, with similar improvements in those with abnormal kidney function (86%), dyslipidaemia (66%) and hypertension (74%). During the 30-day post-operative period, 8% of patients suffered a major complication, and 15% a minor complication, with no mortality seen. Over 3 years follow-up, 13% underwent one or more additional intra-abdominal procedure. Further work by this group has demonstrated improvements in musculoskeletal pain and mobility.

These results have been repeated in many smaller cohorts, e.g. Saudi Arabia and Sweden. In all studies, quality of life was recorded as considerably improved.

Summary

The rising prevalence of morbid obesity in children and adolescents is a growing concern. Increasing evidence is now emerging to suggest that this is associated with significant co-morbidity, which can be reversible. Operative management can help achieve this; however, aggressive holistic management is required to support the success of the surgery alone. Although long-term data is still not available, the above results appear to justify performing surgery in a select patient group. They demonstrate that bariatric surgery can be both a safe and efficacious therapy for treating adolescent obesity and its co-morbidities, and in the right patient, can be life changing.

Further Reading

Alqahtani AR, Elahmedi MO, Al Qahtani A. Co-morbidity resolution in morbidly obese children and adolescents undergoing sleeve gastrectomy. *Surg Obes Relat Dis.* 2014;**10**(5):842–50.

Inge TH, Zeller MH, Jenkins TM, et al. Perioperative outcomes of adolescents undergoing bariatric surgery: the Teen-Longitudinal Assessment of Bariatric Surgery (Teen-LABS) study. *JAMA Pediatr.* 2014;**168**(1):47–53.

Inge TH, Courcoulas AP, Jenkins TM, et al. weight loss and health status 3 years after bariatric surgery in adolescents. Teen-LABS Consortium. *N Engl J Med.* 2016;**374**(2):113–23.

National Obesity Observatory (NOO). *A Simple Guide to Classifying Body Mass Index in Children.* 2011. www.safefood.eu/Professional/Nutrition/Nutrition-News-en/Nutrition-News/July-2011/A-simple-guide-to-classifying-body-mass-index-in-c.aspx (accessed May 2018).

Sachdev P, Makaya T, Marven SS. Bariatric surgery in severely obese adolescents: a single-centre experience. *Arch Dis Child.* 2014;**99**(10):894–8.

Shah AS, D'Alessio D, Ford-Adams ME. et al. Bariatric surgery: a potential treatment for type 2 diabetes in youth. *Diabetes Care.* 2016;**39**(6):934–40.

Index

Printed in the United States
By Bookmasters